FRONTIERS IN RESEARCH OF THE RENIN-ANGIOTENSIN SYSTEM ON HUMAN DISEASE

PROTEASES IN BIOLOGY AND DISEASE

SERIES EDITORS:

NIGEL M. HOOPER, *University of Leeds, Leeds, United Kingdom*

UWE LENDECKEL, *Otto-von-Guericke University, Magdeburg, Germany*

Volume 1
PROTEASES IN TISSUE REMODELLING OF LUNG AND HEART
Edited by Uwe Lendeckel and Nigel M. Hooper

Volume 2
AMINOPEPTIDASES IN BIOLOGY AND DISEASE
Edited in Nigel M. Hooper and Uwe Lendeckel

Volume 3
PROTEASES IN THE BRAIN
Edited by Uwe Lendeckel and Nigel M. Hooper

Volume 4
THE ADAM FAMILY OF PROTEASES
Edited by Nigel M. Hooper and Uwe Lendeckel

Volume 5
PROTEASES IN GASTROINTESTINAL TISSUES
Edited by Uwe Lendeckel and Nigel M. Hooper

Volume 6
INTRAMEMBRANE-CLEAVING PROTEASES (I-CLiPs)
Edited by Nigel M. Hooper and Uwe Lendeckel

Volume 7
FRONTIERS IN RESEARCH OF THE RENIN-ANGIOTENSIN
SYSTEM ON HUMAN DISEASE
Edited by Po Sing Leung

FRONTIERS IN RESEARCH OF THE RENIN-ANGIOTENSIN SYSTEM ON HUMAN DISEASE

Edited by

Po Sing Leung, PhD

Department of Physiology,
Faculty of Medicine,
The Chinese University of Hong Kong,
Shatin, Hong Kong, China

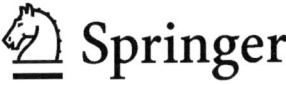 Springer

A C.I.P. Catalogue record for this book is available from the Library of Congress.

ISBN 978-1-4020-6371-8 (HB)
ISBN 978-1-4020-6372-5 (e-book)

Published by Springer,
P.O. Box 17, 3300 AA Dordrecht, The Netherlands.

www.springer.com

Printed on acid-free paper

CONTENTS

Preface vii

Contributors ix

1 Role of ACE, ACE2 and Neprilysin in the Kidney 1
   Mark C. Chappell

2 ACE Inhibition in Heart Failure and Ischaemic Heart Disease 21
   Duncan J. John Campbell

3 Proteases of the Renin-Angiotensin System in Human
   Acute Pancreatitis 55
   R. Pezzilli and L. Fantini

4 The Renin-Angiotensin System in Pancreatic Stellate Cells:
   Implications in the Development and Progression of Type 2
   Diabetes Mellitus 73
   Seung-Hyun Ko, Yu-Bai Ahn, Ki-Ho Song, and Kun-Ho Yoon

5 Renin-Angiotensin System Proteases and the Cardiometabolic
   Syndrome: Pathophysiological, Clinical and Therapeutic Implications .. 87
   Guido Lastra, Camila Manrique, and James R. Sowers

6 The Role of the Renin-Angiotensin System in Hepatic Fibrosis 113
   J.S. Lubel, F.J. Warner, and P.W. Angus

7 The Renin-Angiotensin System in the Breast 135
   *Gavin P. Vinson, Stewart Barker, John R. Puddefoot,
   and Massoumeh Tahmasebi*

8 Role of Local Renin-Angiotensin System in the Carotid Body
   and in Diseases 155
   Man Lung Fung and Po Sing Leung

9 Bone Homeostasis: An Emerging Role
   for the Renin-Angiotensin System 179
   C. Sernia, H. Huang, K. Nguyuen, Y-H. Li, S. Hsu, M. Chen,
   N. Yu, and M. Forwood

10 The Renin-Angiotensin System and its Inhibitors in Human Cancers ... 197
   Lucienne Juillerat-Jeanneret

11 The Skeletal Muscle RAS in Health and Disease 221
   David R. Woods

12 Local Angiotensin Generation and AT$_2$ Receptor Activation 247
   Joep H.M. van Esch and A.H. Jan Danser

13 ADAMs as Mediators of Angiotensin II Actions 273
   A.M. Bourne and W.G. Thomas

Index 303

PREFACE

The circulating renin-angiotensin system (RAS) is a hormonal system that regulates blood pressure, electrolyte and fluid homeostasis. Angiotensin II (Ang II), along with bioactive peptides such as Ang III, Ang IV and Ang (1-7) are the main effector peptides of the RAS. These peptides are the products of the proteolytic actions of renin, angiotensin-converting enzyme (ACE), ACE-2, and other angiotensin-processing peptidases. Such angiotensin peptides exert their functions through their respective angiotensin receptors, namely AT1, AT2, AT4 and AT7 receptors.

In the past decade, it has been recognized that numerous tissues and organs express their own RAS components and peptide activities. Such intrinsic systems are particularly suited for providing autocrine, paracrine or intracrine pathways having local functions that are different from, complementary to and, in some situations even counteracting, the circulating RAS. These local functions include, but are not limited to, cell growth, anti-proliferation, apoptosis, generation of reactive oxygen species, fibrogenesis, hormonal secretion, and vascular tone. The targets of these actions extend beyond the established nervous and cardiovascular systems, and now reach such diverse targets as the bone tissue, carotid body, adipose and liver tissues, and the pancreas. Additionally, local RAS are subject to regulation by various physiological and pathophysiological conditions. Blockade of the RAS thus has the potential to provide extensive and novel strategies for alternative approaches in the treatment of cardiovascular, renal, hepatic, skeletal and pancreatic diseases.

The significance and impact of the RAS in basic research and their clinical implications are reflected by the flourishing publication of original and review research articles; by the appearance of whole issues of journals dedicated to the RAS; and by specialist books on the RAS. In such a rapidly evolving environment, publications that span the spectrum from basic research to the bedside, fill a particularly valuable niche for clinicians and researchers alike. Therefore, the major purpose of this seventh volume of *Proteases in Biology and Disease* series is to provide a topical and timely forum for the critical appraisal of an area of endocrine research that is expanding rapidly. In this book entitled *"Frontiers in Research of the Renin-Angiotensin System on Human Disease"*, a collection of 13 chapters from distinguished and world-class experts in the field has been presented on the contemporary research of the RAS in human disease. In this respect, it is clear that outstanding and stellar work on the novel roles of local RAS and their potential clinical application is being done.in laboratories and clinics across the globe.

In Chapter 1, M.C. Chappell begins with "Role of ACE, ACE2 and Neprilysin in the Kidney". In Chapter 2, D.J. Campbell continues with "ACE Inhibition in Heart Failure and Ischaemic Heart Disease". In Chapter 3, R. Pezzilli and L. Fantini describe "Proteases of the Renin-Angiotensin System in Human Acute Pancreatitis". In Chapter 4, S.H. Ko *et al.* report on "The Renin-Angiotensin System in Pancreatic Stellate Cells: Implications in the Development and Progression of Type 2 Diabetes Mellitus". In Chapter 5, G. Lastra *et al.* review the recent advances in "Renin-Angiotensin System Proteases and the Cardiometabolic Syndrome: Pathophysiological, Clinical and Therapeutic Implications". In Chapter 6, J.S. Lubel *et al.* focus on "The Role of the Renin-Angiotensin System in Hepatic Fibrosis". In Chapter 7, G.P. Vinson *et al.* discuss "The Renin-Angiotensin System in the Breast". In Chapter 8, M.L. Fung and P.S. Leung contribute to "Role of Local Renin-Angiotensin System in the Carotid Body and in Diseases". In Chapter 9, C. Sernia *et al.* concentrate on "Bone Homeostasis: an Emerging Role for the Renin-Angiotensin System". In Chapter 10, L. Juillerat-Jeanneret discusses "The Renin-Angiotensin System and its Inhibitors in Human Cancers". In Chapter 11, D.R. Woods deals with "The Skeletal Muscle RAS in Health and Disease". In Chapter 12, J.H.M. van Esch and A.H. Jan Danser elaborate on "Local Angiotensin Generation and AT2 Receptor Activation". In the last Chapter 13, A.M. Bourne and W.G. Thomas end with "ADAMs as Mediators of Angiotensin II Actions"

Finally, I would like to take this opportunity to express my sincere gratitude to our Series Editors, Uwe Lendeckel and Nigel M. Hooper, for inviting me to do such a great task for Springer: it has been a privilege. I also express my appreciation to my graduate student, Mr. Raymond K.K. Leung, for his skilled assistance on clerical work. This volume should be of general interest to the readership of our "Proteases in Biology and Disease" series, as well as being a comprehensive book for basic scientists, clinicians and newcomers to this field.

Po Sing Leung

Department of Physiology, Faculty of Medicine

The Chinese University of Hong Kong, Hong Kong April 2007

CONTRIBUTORS

Ahn, Yu-Bai   Division of Endocrinology & Metabolism, Department of Internal Medicine, The Catholic University of Korea, Seoul, Korea
e-mail: ybahn@catholic.ac.kr

Angus, Peter W.   Department of Gastroenterology and Hepatology, Austin Health, Studley Road, Heidelberg 3084, Melbourne, Victoria, Australia
e-mail: peter.angus@austin.org.au

Barker, Stewart   School of Biological and Chemical Sciences, Queen Mary University of London, Mile End Road, London E1 4NS, United Kingdom
e-mail: S.Barker@qmul.ac.uk

Bourne, A.M.   Molecular Endocrinology, Baker Heart Research Institute, PO Box 6492 St Kilda Road Central, Melbourne 8008, Victoria, Australia Department of Biochemistry and Molecular Biology, Monash University, Melbourne 3800, Australia
e-mail: allison.bourne@baker.edu.au

Campbell, Duncan J.   St. Vincent's Institute of Medical Research and Department of Medicine, University of Melbourne, Fitzroy, Victoria, Australia
e-mail: dcampbell@svi.edu.au

Chappell, Mark C.   Hypertension and Vascular Disease Center, Department of Physiology and Pharmacology, Molecular Medicine Programme, Wake Forest University School of Medicine, Winston-Salem, NC 27157-1032, USA
e-mail: mchappel@wfubmc.edu

Chen, M.   Department of Physiology & Pharmacology, School of Biomedical Science, University of Queensland, Brisbane, Australia
e-mail: s4012376@student.uq.edu.au

Danser, A.H. Jan   Department of Pharmacology Room EE1418b Erasmus MC Dr. Molewaterplein 50 3015 GE Rotterdam, The Netherlands
e-mail: danser@farma.fgg.eur.nl

Fantini, L.   Department of Internal Medicine and Gastroenterology, Sant'Orsola-Malpighi Hospital, Bologna, Italy
e-mail: lor.fantini@tiscali.it

Forwood, M.   Department of Physiology & Pharmacology, School of Biomedical Science, University of Queensland, Brisbane, Australia
e-mail: m.forwood@uq.edu.au

Fung, Man Lung   Department of Physiology, Faculty of Medicine Building, University of Hong Kong, 21 Sassoon Road, Pokfulam, Hong Kong, The People's Republic of China
e-mail: fungml@hkucc.hku.hk

Hsu, S.   Department of Physiology & Pharmacology, School of Biomedical Science, University of Queensland, Brisbane, Australia
e-mail: s4010346@student.uq.edu.au

Huang, H.   Department of Physiology & Pharmacology, School of Biomedical Science, University of Queensland, Brisbane, Australia
e-mail: hhuang@uq.edu.au

Juillerat-Jeanneret, Lucienne   University Institute of Pathology, Bugnon 25, CH1011 Lausanne, Switzerland
e-mail: lucienne.juillerat@chuv.ch

Ko, Seung-Hyun   Division of Endocrinology and Metabolism, Department of Internal Medicine, The Catholic University of Korea, Seoul, Korea
e-mail: kosh@catholic.ac.kr

Lastra, Guido   Department of Internal Medicine, University of Missouri-Columbia, Columbia, MO 65212, USA
e-mail: lastrag@health.missouri.edu

Leung, Po Sing   Department of Physiology, Chinese University of Hong Kong, Shatin, Hong Kong
e-mail: psleung@cuhk.edu.hk

Li, Y-H.   Department of Physiology & Pharmacology, School of Biomedical Science, University of Queensland, Brisbane, Australia
e-mail: y.li@uq.edu.au

Lubel, J.S.   Department of Gastroenterology, Austin Health, Studley Road, Heidelberg, Melbourne, Victoria, Australia
e-mail: j.lubel@pgrad.unimelb.edu.au

Manrique, Camila   Department of Internal Medicine, University of Missouri-Columbia, Columbia, MO65212, USA
e-mail: manriquec@health.missouri.edu

Nguyuen, K.   Department of Physiology & Pharmacology, School of Biomedical Science, University of Queensland, Brisbane, Australia
e-mail: kima.nguyen@uq.edu.au

Pezzilli, Raffaele   Department of Internal Medicine and Gastroenterology, San'Orsola-Malpighi Hospital, Bologna, Italy
e-mail: pezzilli@aosp.bo.it

Puddefoot, John R.   School of Biological and Chemical Sciences, Queen Mary University of London, Mile End Road, London E1 4NS, United Kingdom
e-mail: J.R.Puddefoot@qmul.ac.uk

Sernia, Conrad   Department of Physiology and Pharmacology, School of Biomedical Science, University of Queensland, Q4072, Brisbane, Australia
e-mail: c.sernia@uq.edu.au

Song, Ki-Ho   Division of Endocrinology & Metabolism, Department of Internal Medicine, The Catholic University of Korea, Seoul, Korea
e-mail: kihos@catholic.ac.kr

Sowers, James R.   Department of Internal Medicine, University of Missouri-Columbia, Columbia, MO65212, USA
e-mail: sowersj@health.missouri.edu

Tahmasebi, Massoumeh   School of Biological and Chemical Sciences, Queen Mary University of London, Mile End Road, London E1 4NS, United Kingdom
e-mail: m.tahmasebi@qmul.ac.uk

Thomas, Walter G.   Molecular Endocrinology, Baker Heart Research Institute, PO Box 6492 St Kilda Road Central, Melbourne 8008, Victoria, Australia
e-mail: walter.thomas@baker.edu.au

van Esch, Joep H.M.   Department of Pharmacology, Erasmus MC, Rotterdam, The Netherlands
e-mail: j.vanesch@erasmusmc.nl

Vinson, Gavin P.   School of Biological and Chemical Sciences, Queen Mary University of London, Mile End Road, London E1 4NS, United Kingdom
e-mail: g.p.vinson@qmul.ac.uk

Warner, F.J.   A.W. Morrow Gastroenterology and Liver Centre, Centenary Institute of Cancer Medicine and Cell Biology, University of Sydney, Sydney, Australia
e-mail: f.warner@centenary.usyd.edu.au

Woods, David R.   Department of Medicine, Royal Victoria Infirmary, Queen Victoria Road, Newcastle, NE1 4LP, U.K.
e-mail: DoctorDRWoods@aol.com

Yoon, Kun-Ho   Division of Endocrinology & Metabolism, Department of Internal Medicine, The Catholic University of Korea, Seoul, Korea
e-mail: yoonk@catholic.ac.kr

Yu, N.   Department of Physiology & Pharmacology, School of Biomedical Science, University of Queensland, Brisbane, Australia
e-mail: s4011639@student.uq.edu.au

CHAPTER 1

ROLE OF ACE, ACE2 AND NEPRILYSIN
IN THE KIDNEY

MARK C. CHAPPELL

Hypertension & Vascular Disease Center, Department of Physiology and Pharmacology, Molecular Medicine Program, Wake Forest University School of Medicine, Winston-Salem, NC 27157-1032, USA

1.   INTRODUCTION

From the initial description of renin activity over a century ago, ongoing study of the renin-angiotensin-aldosterone system (RAAS) continues to yield novel findings that redefine the functional nature of this system, as well as reveal the complexity of the interplay among the various RAAS components. Indeed, the recent discoveries of angiotensin converting enzyme 2 (ACE2) (Crackower *et al* 2002; Donoghue *et al* 2000; Tipnis *et al* 2000); the renin receptor (Nguyen *et al* 2002) and the angiotensin-(1-7) [Ang-(1-7)] receptor (Santos *et al* 2002) represent important examples of our evolving concepts of the RAAS and cardiovascular regulation. Coupled with the emerging view that the RAAS is not defined as simply an endocrine system, these local or tissue systems may exhibit distinct functional and processing pathways (Chappell *et al* 1989; Chappell *et al* 2004; Paul *et al* 2006). The kidney is clearly an important target organ of the circulating RAAS, particularly the actions of Ang II and aldosterone to promote sodium and water reabsorption, as well as their influence on the progression of tissue injury and fibrosis (Harris 1999). The kidney also exhibits a local RAAS that expresses Ang II, Ang-(1-7), and multiple Ang receptor subtypes that mediate the distinct actions of these two peptides in both normal and pathophysiolgocial conditions such as hypertension or diabetes (Burns 2000; Carey & Siragy 2003; Navar *et al* 2000). Figure 1 illustrates one current view of the renal RAAS network that emphasizes the distinct synthetic pathways of Ang II and Ang-(1-7), as well as functional actions mediated by the AT_1, AT_2 and $AT_{(1-7)}$ receptors. Although the emergence of receptor subtypes distinguishes the distinct signaling pathways of Ang II and Ang-(1-7), the post-renin enzymes that form and degrade these peptides must be considered in lieu of the overall regulation of the functional RAAS within the kidney. The inclusion of Ang-(1-12) as a potential intermediate in Ang II formation via a renin-independent pathway reflects the recent

1

Po Sing Leung (ed.), Frontiers in Research of the Renin-Angiotensin System on Human Disease, 1–20.
© 2007 *Springer.*

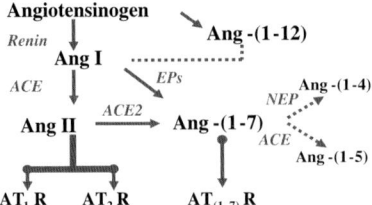

Figure 1. Scheme that depicts the processing pathways involved in the formation and degradation of angiotensin II (Ang II) and Ang-(1-7) within the kidney. Ang II binds to either AT_1 or AT_2 receptor (R) subtypes, while Ang-(1-7) recognizes an AT $_{(1-7)}$ R. ACE, angiotensin converting enzyme; EPs, endopeptidases; NEP, neprilysin

demonstration of endogenous levels of the peptide in the kidney, circulation and other tissues (Nagata *et al* 2006). In this chapter, the roles of ACE2, ACE and the endopeptidase neprilysin in the functional expression of the intrarenal hormones of the RAAS are reviewed.

2.   ANGIOTENSIN CONVRETING ENZYME

ACE may be considered the activation step in the catalytic cascade for the formation of Ang II from Ang I (Fig. 1). Although evidence of non-ACE pathways for biosynthesis of Ang II is evident (Sadjadi *et al* 2005a; Tokuyama *et al* 2002), ACE likely represents the major, if not sole enzyme responsible for Ang II formation under normal physiological conditions in humans and other species. This is not to imply that ACE has no other substrates than Ang I (see below), but that a primary role for ACE is the generation of Ang II. Indeed, the identification of ACE and the characterization of the enzymatic properties must be considered a pivotal achievement in our understanding of the RAAS and cardiovascular disease, as well as leading to the successful development of ACE inhibitors in the treatment for hypertension and renal disease. ACE is a metallopeptidase composed of a single monomeric protein. Somatic ACE contains two catalytic regions designated as the amino (N) and carboxy (C) domains. Selective inhibitors against both catalytic domains of somatic ACE are now available, however, the functional significance of the two domains is presently unknown (Dive *et al* 1999; Georgiadis *et al* 2003). The enzyme cleaves two residues from the carboxy end of various peptides and, hence, its description as a *dipeptidyl*-carboxypepitdase. Within the kidney, somatic ACE is primarily a glycosylphosphatidylinositol-anchored membrane protein and the majority of the enzyme including both catalytic regions faces the extracellular space. ACE is localized throughout the kidney with high concentrations in vascular endothelial cells, proximal tubules and interstitial cells. ACE is also released from the apical surface of epithelial cells into the proximal tubular fluid and likely contributes to the urinary levels of the enzyme (Hattori *et al* 2000). Indeed, the tubular fluid should be considered a distinct intrarenal compartment that contains RAAS processing enzymes and the peptide products may interact with Ang receptors along the entire tubular area of the kidney. The release of ACE from the cell membrane is a specific process as releasing enzymes or "sheddases" have been identified that recognize a unique motif on the stalk region of the enzyme (Beldent et al 1993). The conversion of membrane-bound ACE to a soluble form does not appear to substantially alter the substrate preference or the catalytic properties of the enzyme. Although the significance of this event is not currently understood, enzyme shedding may underlie an endocrine process to transport ACE to more distal areas of the nephron that are deficient in this peptidase activity for the discrete production of Ang II. In this regard, Casarini and colleagues have presented intriguing data that the urinary excretion of the N-terminal domain of ACE may serve as a urinary marker in both humans and experimental hypertensive models (Marques et al 2003).

Extensive evidence suggests that intrarenal ACE participates in the direct formation of Ang II from Ang I. The renal administration of ACE inhibitors reduces interstitial levels of Ang II and attenuates blood pressure. Moreover, in an animal model of tissue-depleted ACE that preserves circulating levels of the enzyme, renal Ang II is significantly reduced (Modrall et al 2003). Interestingly, intrarenal levels of Ang I were also markedly reduced in the tissue ACE null mouse while renal Ang-(1-7) concentrations were maintained (Modrall et al 2003). These data serve to emphasize that ACE participates in the metabolism of other peptide hormones (Skidgel & Erdos 2004). In the case of Ang-(1-7), ACE efficiently metabolizes the peptide to Ang-(1-5), a product which is presently not known to exhibit functional activity (Chappell et al 1998; Deddish et al 1998; Rice et al 2004). We have postulated that the formation of Ang-(1-7), particularly under prolonged activation of the RAAS, is considered to balance or attenuate the constrictor and proliferative actions of Ang II (Chappell & Ferrario 1999; Ferrario et al 2005c). Indeed, Ang-(1-7) exhibits vasodilatory, natriuretic and anti-proliferative actions through the stimulation of nitric oxide and arachidonic acid metabolites (Sampaio et al 2007). Ang-(1-7) abrogates the Ang II-dependent activation of MAP kinase in primary cultures of proximal tubule epithelial cells (Su et al 2006). Moreover, the inhibitory actions of Ang-(1-7) were blocked by the Ang-(1-7) antagonist [D-Ala[7]]-Ang-(1-7) suggesting a receptor mediated pathway distinct from either AT_1 or AT_2 receptor subtypes (Su et al 2006). Similar effects of Ang-(1-7) were originally demonstrated in non-renal cells (Tallant et al 2005a). In the circulation, ACE inhibitors increase circulating levels of Ang-(1-7) and augment the in vivo half life of the peptide by almost 6 fold (Iyer et al 1998; Yamada et al 1998). The urinary excretion of Ang-(1-7) increases in both human and experimental hypertensive models following acute administration of ACE inhibitors (Ferrario et al 1998; Yamada et al 1999). The increased excretion of Ang-(1-7) most likely reflects the reduced intrarenal metabolism of the peptide and the efficient shunting of the Ang I pathway to formation of Ang-(1-7). Our recent studies in isolated sheep proximal tubules reveal that without prior inhibition of ACE, Ang-(1-7) derived from either Ang I or Ang II was rapidly converted to Ang-(1-5) (Shaltout et al 2007). Blockade of Ang-(1-7) partially reverses the beneficial actions of ACE inhibitors on blood pressure in hypertensive rats as an Ang-(1-7) monoclonal antibody or the [D-Ala^7]-Ang-(1-7) antagonist increase blood pressure (Iyer *et al* 1997; Iyer *et al* 2000). Moreover, studies by Benter and colleagues find that the renoprotective effects of exogenous Ang-(1-7) in LNAME-treated SHR were not further improved with the ACE inhibitor captopril (Benter *et al* 2006a).

Apart from Ang II and Ang-(1-7), renal ACE may also participate in the metabolism of other peptides including kinins, substance P and the hematopoietic fragment acetyl-Ser-Asp-Lys-Pro (Ac-SDKP). Bradykinin-(1-9) is very rapidly metabolized by ACE in a two -step process to the inactive fragments bradykinin-(1-7) and bradykinin-(1-5). ACE inhibition is associated with increased circulating and tissue levels of bradykinin-(1-9) and the renal content of kinin is higher in the tissue ACE null mouse (Campbell *et al* 2004). In general, bradykinin is a potent vasodilator and inhibitor of cell growth through stimulation of nitric oxide, as well as exhibiting natriuretic actions within the kidney (Scicli & Carretero 1986). Interestingly, Santos and colleagues have reported that the functional activity of Ang-(1-7), under certain conditions, is dependent on the increased release of bradykinin (Fernandes *et al* 2001). Moreover, the kinin B2 receptor antagonist HOE140 blocked nitric oxide release by the non-peptide Ang-(1-7) agonist AVE0991 (Wiemer *et al* 2002).

Similar to Ang-(1-7), circulating levels of the Ac-SDKP are markedly increased with ACE inhibition and the enzyme cleaves the Lys-Pro bond of the tetrapeptide (Azizi *et al* 1997; Raousseau *et al* 1995). Although current evidence does not support a role for Ac-SDKP in the regulation of blood pressure, the peptide does exhibit potent anti-fibrotic and anti-inflammatory actions (Peng *et al* 2003). Indeed, exogenous administration of Ac-SDKP attenuates proteinuria and improves renal function in several models of renal injury and hypertension (Omata *et al* 2006). Interestingly, Ang-(1-7) and Ac-SDKP may be the only known endogenous substrates that are exclusively cleaved by the N-terminal catalytic domain of human ACE (Raousseau *et al* 1995; Deddish *et al* 1998). Moreover, prolyl (oligo)endopeptidase, an enzyme that processes Ang I or Ang II to Ang-(1-7) in endothelial and neural cells (Chappell *et al* 1990; Santos *et al* 1992), may also convert thymosin-β_2 to Ac-SDKP in plasma and tissue (Cavasin *et al* 2004). The unusual specificity of the N-domain of ACE for Ang-(1-7) and Ac-SDKP suggests an overlap of the activities of these two peptide systems within the kidney as well. Although elucidation of the signaling mechanisms and receptors for Ang-(1-7) and Ac-SDKP is at an early stage, future studies should consider whether there is a basis for the functional similarities between these peptides.

The role of RAAS enzymes including ACE and renin has been primarily emphasized for their catalytic properties; however, compelling evidence now reveals receptor-like properties for these two enzymes. Indeed, a renin receptor was recently cloned by Nyguen and colleagues with significant concentrations of the protein in the glomerulus and vascular smooth muscle cells. (Diez-Freire *et al* 2006; Nguyen *et al* 2002). Receptor-bound renin exhibits increase proteolyitc activity for Ang I formation, but both pro-renin and renin also induce distinct signaling pathways following binding. In isolated mesangial cells, exogenous renin increased TGF-β expression and other matrix proteins including plasminogen activator inhibitor (PAI-1) and fibronectin that was apparently independent of Ang II synthesis (Huang *et al* 2006). ACE inhibitors may also induce cell-specific signaling by inducing conformational changes in membrane-bound ACE without alterations in Ang II or other peptides (Benzing *et al* 1999). Two kinases, c-Jun kinase and MAP kinase kinase 7 associate with the intracellular portion of ACE. Moreover, ACE inhibitors increase the phosphorylation and nuclear trafficking of phosphorylated cJun kinase (Kohlstedt *et al* 2002). This aspect of ACE-dependent activation of various kinases has been demonstrated in human endothelial cells and the question remains as to what extent this occurs in other cells or tissues. In addition, ACE inhibitors or the angiotensin peptides Ang-(1-9) and Ang-(1-7) induce the association of ACE and the bradykinin B2 receptor that prevents the rapid down-regulation of the ligand-receptor complex, thus potentiating the actions of bradykinin (Burckle *et al* 2006; Chen *et al* 2005).

3. ANGIOTENSIN CONVERTING ENZYME 2

Almost 50 years following the discovery of ACE, a new homolog of the enzyme termed ACE2 was identified by two separate groups (Donoghue *et al* 2000; Tipnis *et al* 2000). ACE2 activity is not attenuated by ACE inhibitors nor does the enzyme share the same catalytic properties. In this regard, ACE2 contains a single zinc-dependent catalytic site that corresponds to the C-terminal domain of somatic ACE. ACE2 exhibits carboxypeptidase activity cleaving a single amino acid residue at the carboxyl terminus of various peptides. The original studies assessed Ang I as the peptide substrate for ACE2, given the similar homology to ACE and the existing evidence for ACE-independent pathways; however, ACE2 converted Ang I to the nonapeptide Ang-(1-9) (Donoghue *et al* 2000). This product is currently not known to exhibit functional activity, but may serve as a substrate for the further processing to Ang II or Ang-(1-7) (Li *et al* 2004). The subsequent kinetic studies of over 120 peptides found that the conversion of Ang II to Ang-(1-7) was much preferred over that for Ang I (Vickers *et al* 2002). Indeed, ACE2 exhibits an approximate 500-fold greater kcat/Km for Ang II versus Ang I and has the highest efficiency among the known Ang-(1-7)-forming enzymes (Fig. 2). These studies also revealed that other peptides including apelin 13 and dynorphin are cleaved by ACE2 at a similar or slightly greater efficiency than Ang II (Vickers *et al* 2002). At this time, the majority of studies have focused on the role of ACE2 in the metabolism of angiotensins (see below), principally Ang II to Ang-(1-7), and the role of ACE2 in the processing of apelin or other peptides has not been sufficiently addressed.

Similar to ACE, ACE2 exists in both soluble and membrane-associated forms with high expression in the kidney, heart, brain, lung and testes (Harmer *et al* 2002). Although there is significant circulating ACE activity in various species, plasma levels of ACE2 are quite low, but may vary among species (Elased *et al* 2006; Rice *et al* 2006). Recent studies in the sheep reveal appreciable ACE2 in the plasma, albeit the activity was significantly lower than that for ACE (Fig. 3, inset) (Shaltout *et al* 2007). For this assessment, we compared the enzyme activities using the endogenous substrates for both ACE and ACE2 (Ang I and Ang II, respectively)

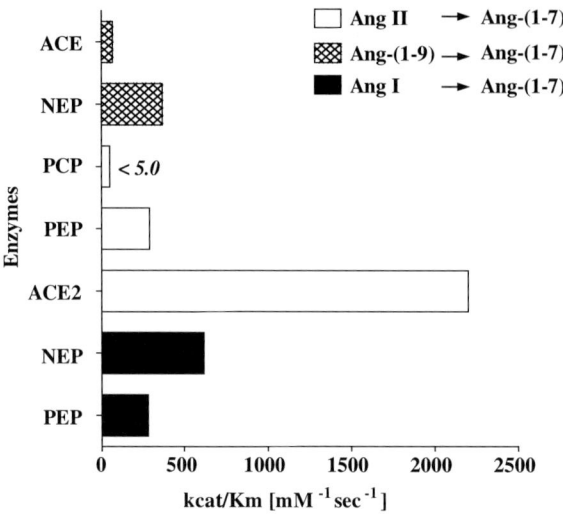

Figure 2. Comparison of the efficiency constants for the formation of Ang-(1-7) from Ang II, Ang-(1-9) and Ang I. Peptidase abbreviations: ACE, angiotensin-converting enzyme; NEP, neprilysin; PCP, prolyl carboxypeptidase; PEP, prolyl (oligo) endopeptidase
Source: Kinetic data from Rice et al 2004 & Welches et al 1993

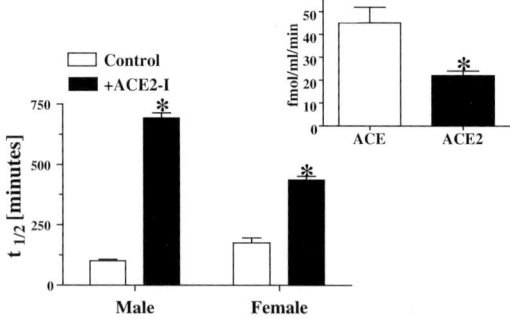

Figure 3. The ACE2 inhibitor MLN-4760 (ACE2-I) increases the half life ($t_{1/2}$) of Ang II in the serum of male and female sheep. Inset: comparison of ACE and ACE2 activities in female serum. ACE and ACE2 were determined by the conversion of Ang I to Ang II and Ang II to Ang-(1-7), respectively, by HPLC analysis in the absence or presence of the ACE2 MLN-4760 and the ACE inhibitor lisinopril. Data are n = 4-5, mean ± SEM;* $P < 0.05$ vs. control

at equimolar concentrations under identical incubation conditions. Interestingly, as shown in Fig. 3, male sheep exhibited higher ACE2 activity than females that likely contributes to the lower half-life ($t_{1/2}$) of serum Ang II in males (Westwood *et al* 2006). Addition of the specific ACE2 inhibitor abolished the conversion of Ang II to Ang-(1-7) as measured by a HPLC-^{125}I-detector and markedly increased the Ang II-[$t_{1/2}$] in both male (6 fold) and female (3 fold) sheep (Fig. 3). These *ex vivo* data in sheep serum demonstrate that circulating ACE2 constitutes a major pathway in the metabolism of Ang II and support the increase in circulating Ang II levels in the ACE2 null mouse (Crackower *et al* 2002). Furthermore, we did not find that soluble ACE2 in the serum contributed to the direct conversion of Ang I to Ang-(1-9) even in the presence of complete ACE inhibition (Shaltout *et al* 2007).

Within the kidney, ACE2 is primarily localized to the apical aspect of the proximal tubule epithelium. Indeed, expression of ACE2 in the renal MDCK cell line revealed exclusive trafficking of the enzyme to the apical side, while the distribution of expressed ACE was different, trafficking to the basolateral and luminal aspects of the cell (Guy *et al* 2005). Consistent with the apical expression of ACE2 in the renal epithelium, we found significant urinary ACE2 activity that converted Ang II to Ang-(1-7), but did not process Ang I to Ang-(1-9) (Shaltout *et al* 2007). The glycosylated form of ACE2 is approximately 120,000 Daltons and the filtration of the enzyme into the tubular fluid is highly unlikely (Shaltout *et al* 2007). In this regard, Lambert and colleagues report that the metallopeptidase ADAM 17 may function as a secretase to release ACE2 from extracellular side of the cell membrane (Lambert *et al* 2005). Interestingly, ADAM 17 does not release ACE suggesting that the regulation for the secretion for ACE and ACE2 is distinct. The localization of ACE2 in the proximal tubule epithelium along with other elements of the RAS (ACE, angiotensinogen, Ang receptors) supports a role for the enzyme in the processing of angiotensin peptides. In the rat kidney, Burns and colleagues found no evidence that ACE2 or other peptidases metabolize Ang II in proximal tubule preparations or in perfused proximal tubule segments isolated from male Sprague Dawley rats (Li *et al* 2004). However, ACE2 activity was clearly evident in the rat tubules as the conversion of exogenous Ang I to Ang-(1-9) was sensitive to the ACE2 peptide inhibitor DX-600 (Li *et al* 2004). Ang-(1-9) was subsequently converted to Ang-(1-7) by ACE, a pathway similar to that reported for Ang I metabolism in isolated cardiomyocytes (Donoghue *et al* 2000). In contrast to the rat, we found that ACE2 was the predominant activity to convert Ang II to Ang-(1-7) in sheep proximal tubules (Shaltout *et al* 2007). The addition of the non-peptide ACE2 inhibitor MLN-4760 significantly attenuated the metabolism of Ang II at early time points. However, as shown in Fig. 4, the significant ACE and neprilysin activities required prior inhibition to protect Ang-(1-7) from rapid degradation in the proximal tubules. We could not demonstrate that ACE2 participated in the direct metabolism of Ang I, particularly under conditions where other enzymatic pathways were blocked (Shaltout *et al* 2007). Indeed, Ang I was directly converted to Ang II and Ang-(1-7) via ACE and neprilysin, respectively. The preferred conversion of Ang II to Ang-(1-7) by ACE2 in the sheep kidney is entirely consistent with kinetic studies on various peptide substrates by the human enzyme (Rice *et al* 2004; Vickers *et al* 2002), as well studies in membrane fractions of mouse kidney and rat renal cortex that demonstrated ACE2-dependent conversion of Ang II to Ang-(1-7) (Elased *et al* 2006; Ferrario *et al* 2005b). An explanation for the discrepancy in the metabolism studies for angiotensin metabolism is not readily apparent; however, if the rat exhibits different kinetic properties for Ang I and Ang II than sheep or human, then the role of ACE2 is likely to be quite different among species. Additionally, these studies have important

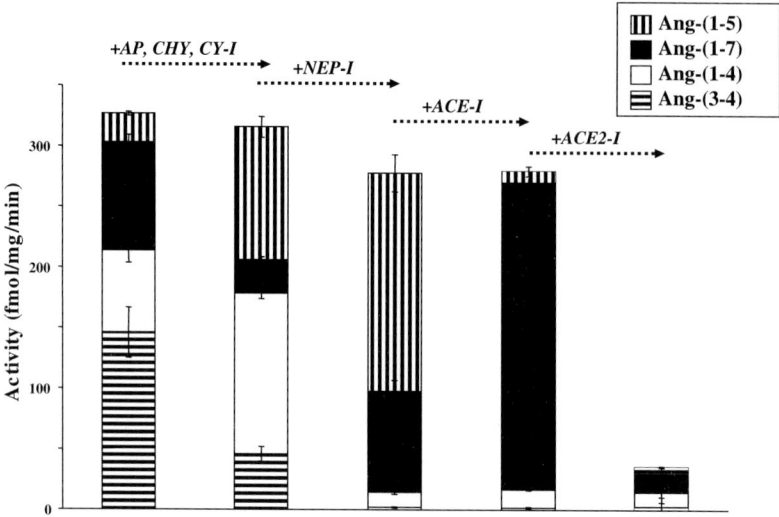

Figure 4. ACE2 inhibition blocks the conversion of Ang II to Ang-(1-7) in isolated proximal tubules from female sheep. Sequential addition of peptidase inhibitors on the formation of Ang II metabolites include: AP, amniopeptidase (amastatin, bestatin); CHY, chymase, carboxypeptidase A (chymostatin, benzyl succinate); CY, cysteine protease (PCMB); NEP, neprilysin (SCH3977), ACE, angiotensin converting enzyme (lisinopril); ACE2 (MLN-4760). Data are n = 4, mean ± SEM

implications on the role of ACE as well, particularly whether ACE is involved in the formation (Li *et al* 2004) or degradation of Ang-(1-7) (Chappell *et al* 1998; Chappell *et al* 2000; Yamada *et al* 1998). Although Campbell and colleague demonstrate significant quantities of endogenous Ang-(1-9) in the rat kidney (Campbell *et al* 1991), chronic ACE inhibition or combined ACE/AT$_1$ blockade (Chappell, unpublished observations) did not attenuate renal Ang-(1-7) levels in the rat. In addition, Ang-(1-7) levels within the kidney were maintained in tissue ACE knockout mice (Modrall *et al* 2003). Thus, these *in vivo* studies do not strongly support an ACE2-ACE cascade leading to the formation of Ang-(1-9) and Ang-(1-7) in the kidney.

The molecular studies utilizing ACE2 knockout mice provide additional evidence for the enzyme's role to balance the expression of Ang II and Ang-(1-7). We originally showed that ACE2 null mice exhibit higher circulating and tissue levels of Ang II (Crackower *et al* 2002). Indeed, the increased ratio of renal Ang II to Ang-(1-7) may contribute to the renal pathologies observed in older ACE2 null mice (Oudit *et al* 2006). Furthermore, the incidence of glomerulosclerosis and proteinuria in the male mice was markedly attenuated by AT$_1$ receptor blockade. Several hypertensive models including the spontaneously hypertensive rat (SHR), stroke-prone SHR and Sabra salt sensitive rat exhibit lower mRNA levels and protein expression for ACE2 in the kidney than normotensive controls (Crackower *et al* 2002; Zhong *et al* 2004), as well as human prehypertensives (Keidar *et al* 2006). Tikellis and colleagues find that renal ACE2 expression is actually higher in the SHR than WKY normotensive controls at day one following birth, similar at 42 days and then dramatically declines in adult SHR by 80 days (Tikellis *et al* 2006). ACE activity, however, was markedly lower in the SHR kidney at all time points measured and declined in both strains at 80 days. Apart from the interesting pattern of development for ACE2 in the kidney, these data emphasize the need to at least consider alterations in both ACE and ACE2 in characterizing the functional output of the RAAS. Moreover, parallel studies to document the changes in renal Ang II and Ang-(1-7) during this developmental period are critical to establish the relevance to altered ACE and ACE2. It is clear that not all hypertensive models exhibit reduced ACE2 in the kidney. Our studies in the male mRen2.Lewis rat, a model of tissue renin expression with increased renal Ang II, found no difference in renal cortical ACE2 activity as compared to the normotensive Lewis strain, although cardiac activity was indeed lower in the hypertensive rats (Ferrario *et al* 2005a; Ferrario *et al* 2005b; Pendergrass *et al* 2006). Chronic blockade with either an ACE inhibitor or AT_1 antagonist increased ACE2 activity in the kidneys of both the mRen2.Lewis and Lewis rats, but enzyme activity was significantly higher in the normotensive strain following treatment (Jessup *et al* 2006). This may reflect the situation where RAAS blockade does not completely reverse the extent of renal injury in the male mRen2.Lewis model. In this regard, the reduced ACE2 and elevated renal Ang II in the injured kidney of albumin-loaded rats was associated with increased NF-κB expression (Takase *et al* 2005). In contrast, ACE2 and its product Ang-(1-7) increase in the kidney of the rat during pregnancy (Brosnihan *et al* 2003). It is well known that the RAAS is activated during pregnancy, yet blood pressure is not altered in normal pregnancy, and it will be of interest to determine whether ACE2 expression within the kidney is altered with pre-eclampsia. Diabetic nephropathy is clearly dependent on an activated RAAS and both ACE inhibitors and AT_1 receptor antagonists are effective in attenuating the progression of injury. Indeed, the renal expression of ACE2 is reduced in the proximal tubules of the streptozotocin-induced model of type I diabetes (Tikellis *et al* 2003; Wysocki *et al* 2006). Moreover, the attenuation of renal injury in this model by ACE inhibition is associated with increased ACE2 expression. A protective role for renal ACE2 is also evident from the findings that chronic ACE2 inhibition in the diabetic *db/db* mice exacerbates the extent of albuminuria almost 3-fold (Ye *et al* 2006). Although angiotensin content was not measured, the *db/db* mice exhibited increased glomerular expression of ACE and reduced ACE2 as compared to the control *db/dm* mice. Interestingly, the localization studies revealed distinct patterns of staining for ACE2 and ACE within the glomerulus – ACE2 in podocytes and ACE in the endothelial cells (Liebau *et al* 2006). Ang-(1-7) or the nonpeptide agonist AVE0991 attenuates proteinuria and improves renal vascular activity in the streptozoticin Type 1 diabetic rat, but did not reverse the urinary excretion of lysozyme, a marker of tubulointerstitial damage (Benter *et al* 2007). Moreover, the ratio of Ang-(1-7) to Ang II formed from exogenous Ang I was lower in glomeruli isolated from the kidneys of diabetic rats, however, the identity of the Ang-(1-7)-forming activity was not determined in this study (Singh *et al* 2005). Thus, in addition to the proximal tubule epithelium, the glomerulus may be a second key site within the kidney where ACE2 may influence the local expression of angiotensin peptides and renal function.

4.   NEPRILYSIN

In the kidney, the endopeptidase neprilysin constitutes significant peptidase activity, particularly within the brush border region of the proximal tubules. Similar to ACE and ACE2, neprilysin is a zinc-dependent metallopeptidase that is anchored to the apical or extracellular region of the membrane, but is apparently resistant to enzymatic shedding. Although neprilysin was initially recognized for its enkephalin-degrading activity and frequently referred to as "enkephalinase", studies now reveal that this enzyme contributes to the metabolism of various peptides with cardiovascular actions including adrenomedullin, angiotensins, kinins, endothelins, substance P and the natriuretic peptides (Skidgel & Erdos 2004). Indeed, the development of neprilysin inhibitors, and more recently, dual or mixed inhibitors that target ACE as well remain potential therapies in cardiovascular disease (Veelken & Schmieder 2002). In general, these dual inhibitors were either equally or more effective in lowering blood pressure and reducing renal injury as compared to monotherapy with an ACE or neprilysin inhibitor (Kubota et al 2003; Tikkanen et al 2002). However, two large clinical trials (OCTAVE, OVERTURE) with the mixed inhibitor omapatrilat revealed an increased incidence of angioedema. Moreover, the drug was no more effective than an ACE inhibitor alone (Kostis et al 2004; Packer et al 2002). A subsequent experimental study has shown that omapatrilat inhibits amniopeptidase P and, although less potent than its actions against ACE and neprilysin, this may further augment the local concentrations of kinins or substance P to exacerbate vascular permeability (Sulpizio et al 2005). In this aspect, the development of more selective inhibitors against ACE and neprilysin may be of clinical benefit.

The rationale for neprilysin inhibition primarily resides in preserving the "cardioprotective" peptides bradykinin and ANP or BNP. However, neprilysin readily metabolizes Ang II to the inactive fragment Ang-(1-4) which undergoes further hydrolysis to the dipeptides Asp-Arg and Val-Tyr. Neprilysin also cleaves endothelin, although it is not clear to what extent reduced intrarenal levels of endothelin are beneficial given the functional diversity of the endothelin A and B receptor subtypes within the kidney (Schiffrin 1999). The additional ACE inhibition would prevent the accumulation of Ang II and further contribute to the protection of kinins, as well as possibly reduce endothelin release. One possible caveat to this approach is that neprilysin is the major Ang-(1-7)-forming activity from Ang I or Ang-(1-9) in the circulation (Campbell et al 1998; Yamamoto et al 1992). Indeed, acute administration of the potent neprilysin inhibitor SCH3977 reduced circulating levels of Ang-(1-7) and increased blood pressure in the SHR chronically treated with the ACE inhibitor lisinoropril (Iyer et al 1997). Although plasma levels of neprilysin are low to non-detectable, the enzyme is appropriately localized to the ectocellular surface of endothelial and smooth muscle cells to contribute to the formation of Ang- (1-7) within the vasculature (Llorens-Cortes et al 1992).

In the kidney, neprilysin may contribute to both the formation as well as the degradation of the Ang-(1-7) (Allred et al 2000). Neprilysin cleaves the Pro^7-Phe^8

bond of Ang I to Ang-(1-7), but the very high levels of the enzyme in the kidney may continue to metabolize Ang-(1-7) at the Tyr^5-Ile^6 bond to form Ang-(1-4) and Ang-(5-7) (Allred *et al* 2000; Chappell *et al* 2001). Indeed, the mixed inhibitor omapatrilat augmented the urinary levels of Ang-(1-7) in both human hypertensives and the SHR model (Ferrario *et al* 2002a; Ferrario *et al* 2002b). The clinical study revealed a strong correlation between the reduction in blood pressure and increased excretion of Ang-(1-7) with the dual peptidase inhibitor (Ferrario *et al* 2002a). Interestingly, chronic treatment of male SHR with omapatrilat (2 weeks, 30 mg/kg daily) was also associated with the increased renal expression of ACE2. As shown in Fig. 5, immunocytochemical studies demonstrate enhanced expression

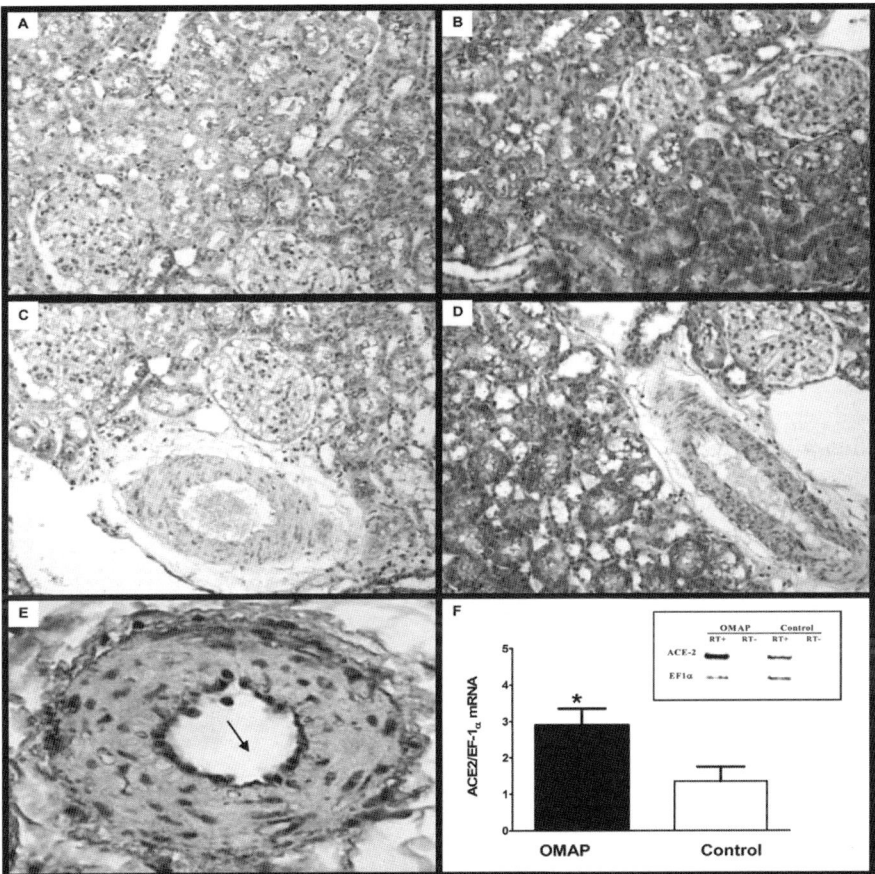

Figure 5. Increased expression of Ang-(1-7) and ACE2 in the renal cortex of SHR following treatment with omapatrilat. Immunocytochemical staining for Ang-(1-7) in control (A) and treated (B) SHR; ACE2 staining in control (C) and treated (D), group. ACE2 staining in renal artery of treated SHR; arrow indicates intimal layer (E). Renal cortical ACE2 mRNA levels are significantly increased 2-fold following omapatrilat treatment (F); inset: ACE2 and EF-1α bands in the presence of the specific RT primers (RT+). Data are n = 7-8, mean ± SEM

of both ACE2 and Ang-(1-7) within the renal cortex of the treated-SHR (Chappell *et al* 2002). Omapatrilat treatment also revealed the renal vascular expression of ACE2 with staining evident in the intimal, medial and adventitial regions of the renal artery (Fig. 5E); vascular staining for the enzyme was undetectable in the untreated SHR group (Fig. 5C). Cortical mRNA of ACE2 expressed as a ratio to EF-1α increased 2-fold suggesting that transcriptional regulation contributes to the enhanced expression of ACE2 within the kidney (Fig. 5F). These studies are of interest as they reveal an additional mechanism of the vasopeptidase inhibitor that may result in the enhanced conversion of Ang II to Ang-(1-7) by ACE2, as well as protecting Ang-(1-7) from both neprilysin- and ACE-dependent degradation within in the kidney. Furthermore, these data suggest an important ability of the dual peptidase inhibitor (as well as the administration of other RAAS inhibitors alone) to restore ACE2 levels in the hypertensive kidney which may mitigate against the Ang II-AT$_1$ receptor axis of the RAAS. Indeed, Raizada and colleagues show that lenti-viral expression of ACE2 has amelioratory effects on blood pressure and cardiac fibrosis in the SHR, although the renal effects of enhanced enzyme activity were not ascertained (Diez-Freire *et al* 2006). Their data clearly demonstrate that ACE2 can markedly alter the balance of an activated RAAS pathway towards a normotensive phenotype. Further study is required to determine the extent that the beneficial actions of increased ACE2 reflect the greater inhibition of Ang II or the increased accumulation of Ang-(1-7) in the kidney or other tissue.

5.   REGULATION OF THE INTRARENAL RAAS

The positive influence of ACE2 in the SHR kidney following blockade of ACE and neprilysin emphasizes the complex regulation of RAAS components within the kidney (see Fig. 6). We have also shown that ACE inhibition alone or AT$_1$ receptor antagonism increases either renal ACE2 mRNA or activity (Igase *et al* 2005; Ferrario *et al* 2005b). Consistent with these data in the intact animal, Gallagher

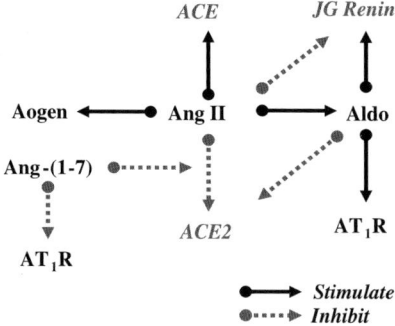

Figure 6. A potential regulatory scheme for the stimulatory and inhibitory pathways of the renin-angiotensin-aldosterone system within the kidney. ACE, angiotensin converting enzymes; Aogen, angiotensinogen; Aldo, aldosterone; AT$_1$R, angiotensin type 1 receptor; JG, juxtaglomerular

and colleagues demonstrate that Ang II directly down regulates ACE2 through activation of the AT_1 receptor (Gallagher *et al* 2006). Although Ang-(1-7) alone did not influence the basal expression of ACE2 in these cells, the peptide attenuated the inhibitory effects of Ang II on ACE2 via a receptor-dependent mechanism (Gallagher *et al* 2006). In contrast to the negative influence on ACE2, Ang II increases ACE expression within the kidney (Harrison-Bernard *et al* 2002; Sadjadi *et al* 2005b). Ang II also positively influences the expression of its precursor protein angiotensinogen (Kobori *et al* 2001; Zhang *et al* 2002), and in selective areas of the kidney, either maintains or up regulates the AT_1 receptor as well (Harrison-Bernard *et al* 2002). This effect on the AT_1 receptor may also lead to increased renal levels of Ang II via receptor mediated uptake and stable sequestration of the circulating peptide (Ingert *et al* 2002). In contrast, Ang-(1-7) can down regulate the AT_1 receptor through stimulation of a cylocoxygenase pathway (Clark *et al* 2003; Clark *et al* 2001). There are few studies on the regulation of the Ang-(1-7) receptor, although chronic ACE or AT_1 blockade reduced *mas* mRNA expression in the renal cortex of the Ren2 Lewis congenic rat (Jessup *et al* 2006). Consistent with the positive feedback concept, the current evidence suggests that aldosterone down regulates ACE2 (Keidar *et al* 2005; Tallant *et al* 2005b) while the mineralo-corticoid increases expression of ACE, AT_1 receptor, renin and intrarenal Ang II (Bayorh *et al* 2006; Klar *et al* 2004; Schiffrin 2006). Thus, the renal RAAS appears to function in a positive regulatory manner on these components to promote or maintain Ang II content. In this regard, ACE2 may serve as an important mechanism to break or reduce the positive gain of the system for Ang II production or enhanced signaling in the kidney. Although Ang II potently reduces juxtaglomerular (JG)-derived release and expression of renin, renin is not suppressed but increases in the collecting duct and distal tubules (Prieto-Carrasquero *et al* 2004). The negative feedback by Ang II on JG renin may also be balanced by renin-independent pathways that contribute to the formation of Ang I. Alternatively, Nagata and colleagues (Nagata *et al* 2006) find significant concentrations of the novel peptide Ang-(1-12) in the kidney and other tissues that may not require renin for the peptide's synthesis (see Fig. 1). The infusion of Ang-(1-12) produced an immediate increase in blood pressure that was abolished by either an ACE inhibitor or an AT_1 receptor antagonist (Nagata *et al* 2006). These data suggest that following formation of Ang-(1-12), the peptide or its intermediate is converted to Ang II by ACE. The elucidation of the enzyme(s) responsible for the formation of Ang-(1-12) and the factors that influence its expression may greatly contribute to our understanding the regulation of the intrarenal RAAS, particularly under pathophysiological conditions.

6. CONCLUSIONS

The majority of experimental studies on the RAAS and the regulation of blood pressure have utilized male animals. As there is overwhelming evidence for sex differences in the extent of hypertension and cardiovascular injury, the consideration of gender in the regulation of the renal RAAS enzyme cascade should be carefully considered (Bachmann *et al* 1991; Brosnihan *et al* 1999; Reckelhoff *et al* 2000). For example, the presence of renal damage in the male ACE2 knockout mice was not evident in the estrogen replete female littermates and possibly there is greater expression of RAAS components in the males with the loss of ACE2 (Oudit *et al* 2006). We and others have shown that estrogen depletion is associated with altered expression of renin, AT_1 receptors, ACE and NOS isoforms, as well as exacerbates hypertension and salt-sensitive renal injury (Bayorh *et al* 2001; Brosnihan *et al* 1997; Chappell *et al* 2003; Chappell *et al* 2006; Harrison-Bernard *et al* 2003; Roesch *et al* 2000; Yamaleyeva *et al* 2007). Moreover, in lieu of the negative outcomes for estrogen or combined hormone replacement in older women (HERS, WHI), the influence of aging on the response of the intrarenal RAAS and other systems may be of equal importance. Clearly, understanding the regulation and interplay of ACE, ACE2 and neprilysin within the kidney, as well as other areas including the heart, brain and vascular beds are critical to treating the burgeoning problem of cardiovascular disease.

ACKNOWLEDGEMENTS

These studies were supported in part by grants from the National Institute of Health grants (HL-56973 and HL-51952) and the American Heart Association (AHA-151521 and AHA-355741). An unrestricted grant from the Unifi Corporation (Greensboro, NC) and the Farley-Hudson Foundation (Jacksonville, NC) is also acknowledged.

REFERENCES

Allred AJ, Diz DI, Ferrario CM, Chappell MC, 2000, Pathways for angiotensin-(1-7) metabolism in pulmonary and renal tissues. *Am J Physiol* **279**: F841–F850

Azizi M, Ezan E, Nicolet L, Grognet J-M, Menard J, 1997, High plasma level of *N*-Acetyl-Seryl-Aspartyl-Lysyl-Proline: A new marker of chronic angiotensin-converting enzyme inhibition. *Hypertension* **30**: 1015–1019

Bachmann J, Feldmer M, Ganten U, Stock G, Ganten D, 1991, Sexual dimorphism of blood pressure: Possible role of the renin-angiotensin system. *J. Steroid Biochem.* **40**: 511–515

Bayorh MA, Mann G, Walton M, Eatman D, 2006, Effects of enalapril, tempol, and eplerenone on salt-induced hypertension in Dahl salt-sensitive rats. *Clin and Exper Hypertension* **28**: 121–32

Bayorh MA, Socci RR, Eatman D, Wang M, Thierry-Palmer M, 2001, The role of gender in salt-induced hypertension. *Clin and Exper Hypertension* **23**: 241–256

Beldent V, Michaud A, Wei L, Chauvet M-T, Corvol P, 1993, Proteolytic release of human angiotensin-converting enzyme: localization of the cleavage site. *J Biol Chem* **268**: 26428–26434

Benter IF, Yousif MHM, Anim JT, Cojocel C, Diz DI, 2006, Angiotensin-(1-7) prevents development of severe hypertension and end-organ damage in spontaneously hypertensive rats treated with L-NAME. *Am J Physiol* **290**: H684–H691

Benter IF, Yousif MHM, Cojocel C, Al-Maghrebi M, Diz DI, 2007, Angiotensin-(1-7) prevents diabetes-induced cardiovascular dysfunction. *Am J Physiol* **292**: H666–H672

Benzing T, Fleming I, Blaukat A, Muller-Esterl W, Busse R, 1999, Angiotensin-converting enzyme inhibitor ramiprilat interferes with the sequestration of the B2 kinin receptor within the plasma membrane of native endothelial cells. *Circulation* **99**: 2034–2040

Brosnihan KB, Li P, Ganten D, Ferrario CM, 1997, Estrogen protects transgenic hypertensive rats by shifting the vasoconstrictor-vasodilator balance of RAS. *Am J Physiol* 273: R1908–R1915

Brosnihan KB, Senanayake PS, Li P, Ferrario CM, 1999, Bi-directional actions of estrogen on the renin-angiotensin system. *Braz. J. Med. Biol. Res.* 32: 373–381

Brosnihan KB, Neves LA, Joyner J, Averill DB, Chappell MC, Penninger JM, Ferrario CM, 2003, Enhanced renal immunocytochemical expression of ANG-(1-7) and ACE2 during pregnancy. *Hypertension* 42: 749–753

Burckle CA, Danser AHJ, Muller D, Garrelds IM, Gasc JM, Popova E, Pleham R, Peters J, Bader M, Nguyen G, 2006, Elevated blood pressure and heart rate in human renin receptor transgenic rats. *Hypertension* 47: 552–556

Burns KD, 2000, Angiotensin II and its receptors in the diabetic kidney. *American Journal of Kidney Diseases* 36: 449–467

Campbell DJ, Alexiou T, Xiao HD, Fuchs S, McKinley MJ, Corvol P, Bernstein KE, 2004, Effect of reduced angiotensin-converting enzyme gene expression and angiotensin-converting enzyme inhibition on angiotensin and bradykinin peptide levels in mice. *Hypertension* 43: 854–859

Campbell DJ, Anastasopoulos F, Duncan AM, James GM, Kladis A, Briscoe TA, 1998, Effects of neutral endopeptidase inhibition and combined angiotensin converting enzyme and neutral endopeptidase inhibition on angiotensin and bradykinin peptides in rats. *Journal of Pharmacology & Experimental. Therapeutics.* 287: 567–577

Campbell DJ, Lawrence AC, Towrie A, Kladis A, Valentijn AJ, 1991, Differential regulation of angiotensin peptide levels in plasma and kidney of the rat. *Hypertension* 18: 763–773

Carey RM, Siragy HM, 2003, Newly recognized components of the Renin-Angiotensin system: potential roles in cardiovascular and renal regulation. *Endocr. Rev* 24: 261–271

Cavasin MA, Nour-Eddine R, Yang X-P, Carretero OA, 2004, Prolyl oligopeptidase is involved in release of the antifibrotic peptide Ac-SDKP. *Hypertension* 43: 1140–1145

Chappell MC, Brosnihan KB, Diz DI, Ferrario CM, 1989, Angiotensin-(1-7) is an endogenous peptide in the rat brain: evidence for differential processing of angiotensin peptides. *J Biol Chem* 264: 16518–16523

Chappell MC, Tallant EA, Brosnihan KB, Ferrario CM, 1990, Processing of angiotensin peptides by NG108-15 neuroblastoma X glioma hybrid cell line. *Peptides* 11: 375–380

Chappell MC, Pirro NT, Sykes A, Ferrario CM, 1998, Metabolism of angiotensin-(1-7) by angiotensin converting enzyme. *Hypertension* 31: 362–367

Chappell MC, Ferrario CM, 1999, Angiotensin-(1-7) in hypertension. *Curr. Opin. Nephrol. Hypertens.* 88: 231–235

Chappell MC, Gomez MN, Pirro NT, Ferrario CM, 2000, Release of angiotensin-(1-7) from the rat hindlimb: influence of angiotensin-converting enzyme inhibition. *Hypertension* 35: 348–352

Chappell MC, Allred AJ, Ferrario CM, 2001, Pathways of angiotensin-(1-7) metabolism in the kidney. *Nephrol Dial Transplant* 16: 22–26

Chappell MC, Jung F, Gallagher PE, Averill DB, Crackower MA, Penninger JM, Ferrario CM, 2002, Omapatrilat treatment is associated with increased ACE-2 and angiotensin-(1-7) in spontaneously hypertensive rats. *Hypertension* 40: 409 [Abstract]

Chappell MC, Gallagher PE, Averill DB, Ferrario CM, Brosnihan KB, 2003, Estrogen or the AT1 antagonist olmesartan reverses the development of profound hypertension in the congenic mRen2.Lewis rat. *Hypertension* 42: 781–786

Chappell MC, Modrall JG, Diz DI, Ferrario CM, 2004, Novel aspects of the renal renin-angiotensin system: angiotensin-(1-7), ACE2 and blood pressure regulation. In *Kidney and Blood Pressure Regulation*, ed. H Suzuki, T Saruta,77–89. Basel, Karger

Chappell MC, Yamaleyeva LM, Westwood BM, 2006, Estrogen and salt sensitivity in the female mRen(2).Lewis rat. *Am J Physiol* 291: R1557–R1563

Chen Z, Tan F, Erdos EG, Deddish PA, 2005, Hydrolysis of angiotensin peptides by human angiotensin I-converting enzyme and the resensitization of B_2 kinin receptors. *Hypertension* 46: 1368–1373

Clark MA, Diz DI, Tallant EA, 2001, Angiotensin-(1-7) downregulates the angiotensin II type 1 receptor in vascular smooth muscle cells. *Hypertension* 37: 1141–1146

Clark MA, Tallant EA, Tommasi EN, Bosch SM, Diz DI, 2003, Angiotensin-(1-7) reduces renal angiotensin II receptors through a cylocoxygenase dependent pathway. *J. Cardiovasc. Pharmacol.***41**: 276–283

Crackower MA, Sarao R, Oudit GY, Yagil C, Kozieradzki I Oliveira-dos-Santos AJ, da Costa J, Zhang L, Pei Y, Scholey J, Bray MR, Backx PH, Chappell MC, Yagil Y, Penninger JM, 2002, Angiotensin-converting enzyme 2 is an essential regulator of heart function. *Nature* **417**: 822–828

Deddish PA, Marcic B, Jackman HL, Wang H-Z, Skidgel RA, Erdos EG, 1998, N-domain specific substrate and C-domain inhibitors of angiotensin converting enzyme. *Hypertension* **31**: 912–917

Diez-Freire C, Vasquez J, Correa de Adjounian MF, Ferrari MFR, Yuan L, Silver X, Torres R, Raizada MK, 2006, ACE2 gene transfer attenuates hypertension-linked pathophysiological changes in the SHR. *Physiol Genomics* **27**: 12–19

Dive V, Cotton J, Yiotakis A, Michaud A, Vassiliou S, Jiracek J, Vazeux G, Chauvet MT, Cuniasse P, Corvol P, 1999, RXP 407, a phosphinic peptide, is a potent inhibitor of angiotensin I converting enzyme able to differentiate between its two active sites. *Proc. Natl. Acad. Sci. USA* **96**: 4330–4335

Donoghue M, Hsieh F, Baronas E, Godbout K, Gosselin M, Stagliano N, Donovan M, Woolf B, Robinson K, Jeyaseelan R, Breitbart RE, Acton S, 2000, A novel angiotensin-converting enzyme-related carboxypeptidase (ACE2) converts angiotensin I to angiotensin 1-9. *Circ Res* **87**: E1–E9

Elased KM, Cunha TS, Gurley SB, Coffman TM, Morris M, 2006, New mass spectrometric assay for angiotensin-converting enzyme 2 activity. *Hypertension* **47**: 1010–1017

Fernandes L, Fortes ZB, Nigro D, Tostes RC, Santos RA, Carvalho MHC, 2001, Potentiation of bradykinin by angiotensin-(1-7) on arterioles of spontaneously hypertensive rats studied in vivo. *Hypertension* **37**: 703–709

Ferrario CM, Martell N, Yunis C, Flack JM, Chappell MC, Brosnihan KB, Dean RH, Fernandez A, Novikov S, Pinillas C, Luque M, 1998, Characterization of angiotensin-(1-7) in the urine of normal and essential hypertensive subjects. *Am. J. Hypertens.* **11**: 137–146

Ferrario CM, Smith RD, Brosnihan KB, Chappell MC, Campese VM, Vesterqvist O, Liao W, Ruddy MC, Grim CE, 2002a, Effects of omapatrilat on the renin angiotensin system in salt sensitive hypertension. *Am J Hypertens* **15**: 557–564

Ferrario CM, Averill DA, Chappell MC, Brosnihan KB, Diz DI, 2002b, Vasopeptidase inhibition and angiotensin-(1-7) in the spontaneously hypertensive rat. *Kidney Int.* **62**: 1349–57

Ferrario CM, Jessup JA, Chappell MC, Averill DB, Brosnihan KB, Gallagher PE, 2005a, Effect of angiotensin converting enzyme inhibition and angiotensin II receptor blockers on cardiac angiotensin converting enzyme 2. *Circulation* **111**: 2605–2610

Ferrario CM, Jessup JA, Gallagher PE, Averill DB, Brosnihan KB, Chappell MC. 2005b. Effects of renin angiotensin system blockade on renal angiotensin-(1-7) forming enzymes and receptors. *Kidney Int.* **68**: 2189–2196

Ferrario CM, Trask AJ, Jessup JA. 2006. Advances in biochemical and functional roles of angiotensin converting enzyme 2 and angiotensin-(1-7) in the regulation of cardiovascular function. *Am J Physiol* **289**: H2281–H2290

Gallagher PE, Chappell MC, Ferrario CM, Tallant EM, 2006, Distinct roles for Ang II and ANG-(1-7) in the regulation of angiotensin-converting enzyme 2 in rat astrocytes. *Am J Physiol* **290**: C420–C426

Georgiadis D, Beau F, Czarny B, Cotton J, Yiotakis A, Dive V, 2003, Roles of the two active sites of somatic angiotensin-converting enzyme in the cleavage of angiotensin I and bradykinin: insights from selective inhibitors. *Circ Res* **93**: 148–154

Guy JL, Lambert DW, Warner FJ, Hooper NM, Turner AJ, 2005, Membrane-associated zinc peptidase families: comparing ACE and ACE2. *Biochim Biophys Acta* **1751**: 2–8

Harmer D, Gilbert M, Borman R, Clark KL, 2002, Quantitative mRNA expression profiling of ACE 2, a novel homologue of angiotensin converting enzyme. *FEBS Lett.* **532**: 107–110

Harris RC, 1999, Potential mechanisms and physiologic actions of intracellular angiotensin II. *Am J Med. Sci.* **318**: 374–389

Harrison-Bernard LM, Zhou J, Kobori H, Ohishi M, Navar LG, 2002, Intrarenal AT$_1$ receptor and ACE binding in ANG II-induced hypertensive rats. *Am J Physiol* **281**: F19–F25

Harrison-Bernard LM, Schulman IH, Raij L, 2003, Postovariectomy hypertension is linked to increased renal AT1 receptor and salt sensitivity. *Hypertension* **42**: 1157–1163

Hattori MA, Del Ben GL, Carmona AK, Casarini DE, 2000, Angiotensin I-converting enzyme isoforms (high and low molecular weight) in urine of premature and full-term infants. *Hypertension* **35**: 1284–1290

Huang Y, Wongamorntham S, Kasting J, McQuillan D, Owens RT Yu L, Noble NA, Border W, 2006, Renin increases mesangial cell transforming growth factor-*B*1 matrix proteins through receptor-mediated, angiotensin II-independent mechanisms. *Kid. Int.* **69**: 105–113

Igase M, Strawn WB, Gallagher PE, Geary RL, Ferrario CM, 2005, Angiotensin II AT1 receptors regulate ace2 and angiotensin-(1-7) expression in aorta of spontaneously hypertensive rats. *Am J Physiol* **289**: H1013–H1019

Ingert C, Grima M, Coquard C, Barthelmebs M, Imbs J-L, 2002, Contribution of angiotensin II internalization to intrarenal angiotensin II levels in rats. *Am J Physiol* **283**: 1003–1110

Iyer SN, Ferrario CM, Chappell MC, 1998, Angiotensin-(1-7) contributes to the antihypertensive effects of blockade of the renin-angiotensin system. *Hypertension* **31**: 356–361

Iyer SN, Yamada K, Diz DI, Ferrario CM, Chappell MC, 2000, Evidence that prostaglandins mediate the antihypertensive actions of angiotensin-(1-7) during chronic blockade of the renin-angiotensin system. *J. Cardiovasc. Pharmacol.* **36**: 109–217

Jessup JA, Gallagher PE, Averill DB, Brosnihan KB, Tallant EA, Chappell MC, Ferrario CM, 2006, Effect of angiotensin II blockade on a new congenic model of hypertension derived from transgenic Ren-2 rats. *Am J Physiol* **291**: H2166–H2172

Keidar S, Gamliel-Lazarovich A, Kaplan M, Pavlotzky E, Hamoud S, Hayek T, Karry R, Abassi Z, 2005, Mineralocorticoid receptor blocker increases angiotensin-converting enzyme 2 activity in congestive heart failure patients. Circ Res **97**: 946–953

Keidar S, Strizevsky A, Raz A, Gamliel-Lazarovich A, 2006, ACE2 activity is increased in monocyte-derived macrophages from prehypertensive subjects. *Nephrol Dial Transplant*: 1–5

Klar J, Vitzhum H, Kurtz A, 2004, Aldosterone enhances renin expression in juxtaglomerular cells. A J Physiol 286: F349–F355

Kobori H, Harrison-Bernard LM, Navar LG, 2001, Expression of angiotensinogen mRNA and protein in angiotensin II-dependent hypertension. *J Am Soc Nephrol* **12**: 431–439

Kohlstedt K, Shoghi F, Muller-Esterl W, Busse R, Fleming I, 2002, CK2 phosphorylates the angiotensin-converting enzyme and regulates its retention in the endothelial cell plasma membrane. *Circ Res.* **91**: 749–756

Kostis JB, Packer M, Black HR, Schmieder R, Henry D, Levy E, 2004, Omapatrilat and Enalapril in Patients With Hypertension: The Omapatrilat Cardiovascular Treatment vs. Enalapril (OCTAVE) Trial. *Am J Hypertens* **17**: 111–121

Kubota E, Dean RG, Hubner RA, Casley DJ, Johnston CI, Burrell LM, 2003, Differential tissue and enzyme inhibitory effects of the vasopeptidase inhibitor omapatrilat in the rat. *Clin Sci* **105**: 339–345

Lambert DW, Yarski M, Warner FJ, Thornhill P, Parkin ET, Smith AI, Hooper NM, Turner AJ, 2005, Tumor necrosis factor-a convertase (ADAM17) mediates regulated ectodomain shedding of the severe-acute respiratory syndrome-coronavirus (SARS-Co-V) receptor, angiotensin-converting enzyme-2 (ACE2). *J Biol Chem* **280**: 30113–30119

Li N, Zimpelmann J, Cheng K, Wilkins JA, Burns KD, 2004, The role of angiotensin converting enzyme 2 in the generation of angiotensin 1-7 by rat proximal tubules. *Am J Physiol* **288**: F353–F362

Liebau MC, Lang D, Bohm J, Endlich N, Bek MJ, Witherden I, Mathieson PW, Saleem MA, Pavenstadt H, Fischer KG, 2006, Functional expression of the renin-angiotensin system in human podocytes. *Am J Physiol* **90**: F710–F719

Llorens-Cortes C, Huang H, Vicart P, Gasc J-M, Paulin D, Corvol P, 1992, Identification and characterization of neutral endopeptidase in endothelial cells from venous or arterial origins. *J Biol Chem* **267**: 14012–14018

Marques GDM, Quinto BMR, Plavinik FL, Krieger JE, Marson O, Casarini DE, 2003, N-domain angiotensin-I-converting enzyme with 80 kDa as a possible genetic marker of hypertension. *Hypertension* **42**: 693–701

Modrall JG, Sadjadi J, Brosnihan KB, Gallagher PE, Ya C-H, Bernstein KE, Chappell MC. 2003. Depletion of tissue ace differentially influences the intrarenal and urinary expression of angiotensins. *Hypertension* **43**: 4849–4853

Nagata S, Kato J, Sasaki K, Minamino N, Eto T, Kitamura K, 2006, Isolation and identification of proangiotensin-12, a possible component of the renin-angiotensin system. *Biochem Biophys Res Comm* **350**: 1026–1031

Navar LG, Harrison-Bernard LM, Nishiyama A, Kobori H, 2002, Regulation of intrarenal angiotensin II in hypertension. *Hypertension* **39**: 316–322

Nguyen G, Delarue F, Burckle C, Bouzhir L, Giller T, Sraer JD. 2002. Pivotal role of the renin/prorenin receptor in angiotensin II production and cellular responses to renin. *J Clin Invest* **109**: 1417–1427

Omata M, Taniguchi H, Koya D, Kanasaki K, Sho R, KatoY, Kojima R, Haneda M, Inomata N, 2006, N-Acetyl-Seryl-Aspartyl-Lysyl-Proline ameliorates the progression of renal dysfunction and fibrosis and WKY rats with established anti-glomerular basement membrane nephritis. *J Am Soc Nephrol* **17**: 674–685

Oudit GY, Herzenberg AM, Kassiri Z, Wong D, Reich H, Khokha R, Crackower MA, Backx PH, Penninger JM, Scholey JW, 2006, Loss of angiotensin-converting enzyme-2 leads to the late development of angiotensin II-dependent glomerulosclerosis. *Am J Pathol* **168**: 1808–1820

Packer M, Califf RM, Konstam MA, Krum H, McMurray JJ, Rouleau JL, Swedberg K, 2002, Comparison of omapatrilat and enalapril in patients with chronic heart failure. The omapatrilat versus enalapril randomized trial of utility in reducing events (OVERTURE). *Circulation* **106**: 920–926

Paul M, Mehr AP, Kreutz R. 2006. Physiology of local renin-angiotensin systems. *Physiol Rev* **86**: 747–803

Pendergrass KD, Averill DB, Ferrario CM, Diz DI, Chappell MC, 2006, Differential expression of nuclear AT1 receptors and angiotensin II within the kidney of the male congenic mRen2.Lewis rat. *Am J Physiol Renal Physiol* **290**: F1497–F1506

Peng H, Carretero OA, Brigstock DR, Oja-Tebbe N, Rhaleb N-E, 2003, Ac-SDKP reverses cardiac fibrosis in rats with renovascular hypertension. *Hypertension* **42**: 1164–1170

Prieto-Carrasquero MC, Harrison-Bernard LM, Kobori H, Ozawa Y, Hering-Smith KS, Hamm LL, Navar LG, 2004, Enhancement of collecting duct renin in angiotensin II-dependent hypertensive rats. *Hypertension* **44**: 223–229

Raousseau A, Michaud A, Chauvet M-T, Lenfant M, Corvol P, 1995, The hemoregulatory peptide N-acetyl-Ser-Asp-Lys-Pro is a natural and specific substrate of the N-terminal active site of human angiotensin-converting enzyme. *J. Biol. Chem.* **270**: 3656–3661

Reckelhoff JF, Zhang H, Srivastava K, 2000, Gender differences in development of hypertension in spontaneously hypertensive rats: role of the renin-angiotensin system. *Hypertension* **35**: 48048–3

Rice GI, Jones AL, Grant PJ, Carter AM, Turner AJ, Hooper NM, 2006, Circulating activities of angiotensin-converting enzyme, its homolog, angiotensin-converting enzyme 2, and neprilysin in a family study. *Hypertension* **48**: 914–920

Rice GI, Thomas DA, Grant PJ, Turner AJ, Hooper NM, 2004, Evaluation of angiotensin-converting enzyme (ACE), its homologue ACE2 and neprilysin in angiotensin peptide metabolism. *Biochem J* **383**: 45–51

Roesch DM, Tian Y, Zheng W, Shi M, Verbalis JG, Sandberg K, 2000, Estradiol attenuates angiotensin-induced aldosterone secretion in ovariectomized rats. *Endocrinology* **141**: 4629–4636

Sadjadi J, Kramer GL, Yu C, Welborn MB, Chappell MC, Modrall JG, 2005a, Angiotensin converting enzyme-independent angiotensin II production by chymase is up-regulated in the ischemic kidney in renovascular hypertension. *J Surg Res* **127**: 65–69

Sadjadi J, Kramer GL, Yu CH, Welborn MB, Modrall JG, 2005b, Angiotensin II exerts positive feedback on the intrarenal renin-angiotensin system by an angiotensin converting enzyme-dependent mechanism. *J Surg Res* **129**: 272–277

Sampaio WO, dos Santos RA, Faria-Silva R, de Mata Machado LT, Schiffrin EL, Touyz RM, 2007, Angiotensin-(1-7) through receptor mas mediates endothelial nitric oxide synthase activation via Akt-dependent pathways. *Hypertension* **49**: 185–192

Santos RA, Silva ACS, Maric C, Speth R, Machado RP de Buhr I, Heringer-Walther S, Pinheiro SVB, Lopes MT, Bader M, Mendes EP, Lemos VS, Campagnole-Santos MJ, Schultheiss HP, Speth R, Walther T, 2003, Angiotensin-(1-7) is an endogenous ligand for the G protein-coupled receptor Mas. *Proc Natl Acad Sci* **100**: 8258–8263

Santos RAS, Brosnihan KB, Jacobsen DW, DiCorleto PE, Ferrario CM, 1992, Production of angiotensin-(1-7) by human vascular endothelium. *Hypertension* **19**: II-56-II-61

Schiffrin EL, 1999, Role of endothelin-1 in hypertension. *Hypertension* **34**: 876–881

Schiffrin EL, 2006, Effects of aldosterone on the vasculature. *Hypertension* **47**: 312–318

Scicli AG, Carretero OA, 1986, Renal kallikrein-kinin system. *Kidney Int.* **29**: 120–130

Shaltout HA, Westwood B, Averill DB, Ferrario CM, Figueroa J, Diz DI, Rose J, Chappell MC, 2007, Angiotensin Metabolism in Renal Proximal Tubules, Urine and Serum of Sheep: Evidence for ACE2-Dependent Processing of Angiotensin II. *Am J Physiol* **292**: F82–F91

Singh R, Singh A, Leehey DJ, 2005, A novel mechanism for angiotensin II formation in streptozoticin-diabetic rat glomeruli. *Am J Physiol* **288**: F1183–F1190

Skidgel RA, Erdos EG. 2004. Angiotensin converting enzyme (ACE) and neprilysin hydrolyze neuropeptides: a brief history, the beginning and follow-ups to early studies. *Peptides* **25**: 521–525

Su Z, Zimpelmann J, Burns KD, 2006, Angiotensin-(1-7) inhibits angiotensin II-stimulated phosphorylation of MAP kinases in proximal tubular cells. *Kidney Int.* **69**: 2212–2218

Sulpizio AC, Pullen MA, Edwards RM, Louttit JB, West R, Brooks DP, 2005, Mechanism of vasopeptidase inhibitor-induced plasma extravasation: Comparison of omapatrilat and the novel neutral endopeptidase 24.11/angiotensin-converting enzyme inhibitor GW796406. *J Pharm Exp Therapeutics* **315**: 1306–1313

Takase O, Marumo T, Imai N, Hirahashi J, Takayanagi A, Hishikawa K, Hayashi M, Shimizu N, Fujita T, Saruta T, 2005, NF-kappaB-dependent increase in intrarenal angiotensin II induced by proteinuria. *Kidney Int* **68**: 464–473

Tallant EA, Ferrario CM, Gallagher PE, 2005a, Angiotensin-(1-7) inhibits growth of cardiac myocytes through activation of the *mas* receptor. *Am J Physiol* **289**: H1560–H1566

Tallant EA, Ferrario CM, Gallagher PE, 2005b, Differential regulation of cardiac angiotensin converting enzyme 2 (ACE2) and ACE by aldosterone. **46**: 886 [Abstract]

Tikellis C, Johnston CI, Forbes JM, Burns WC, Burrell LM Risvanis J, Cooper ME, 2003, Characterization of renal Angiotensin-converting enzyme 2 in diabetic nephropathy. *Hypertension* **41**: 392–397

Tikellis C, Cooper ME, Bialkowski K, Johnston CI, Burns WC, Lew RA, Smith AI, Thomas MC, 2006, Developmental expression of ACE2 in the SHR kidney: A role in hypertension? *Kidney Int* **70**: 34–41

Tikkanen I, Tikkanen T, Cao Z, Allen TJ, Davis BJ, Lassila M, Casley D, Johnston CI, Burrell LM, Cooper ME, 2002, Combined inhibition of neutral endopeptidase with angiotensin converting enzyme or endothelin converting enzyme in experimental diabetes. *J Hypertens* **20**: 707–714

Tipnis SR, Hooper NM, Hyde R, Karran E, Christie G, Turner AJ, 2000, A human homolog of angiotensin-converting enzyme. Cloning and functional expression as a captopril-insensitive carboxypeptidase. *J Biol Chem* **275**: 33238–33243

Tokuyama H, Hayashi K, Matsuda H, Kubota E, Honda M, Okubo K, Takamatsu I, Tatematsu S, Ozawa Y, Wakino S, Saruta T, 2002, Differential regulation of elevated renal angiotensin II in chronic renal ischemia. *Hypertension* **40**: 34–40

Veelken R, Schmieder RE, 2002, Neutral endopeptidase inhibition: the potential of the new therapeutic approach in cardiovascular disease evolves. *J Hypertens* **20**: 599–603

Vickers C, Hales P, Kaushik V, Dick L, Gavin J, Tang J, Godbout K, Parsons T, Baronas E, Hsieh F, Acton S, Patane M, Nichols A, Tummino P, 2002, Hydrolysis of biological peptides by human angiotensin-converting enzyme-related carboxypeptidase. *J Biol Chem* **277**: 14838–14843

Welches WR, Brosnihan KB, Ferrario CM, 1993, A comparison of the properties, and enzymatic activity of three angiotensin processing enzymes: angiotensin converting enzyme, prolyl endopeptidase and neutral endopeptidase 24.11. *Life Sci.* **52**: 1461–1470

Westwood BM, Figueroa J, Rose JM, Chappell MC, 2006, Distinct gender differences in the ACE2-dependent metabolism of angiotensin II in the serum of sheep. *Hypertension* **48**: 46 [Abstract]

Wiemer G, Dobrucki LW, Louka FR, Malinski T, Heitsch H, 2002, AVE 0991, a nonpeptide mimic of the effects of angiotensin-(1-7) on the endothelium. *Hypertension* **40**: 847–852

Wysocki J, Ye M, Soler MJ, Gurley SB, Xiao HD, Bernstein KE, Coffman TM, Chen S, Batlle D, 2006, ACE and ACE2 activity in diabetic mice. *Diabetes* **55**: 2132–2139

Yamada K, Iyer SN, Chappell MC, Ganten D, Ferrario CM, 1998, Converting enzyme determines the plasma clearance of angiotensin-(1-7). *Hypertension* **98**: 496–502

Yamada K, Iyer SN, Chappell MC, Brosnihan KB, Fukuhara M, Ferrario CM, 1999, Differential response of angiotensin peptides in the urine of hypertensive animals. *Regul. Pept.* **80**: 57–66

Yamaleyeva LM, Gallagher PE, Vinsant S, Chappell MC, 2007, Discoordinate regulation of renal nitric oxide synthase isoforms in ovariectomized mREN2.Lewis rats. *Am J Physiol* **292**: R819–R826

Yamamoto K, Chappell MC, Brosnihan KB, Ferrario CM, 1992, In vivo metabolism of angiotensin I by neutral endopeptidase (EC 3.4.24.11) in spontaneously hypertensive rats. *Hypertension* **19**: 692–696

Ye M, Wysocki J, William J, Soler MJ, Cokic I, Batlle D, 2006, Glomerular localization and expression of angiotensin-converting enzyme 2 and angiotensin-converting enzyme: Implications for albuminemia in diabetes. *J Am Soc Nephrol* **17**: 3067–3075

Zhang SL, To C, Chen X, Filep JG, Tang SS, Ingelfinger JR, Chan JS, 2002, Essential role(s) of the intrarenal renin-angiotensin system in transforming growth factor-beta1 gene expression and induction of hypertrophy of rat kidney proximal tubular cells in high glucose. *J Am Soc. Nephrol.* **13**: 302–312

Zhong JC, Huang DY, Yang YM, Li YF, Liu GF, Song XH, Du K, 2004, Upregulation of angiotensin-converting enzyme 2 by all-trans retinoic acid in spontaneously hypertensive rats. *Hypertension* **44**: 907–912

CHAPTER 2

ACE INHIBITION IN HEART FAILURE
AND ISCHAEMIC HEART DISEASE

DUNCAN J. JOHN CAMPBELL

St. Vincent's Institute of Medical Research and Department of Medicine, University of Melbourne, Fitzroy, Victoria, Australia

1.   INTRODUCTION

Angiotensin converting enzyme (dipeptidyl carboxypeptidase I, kininase II, EC 3.4.15.1, ACE) plays a major role in the metabolism of many different peptides, including angiotensin (Ang) I, bradykinin, kallidin, and *N*-acetyl-seryl-aspartyl-lysyl-proline (AcSDKP). ACE inhibitors are established therapy for heart failure and ischaemic heart disease, and alterations of Ang II, bradykinin, kallidin, and AcSDKP peptide levels are implicated in the mechanisms of this therapy. This chapter briefly describes the renin angiotensin, kallikrein kinin, and AcSDKP systems, and their role in cardiovascular physiology and disease. The role of ACE inhibition in treatment and prevention of heart failure and ischaemic heart disease is summarised, and the possible mechanisms of the therapeutic benefits of ACE inhibitors are described. This is not an exhaustive review, but focuses on those aspects most relevant to the clinical application of ACE inhibitors.

2.   THE CARDIAC RENIN-ANGIOTENSIN SYSTEM (RAS)

2.1.   Pathways of Ang Peptide Formation and Metabolism

Figure 1 shows an outline of the pathways of Ang peptide formation and metabolism. In addition to the classical pathway involving renin and ACE, alternative pathways have been proposed (Campbell 2006). There remain many questions concerning the mechanisms of Ang peptide formation in discrete tissue compartments such as the heart. Serine proteases, for example, may form Ang II by processes independent of renin at sites of inflammation or coagulation, where kallikrein and/or cathepsin G may be active.

Po Sing Leung (ed.), Frontiers in Research of the Renin-Angiotensin System on Human Disease, 21–54.
© 2007 *Springer.*

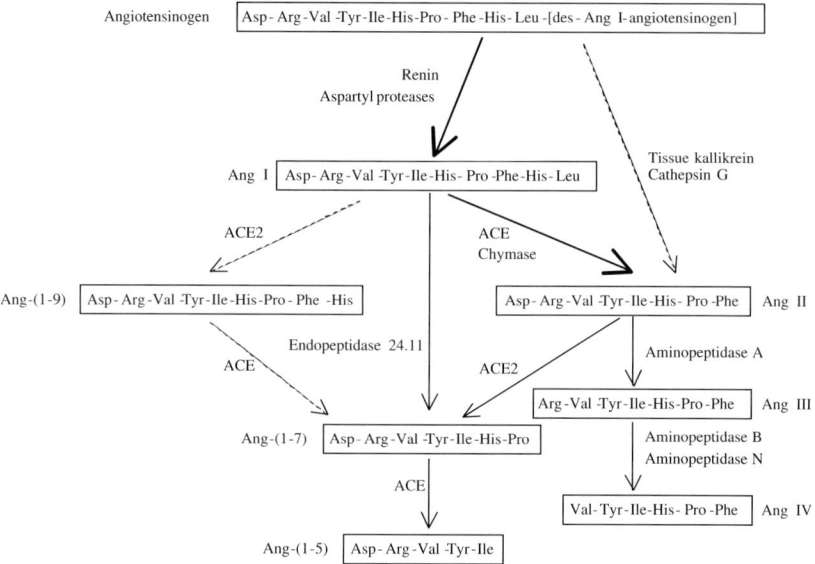

Figure 1. Pathways of Ang peptide formation and metabolism. Adapted from (Campbell 2006)

2.2.   Renin and Angiotensinogen

Studies of nephrectomised animals show the main mechanism of Ang peptide formation in the heart involves kidney-derived renin (Campbell *et al* 1993; Danser *et al* 1994). Renin messenger RNA (mRNA) levels in the heart are very low or undetectable (De Mello *et al* 2000). Cardiac renin expression may, however, be induced by myocardial infarction and macrophages and myofibroblasts may express renin at the site of repair (Sun *et al* 2001). All Ang peptides are derived from angiotensinogen. Although angiotensinogen may be produced in low levels in the heart (Dostal *et al* 1999; Paul *et al* 2006), plasma is the main source of angiotensinogen for Ang peptide formation in the heart.

2.3.   ACE

ACE is a membrane-bound zinc-containing metallopeptidase, some of which is cleaved from membranes and released as soluble ACE found in plasma and other fluids (Erdos 1990). ACE has two catalytic domains with differential substrate specificities and susceptibility to ACE inhibitors (Wei *et al* 1991; Wei *et al* 1992; Jaspard *et al* 1993). Table 1 lists the many substrates of ACE. Those ACE substrates most related to cardiac function are Ang I, the bradykinin and kallidin peptides, and AcSDKP. Both catalytic domains of ACE posses dipeptidyl carboxypeptidase and endopeptidase activities and can cleave Ang I, bradykinin-(1-9), bradykinin-(1-7), and substance P. However, the *N*-terminal catalytic domain cleaves of lutein-

Table 1. Substrates of ACE

Angiotensin I and angiotensin-(1-7)
Bradykinin-(1-9), bradykinin-(1-8), and bradykinin-(1-7)
Lys^0-bradykinin-(1-9) (kallidin), Lys^0-bradykinin-(1-8), and Lys^0-bradykinin-(1-7)
Substance P
N-acetyl-seryl-aspartyl-lysyl-proline (AcSDKP)
Chemotactic peptide
Neurotensin
Luteinising hormone-releasing hormone (LH-RH)
Enkephalins
Cholecystokinin
Gastrin

Adapted from (Ehlers et al 1990; Erdos 1990; Hooper 1991; Rieger et al 1993)

ising hormone-releasing hormone (LH-RH) and AcSDKP more efficiently than the *C*-terminal domain (Jaspard *et al* 1993; Rousseau *et al* 1995).

The two catalytic domains of ACE interact differently with ACE inhibitors. Captopril, enalapril, lisinopril, and trandolapril are all highly potent inhibitors of both domains. Whereas trandolapril, lisinopril and enalapril show preference for the *C*-terminal catalytic domain, captopril shows preference for the *N*-terminal catalytic domain (Wei *et al* 1992).

ACE has a widespread tissue distribution, including vascular endothelium and smooth muscle cells, the brush border of proximal tubule cells of the kidney, and the brain (Erdos 1990). ACE is expressed by the endothelium of the coronary vasculature, and by the endocardium and epicardium, but not by the valves in the human heart (Dostal *et al* 1999). ACE is also expressed by cardiac fibroblasts, and fibroblast expression of ACE is increased in the border zone of myocardial infarction (Dostal *et al* 1999; Burrell *et al* 2005). Cardiac ACE expression is up-regulated in heart failure (Hirsch *et al* 1991; Studer *et al* 1994).

2.4. Ang Receptors

Many different cell types express Ang receptors in the heart. The type 1 Ang (AT_1) receptor is expressed by coronary smooth muscle and endothelial cells, cardiomyocytes, fibroblasts, nerves, and conduction tissue (Regitz-Zagrosek *et al* 1998). AT_2 receptors are expressed by fibroblasts and endothelial cells (Regitz-Zagrosek *et al* 1998). In heart failure, cardiomyocyte AT_1 receptor expression may be down-regulated, whereas fibroblast expression of both AT_1 and AT_2 receptors is increased (Ohkubo *et al* 1997).

The AT_1 receptor mediates most of the known actions of Ang II. There is continuing uncertainty about the role of the AT_2 receptor, which may mediate actions of Ang II in the vasculature and heart that differ from those of the AT_1 receptor (Carey *et al* 2001; Voros *et al* 2006). The AT_2 receptor is described further by Danser in chapter 3 of this volume.

2.5.   Mast Cell Chymase

Human heart chymase was initially discovered in homogenates of human heart and proposed to be the major pathway of conversion of Ang I to Ang II in the heart (Urata *et al* 1990). Given that chymase is not inhibited by ACE inhibitors, it represented a potential pathway of continued Ang II formation in patients taking ACE inhibitor therapy (Dell'Italia *et al* 2002), and thereby provided a rationale for a possible superiority of AT_1 receptor blocker (ARB) therapy over ACE inhibitor therapy. However, studies of the effects of ACE inhibition in rats, mice, and humans, and of ACE gene knockout in mice, show ACE is the dominant pathway of Ang II formation in the heart (Campbell *et al* 1994; Campbell *et al* 1999; Zeitz *et al* 2003; Campbell *et al* 2004a).

2.6.   ACE-related Carboxypeptidase (ACE2)

ACE-related carboxypeptidase (ACE2), like ACE, is a membrane-associated and secreted metalloprotease expressed predominantly on endothelium (Donoghue *et al* 2000; Tipnis *et al* 2000; Hamming *et al* 2004). ACE2 is expressed in all human tissues, with relatively high levels in renal and cardiovascular tissues, and also in the gut (Harmer *et al* 2002). In contrast to the dipeptidyl carboxypeptidase activity of ACE, ACE2 cleaves Ang I to Ang-(1-9) and also cleaves ANG II to Ang-(1-7). ACE2 is not inhibited by ACE inhibitors.

Kinetic considerations make it unlikely that ACE2 contributes to Ang I metabolism *in vivo* (Jaspard *et al* 1993; Vickers *et al* 2002). ACE and ACE2 have similar K_m for Ang I (16 and 6.9 µmol/L, respectively) but the K_{cat} for ACE (40 s^{-1}) is approximately 1000-fold higher than that for ACE2 (0.034 s^{-1}), such that the K_{cat}/K_m ratio is approximately 500-fold higher for ACE (2.5 x 10^6 L/mol per s) than for ACE2 (4.9 x 10^3 L/mol per s). By contrast, the K_m (2 µmol/L), K_{cat} (3.5 s^{-1}), and K_{cat}/K_m ratio (1.8 x 10^6 L/mol per s) of ACE2 for Ang II (Vickers *et al* 2002) make it more likely to participate in Ang II metabolism.

Initial genetic studies suggested an important role for ACE2 in Ang peptide metabolism in the heart. The ACE2 gene knockout mouse was reported to have a cardiomyopathic phenotype associated with increased Ang II levels in plasma, heart, and kidney. Additionally, the cardiomyopathic phenotype was ameliorated by concomitant ACE gene knockout, suggesting that altered Ang peptide metabolism contributed to the phenotype (Crackower *et al* 2002). In subsequent studies the ACE2 gene knockout mouse had a normal cardiac phenotype, although it had an enhanced pressor response to Ang II administration (Gurley *et al* 2006).

ACE2 activity is reported to be increased in the hearts of patients with heart failure (Zisman *et al* 2003). However, measurement of Ang peptides in coronary venous blood of patients with heart failure or ischaemic heart disease does not support an important role for ACE2 in either Ang I or Ang II metabolism in the human heart (Campbell *et al* 2004b). Elucidation of the role of ACE2 in Ang II metabolism must await the development of specific ACE2 inhibitors.

2.7.   Effects of the RAS on the Heart and Vasculature

2.7.1.   Actions of Ang II

Both systemic and local actions of Ang II impact on the heart. Systemic actions of Ang II include its vasoconstrictor action to increase blood pressure and the stimulation of aldosterone secretion. Increased aldosterone levels may produce hypokalaemia and contribute to cardiac fibrosis (Brilla et al 1993).

Local cardiac actions of Ang II include inotropic and hypertrophic effects, and cardiac remodelling (Paul et al 2006). AT$_1$ receptor stimulation induces both myocyte hypertrophy and collagen synthesis (Regitz-Zagrosek et al 1998). Moreover, Ang II may contribute to oxidative stress, inflammation, and thrombosis (Dzau 2001; Duprez 2006). AT$_1$-mediated NADPH oxidase activation leads to generation of reactive oxygen species, widely implicated in vascular inflammation and fibrosis (Li et al 2004; Mehta et al 2007). Ang II also activates gene transcription factors involved in vascular inflammation and remodelling (Oettgen 2006). Ang II and its metabolite Ang IV may promote thrombosis by stimulating plasminogen activator inhibitor type 1 (PAI-1) and PAI-2 production by the vasculature (Van Leeuwen et al 1994; Feener et al 1995; Kerins et al 1995). Additionally, Ang II may promote thrombosis by activation of nuclear factor κB-dependent proinflammatory genes and accelerating vascular expression of tissue factor (Dielis et al 2005).

Ang II stimulates endothelin release (Kohno et al 1992; Moreau et al 1997) and endothelin blockade prevents some of the cardiovascular actions of Ang II (Webb et al 1992; Rajagopalan et al 1997; Herizi et al 1998).

2.7.2.   Actions of Ang-(1-7)

Ang-(1-7) is a biologically active peptide (Ferrario et al 1991). The main pathway of Ang-(1-7) formation is by cleavage of Ang I by neutral endopeptidase (NEP, endopeptidase 24.11) (Yamamoto et al 1992; Duncan et al 1999) (Fig. 1). Ang-(1-7) may also be formed by ACE2 cleavage of Ang II, but the significance of this pathway remains to be established.

Many actions of Ang-(1-7) are contrary to those of Ang II, and Ang-(1-7) is proposed to function as a counter-regulatory hormone in blood pressure control, and in other cardiovascular actions of Ang II. Ang-(1-7) reduces blood pressure and produces endothelium-dependent vasodilatation (Benter et al 1993; Pörsti et al 1994; Benter et al 1995; Nakamoto et al 1995; Brosnihan et al 1996; Le Tran et al 1997), actions that may be due in part to potentiation by Ang-(1-7) of the hypotensive effects of kinins (Paula et al 1995; Lima et al 1997) and/or to stimulation of vascular prostaglandin production (Benter et al 1993; Paula et al 1995). In support of a role for kinin-mediated nitric oxide production in its vasodilator effects, Ang-(1-7) induced vasodilatation and hypotension were attenuated by nitric oxide synthase (NOS) inhibition (Pörsti et al 1994; Gorelik et al 1998), by the type 2 bradykinin (B$_2$) receptor antagonist icatibant (Pörsti et al 1994; Abbas et al 1997; Lima et al 1997; Gorelik et al 1998), and also by

AT_2 receptor antagonism (Lima *et al* 1997). Moreover, Ang-(1-7) stimulation of nitric oxide release from coronary vessels was blocked by icatibant (Brosnihan *et al* 1996).

High concentrations of Ang-(1-7) inhibit ACE, leading to the suggestion that Ang-(1-7) potentiates the effects of bradykinin through ACE inhibition (Li *et al* 1997). However, the IC_{50} for Ang-(1-7) inhibition of ACE was 650 nmol/L and it is unlikely endogenous Ang-(1-7) levels would be sufficient to produce this effect. Ang-(1-7), like other ACE inhibitors, may potentiate the actions of a B_2 receptor agonist by an indirect mechanism that is independent of bradykinin hydrolysis (Deddish *et al* 1998), possibly by sensitisation of the B_2 receptor (Marcic *et al* 1999). This mechanism of potentiation of kinin-induced hypotension by Ang-(1-7) is unlikely to operate *in vivo*, however, because micromolar concentrations of Ang-(1-7) were required to produce this effect (Deddish *et al* 1998).

Plasma Ang-(1-7) levels are less than Ang II levels, except during ACE inhibition when Ang-(1-7) levels increase several-fold, in parallel with the increase in Ang I levels (Lawrence *et al* 1990; Menard *et al* 1997). Tissue levels of Ang-(1-7) are very low or undetectable, even with ACE inhibition (Campbell *et al* 1993; 1994). There is, therefore, uncertainty whether Ang-(1-7) levels are sufficient to play a role in cardiovascular physiology and disease states in humans.

3.   THE CARDIAC KALLIKREIN KININ SYSTEM (KKS)

3.1.   Pathways of Kinin Peptide Formation and Metabolism

Figure 2 shows an outline of the pathways of kinin peptide formation. A proportion of kininogens is hydroxylated on Pro^3 of the bradykinin sequence, leading to the formation of hydroxylated kinin peptides.

3.2.   Kallikreins and Kininogens

The kininogens are the sole precursors of the kinin peptides and are coded by a single gene. Differential splicing of the initial mRNA transcript produces two different mRNA coding for either high or low molecular weight kininogen. Each is a glycoprotein that contains the kinin sequence in its mid portion. Tissue kallikrein and plasma kallikrein are both serine proteases. Whereas a single gene codes for plasma kallikrein there is a large family of tissue kallikrein genes, although KLK1 is the only tissue kallikrein known to generate kinin peptides (Yousef *et al* 2001). Kininogens and tissue kallikrein are expressed in many different tissues. Plasma kallikrein is predominantly expressed in liver, although recent studies suggest expression of plasma kallikrein in the brain (Takano *et al* 1999).

In humans, plasma kallikrein forms bradykinin from high molecular weight kininogen, whereas tissue kallikrein forms kallidin from high or low molecular weight kininogens (Fig. 3). By contrast, both plasma and tissue kallikrein generate

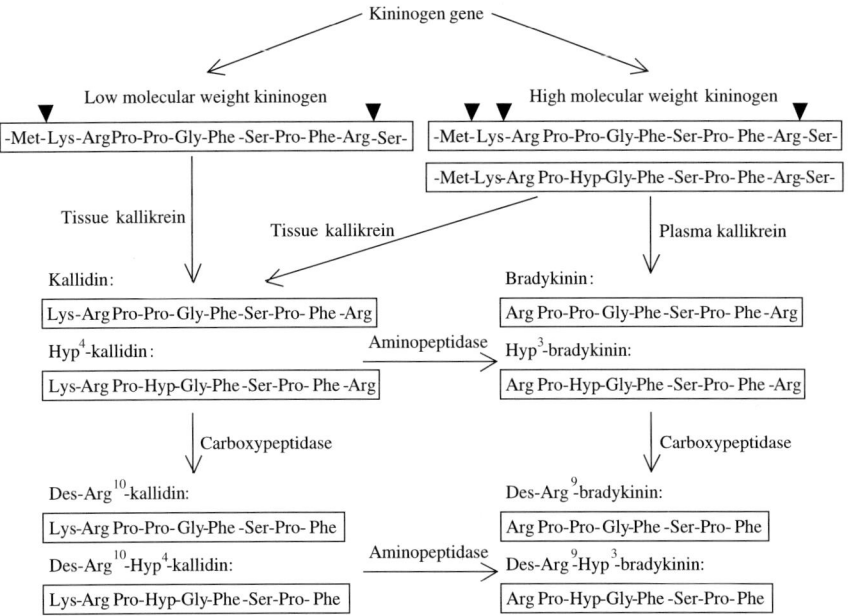

Figure 2. An outline of the formation of kallidin and bradykinin peptides in humans. A proportion of high molecular weight kininogen is hydroxylated on Pro^3 of the bradykinin sequence, giving rise to both hydroxylated and non-hydroxylated peptides. Adapted from (Campbell 2003)

bradykinin in rodents (Bhoola *et al* 1992). Bradykinin may also be generated by aminopeptidase-mediated cleavage of kallidin.

Alternative pathways of kinin formation involving enzymes other than kallikreins may operate in disease states. Although low molecular weight kininogen is a poor substrate for plasma kallikrein, it will form bradykinin in the presence of neutrophil elastase which, by cleaving a fragment from low molecular weight kininogen, renders it much more susceptible to cleavage by plasma kallikrein (Sato *et al* 1988). Moreover, the combination of mast cell tryptase and neutrophil elastase releases bradykinin from oxidized kininogens that are resistant to cleavage by kallikreins (Kozik *et al* 1998).

Kinin production *in vivo* is controlled in part by endogenous inhibitors of the kallikrein enzymes. The main inhibitors of plasma kallikrein are C1 inhibitor, α_2-macroglobulin and antithrombin III (Bhoola *et al* 1992). An important inhibitor of tissue kallikrein is kallistatin, although the function of kallistatin *in vivo* is uncertain (Chao *et al* 1996).

All components of a functional KKS are expressed in the heart (Spillmann *et al* 2006). The heart and vasculature express tissue kallikrein (Oza *et al* 1990; Xiong *et al* 1990; Nolly *et al* 1992; Nolly *et al* 1994). In addition, plasma kallikrein, a member of the contact system, generates bradykinin at the endothelial surface of blood vessels (Campbell 2003).

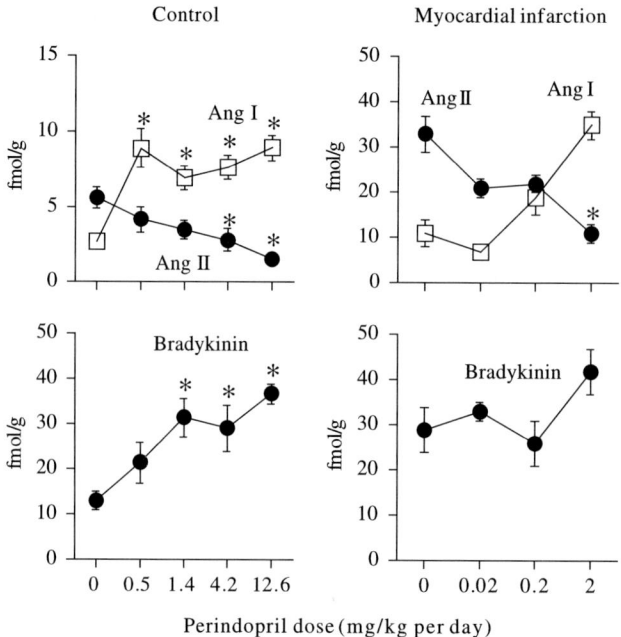

Figure 3. Dose related effects of the ACE inhibitor perindopril on Ang II, Ang I, and bradykinin levels in the cardiac ventricles of control rats and rats with myocardial infarction. *, $P < 0.05$ compared to 0 mg/kg per day perindopril. Data adapted from (Campbell et al 1994; Duncan et al 1996)

3.3.   Kinin Receptors

Kinins act via two types of kinin receptor, the B_1 and the B_2 receptors. The B_2 receptor normally predominates, whereas the B_1 receptor is induced by tissue injury. The KKS generates 8 bioactive kinin peptides: bradykinin, Hyp^3-bradykinin, kallidin, and Hyp^4-kallidin act on the B_2 receptor, whereas their carboxypeptidase metabolites des-Arg^9-bradykinin, des-Arg^9-Hyp^3-bradykinin, des-Arg^{10}-kallidin, and des-Arg^{10}-Hyp^4-kallidin act on the B_1 receptor. Hydroxylated kinins have similar biological activity to non-hydroxylated kinins.

Of particular interest is the recent report that the human B_2 receptor is activated by both plasma and tissue kallikrein (Hecquet *et al* 2000). Cathepsin G and trypsin similarly activate the B_2 receptor and activation is blocked by icatibant. Thus, the B_2 receptor may belong to a new group of serine-protease-activated receptors (Hecquet *et al* 2000).

3.4.   Kinin Metabolism

ACE is one of many enzymes that metabolise kinin peptides (Campbell 2003) and the efficiency of metabolism is an important determinant of their levels in blood and tissues. Consequently, inhibition of any single enzyme that contributes to kinin metabolism causes only a modest increase in kinin levels.

3.5.   Effects of the KKS on the Heart and Vasculature

Kinin peptides have a broad spectrum of activities and both systemic and local cardiac actions impact on the heart (Bhoola *et al* 1992). Kinin peptides act through many different second messenger systems, in particular nitric oxide and prostaglandins (Bhoola *et al* 1992). The B_2 receptor participates in an inhibitory interaction with endothelial NOS (eNOS) that is reversed by bradykinin (Ju *et al* 1998). This interaction may recruit eNOS to the B_2 receptor and allow for effective coupling of bradykinin signalling to the nitric oxide pathway. Kinins are potent vasodilators and promote diuresis and natriuresis. Kinins in high concentration also participate in the cardinal features of inflammation, producing vascular permeability, neutrophil chemotaxis and pain (Bhoola *et al* 1992).

Cardiac bradykinin levels are increased during the acute phase of myocardial infarction in rats (Duncan *et al* 1997). By contrast, we found decreased kallidin levels in coronary sinus blood of subjects with heart failure, suggesting down-regulation of the cardiac KKS in heart failure (Duncan *et al* 2000).

There is a large body of evidence demonstrating anti-hypertrophic and cardio-protective actions of the KKS (Griol-Charhbili *et al* 2005; Koch *et al* 2006; Park *et al* 2006; Spillmann *et al* 2006). The cardioprotective effects of bradykinin included the reduction of arrhythmias, reduction of lactate, lactate dehydrogenase, and creatine kinase release, and increase in myocardial contractility and myocardial levels of glycogen, adenosine triphosphate and creatine phosphate during post-ischaemic reperfusion of the isolated working rat heart (Linz *et al* 1992). Moreover, bradykinin suppressed endothelin release from the post-ischaemic rat heart (Brunner *et al* 1996). Kinins protect against ischaemia-reperfusion injury by decreasing endothelial adherence of leukocytes, leading to attenuation of post-ischaemic leukocyte adherence, attenuation of disruption of the microvascular barrier and reduced tissue injury (Shigematsu *et al* 1999). Many of the actions of kinins counteract those of Ang II, by causing endothelium-dependent vasodilatation through endothelial release of nitric oxide and prostacyclin (Pelc *et al* 1991; Lamontagne *et al* 1992; Gallagher *et al* 1998). Kinins also counteract the hypertrophic actions of Ang II and reduce collagen formation (Gallagher *et al* 1998; Ritchie *et al* 1998).

Administration of kinin receptor antagonists indicates a role for endogenous kinins in the regulation of the coronary vasculature and in the myocardial response to myocardial infarction. Icatibant reduced flow-dependent vasodilatation of human coronary arteries, indicating a role for kinins in the regulation of coronary vascu-lature (Groves *et al* 1995). Icatibant enhanced myocardial interstitial deposition of collagen following myocardial infarction in the rat, indicating a role for endogenous kinins in the modulation of collagen deposition; however, icatibant did not modify morphological and molecular markers of cardiomyocyte hypertrophy (Wollert *et al* 1997). Kinins participate in the process of ischaemic preconditioning, and have also been shown to limit reperfusion injury (Baxter *et al* 2002). Kinins may also protect against thrombosis by stimulating endothelial release of nitric oxide, prosta-cyclin, and tissue plasminogen activator (Dielis *et al* 2005). New properties of kinin peptides are being discovered. For example, B_1 receptors may have an important role in angiogenesis (Emanueli *et al* 2002).

4. ACSDKP

4.1. AcSDKP Formation

AcSDKP is an inhibitor of pluripotent haemopoietic stem cell proliferation (Lenfant *et al* 1989; Bonnet *et al* 1993), and is normally present in human plasma and mononuclear cells (Pradelles *et al* 1990). AcSDKP is released from its precursor thymosin-ß₄ by prolyl oligopeptidase (Cavasin *et al* 2004) and it is cleaved to an inactive form by the dipeptidyl carboxypeptidase activity of the *N*-terminal catalytic domain of ACE (Rousseau *et al* 1995). AcSDKP has a 4.5 min half-life in the circulation and is probably released continuously (Azizi *et al* 1997). The importance of ACE in AcSDKP metabolism is shown by the 5-fold increase in AcSDKP plasma levels that accompany ACE inhibition (Azizi *et al* 1997).

4.2. Functions of AcSDKP in the Heart

AcSDKP inhibits DNA and collagen synthesis by cardiac fibroblasts (Rhaleb *et al* 2001), and both prevents and reverses myocardial inflammation and fibrosis in rats with heart failure after myocardial infarction (Yang *et al* 2004). AcSDKP and thymosin-ß₄ stimulate coronary vasculogenesis and angiogenesis (Wang *et al* 2004; Smart *et al* 2007), and AcSDKP increases myocardial capillary density in rats with myocardial infarction (Wang *et al* 2004).

5. ACE INHIBITION IN HEART FAILURE AND ISCHAEMIC HEART DISEASE

Many clinical trials demonstrate the therapeutic benefit of ACE inhibition in heart failure and ischaemic heart disease. It is of note, however, that the effects of ACE inhibitors are dose related. Large clinical trials, by necessity, use only one dose of any drug. The results of such trials are just as much a measure of the effect of the dose as they are a measure of the effect of the drug. Use of a less than optimal dose may fail to reveal a drug's true therapeutic potential. This is of particular concern in a head-to-head comparison of two active drugs, where the result may be more due to choice of dose than to choice of drug. Clinicians should strive to achieve drug doses that have proven to be of benefit in clinical trials. At present, a large proportion of patients receiving ACE inhibitor therapy are receiving less than optimal doses (Lenzen *et al* 2005). Measurement of plasma Ang peptide levels is not feasible for the monitoring of ACE inhibitor therapy, but measurement of plasma AcSDKP levels may assist in this regard (Struthers *et al* 1999).

5.1. ACE Inhibition in Heart Failure

Heart failure is associated with neurohormonal activation that includes increased renin, Ang II, and aldosterone levels, and activation of the sympathetic nervous system (Francis *et al* 1993). Increased Ang II, aldosterone, noradrenaline, and adrenaline levels predict increased mortality in heart failure patients (Swedberg *et al* 1990). Therapies that counteract the effects of RAS and sympathetic nervous system activation are the cornerstone of heart failure therapy (Hunt *et al* 2001; Swedberg *et al* 2005).

Acute ACE inhibition in heart failure patients promotes arterio- and veno-dilatation, with reduction in both afterload and preload, and an associated increase in cardiac output, stroke volume, and stroke work index, along with a decrease in pulmonary capillary wedge pressure, indicating improved left ventricular (LV) function (Gavras *et al* 1978; Ader *et al* 1980). The Cooperative North Scandinavian Enalapril Survival Study (CONSENSUS) demonstrated reduced mortality and improved symptoms with enalapril therapy in patients with severe heart failure (The CONSENSUS Trial Study Group 1987). Moreover, mortality was lower with enalapril therapy than with hydralazine-isosorbide dinitrate therapy in the second Veterans Administration Cooperative Vasodilator-Heart Failure Trial (V-HeFT II) (Cohn *et al* 1991). The Studies of Left Ventricular Dysfunction (SOLVD) confirmed the survival benefits of enalapril therapy in patients with reduced LV ejection fraction and heat failure (The SOLVD Investigators 1991) and also demonstrated the prevention of heart failure in asymptomatic subjects with reduced LV ejection fraction (The SOLVD Investigators 1992).

ACE inhibition improves survival, symptoms, and functional capacity, and reduces hospitalisation in patients with moderate and severe heart failure and LV systolic dysfunction (Flather *et al* 2000; Abdulla *et al* 2004). ACE inhibition is recommended as first-line therapy in patients with a reduced LV ejection fraction with or without symptoms, and should be up-titrated to the doses shown to be effective in clinical trials (Hunt *et al* 2001; Swedberg *et al* 2005).

5.2.   ACE Inhibition After Myocardial Infarction

Although the patients recruited to the CONSENSUS, V-HeFT II, and SOVD studies had reduced LV ejection fraction due most often to ischaemic heart disease, they were enrolled several months or more after a myocardial infarction. Studies in rats demonstrated survival advantage of ACE inhibitor therapy commenced 14 days after myocardial infarction (Pfeffer *et al* 1985b). Additionally, ACE inhibition reduced arterial pressure and total peripheral resistance, attenuated LV remodelling, prevented deterioration in cardiac output and stroke volume index, and prevented the increase in LV volume, LV chamber stiffness and LV end diastolic pressure in rats with myocardial infarction (Pfeffer *et al* 1985a).

These benefits of ACE inhibition in rats with myocardial infarction were confirmed in patients. The Survival and Ventricular Enlargement (SAVE) trial showed reduced mortality with ACE inhibitor therapy when commenced 3-16 days after myocardial infarction in patients with asymptomatic LV dysfunction (Pfeffer *et al* 1992). In addition, ACE inhibitor therapy reduced the incidence of both fatal and nonfatal major cardiovascular events, including the development of severe heart failure and recurrent myocardial infarction.

The benefits of ACE inhibitor therapy after myocardial infarction were confirmed in the Acute Infarction Ramipril Efficacy (AIRE) and the Trandolapril Cardiac Evaluation (TRACE) studies (The Acute Infarction Ramipril Efficacy (AIRE) Study Investigators 1993; Kober *et al* 1995). The AIRE study recruited patients 2-9 days after myocardial infarction who had shown clinical evidence of heart failure at any time. The TRACE study recruited patients 3-7 days after myocardial infarction who had a LV ejection fraction $\leq 35\%$. Both the AIRE and TRACE studies showed survival advantage with ACE inhibitor therapy and the TRACE study showed less development of severe heart failure. Other large clinical trails confirmed the benefits of ACE inhibition after myocardial infarction (GISSI-3 Gruppo 1994; ISIS-4 Collaborative Group 1995).

In addition to mortality benefit and reduction of severe heart failure, ACE inhibition after myocardial infarction attenuates LV remodelling, LV enlargement and increase in LV mass, and improves LV ejection fraction after myocardial infarction (Pfeffer *et al* 1988; Sharpe *et al* 1991; Sogaard *et al* 1993; Johnson *et al* 1997).

By contrast, the CONSENSUS II trial found the commencement of ACE inhibitor therapy within 24 hours of myocardial infarction did not improve survival (Swedberg *et al* 1992). The failure of ACE inhibition to improve outcomes in the CONSENSUS II trial may have been due to its protocol. ACE inhibitor treatment was started with intravenous infusion of 1 mg enalaprilat within 24 hours after the onset of chest pain, followed by administration of oral enalapril. Intravascular administration of ACE inhibitor had a negative inotropic effect in several human studies (Foult *et al* 1988; Haber *et al* 1994; Zeitz *et al* 2003), although not in another (Friedrich *et al* 1994). Thus, the failure of ACE inhibitor therapy to produce benefit in the CONSENSUS II trial may have been due to the negative inotropic effect of intravenously administered enalaprilat, in addition to its administration within 24 hours of chest pain.

Current European Society of Cardiology guidelines recommend the initiation of ACE inhibitors after the acute phase of myocardial infarction in patients with signs or symptoms of heart failure, even if transient, to improve survival and to reduce re-infarctions and hospitalisations for heart failure (Swedberg *et al* 2005).

5.3.   ACE Inhibition in Stable Vascular Disease

Two large-scale clinical trials demonstrated the benefits of ACE inhibition in patients with stable vascular disease or at high risk of vascular disease. These were the Heart Outcomes Prevention Evaluation (HOPE) study (The Heart Outcomes Prevention Evaluation Study Investigators 2000) and The European Trial on Reduction of Cardiac Events with Perindopril in Stable Coronary Artery Disease (EUROPA) study (The European Trial on Reduction of Cardiac Events with Perindopril in Stable Coronary Artery Disease Investigators 2003).

The HOPE study was based on emerging evidence that ACE inhibition reduced the risk of myocardial infarction in patients with low ejection fraction (Pfeffer *et al* 1992; Yusuf *et al* 1992; Lonn *et al* 1994). It examined the effects of addition of 10 mg ramipril to standard therapy in patients aged at least 55 years with a history of coronary artery disease, stroke, peripheral vascular disease, or diabetes, plus at least one other cardiovascular risk factor (hypertension, elevated total cholesterol level, low high-density lipoprotein cholesterol level, cigarette smoking, or microalbuminuria). Patients were excluded if they had heart failure, were known to have a low ejection fraction, were taking an ACE inhibitor or vitamin E, had uncontrolled hypertension or overt nephropathy, or had had a myocardial infarction or stroke within 4 weeks before the study began. During a mean follow-up of 5 years ramipril reduced the primary outcome (composite of myocardial infarction, stroke, or death from cardio-vascular causes) from 17.8% to 14.0% (relative risk 0.78, 95% confidence interval 0.70 to 0.86; P < 0.001). Treatment with ramipril reduced the rates of death from cardiovascular causes and all-cause mortality, myocardial infarction, revascularisation procedures, cardiac arrest, heart failure, and complications related to diabetes.

The EUROPA study examined the effects of addition of 8 mg perindopril to standard therapy in patients with previous myocardial infarction, angiographic evidence of coronary heart disease, coronary revascularization, or a positive stress test. Past history of heart failure was recorded in 1.3% of subjects, but none had clinical signs of heart failure, with 10% in New York Heart Association class I and none in class II or higher. During a mean follow-up of 4.2 years, perindopril reduced the primary outcome (composite of cardiovascular death, non-fatal myocardial infarction, cardiac arrest with successful resuscitation) from 9.9% to 8.0% (relative risk 0.80, 95% confidence interval 0.71 to 0.91; P<0.001). The main contributor to this reduction in the primary outcome was the reduction in non-fatal myocardial infarction. Perindopril also reduced the incidence of heart failure requiring hospitalisation.

By contrast, the Prevention of Events with Angiotensin Converting Enzyme Inhibition (PEACE) study failed to show an effect of ACE inhibition on its primary endpoint (The PEACE Trial Investigators 2004). The PEACE study examined the effects of addition of 4 mg trandolapril to standard therapy on cardiovascular events in patients with stable coronary heart disease and preserved LV function. During a median follow-up of 4.8 years, trandolapril produced non-statistically significant reductions in the primary endpoint (composite of cardiovascular death, myocardial infarction, and coronary revascularization) from 22.5% to 21.9%, and in cardiovascular death and non-fatal myocardial infarction from 8.5% to 8.3%, although trandolapril reduced hospitalisation or death due to heart failure from 3.7% to 2.8%. Participants in the PEACE study were at lower risk of cardiovascular events than those in the HOPE and EUROPA studies. The baseline blood pressure of PEACE participants was less than that of patients in the HOPE and EUROPA studies, and was similar to the level achieved with active therapy in the HOPE and EUROPA studies. In addition, PEACE participants received more intensive management of risk factors than did those in the HOPE and EUROPA studies, with 70% of PEACE participants receiving lipid lowering therapy (29% in HOPE, 56% in EUROPA), and 72% had undergone coronary revascularization before enrollment (40% in HOPE, 54% in EUROPA). Thus, PEACE participants had an event rate similar to that of the general population (1.6% annualised rate of death), and the more aggressive management of their risk factors may have negated any potential benefit from ACE inhibitor therapy.

There has been debate about the reasons for the failure of the PEACE study to show an effect of trandolapril on the primary endpoint (Pitt 2004; Fox *et al* 2006a). Although the dose and type of ACE inhibitor may be implicated, the most likely explanation is the low event rate in its relatively low risk population (necessitating the inclusion of revascularisation as part of the primary endpoint), such that the study did not have sufficient statistical power to achieve its aim. The Ischemia Management with Accupril post bypass Graft via Inhibition of angiotensin converting enzyme (IMAGINE) study similarly showed a lack of benefit from 40 mg quinapril in optimally treated low-risk patients after coronary artery bypass grafting (Keuper *et al* 2005).

Pooled analysis of the HOPE, EUROPA, and PEACE trials showed ACE inhibition reduced all cause and cardiovascular mortality, non-fatal myocardial infarction, stroke, heart failure, and coronary artery bypass surgery, leading to the recommendation that ACE inhibitors be considered in all patients with atherosclerosis (Dagenais *et al* 2006). A meta-analysis of the HOPE, EUROPA, PEACE, and other studies came to a similar conclusion (Al-Mallah *et al* 2006). However, the number needed to treat for 4.4 years to prevent either one death, one non-fatal myocardial infarction, or one coronary revascularisation procedure was 100 (Al-Mallah *et al* 2006). Current European Society of Cardiology guidelines state: "ACE inhibition is well established in the treatment of heart failure or LV dysfunction and in the treatment of diabetic patients. Thus, it is appropriate to consider ACE inhibitors for the treatment of patients with stable angina pectoris and co-existing hypertension, diabetes, heart failure, asymptomatic LV dysfunction and post-myocardial infarction. In angina patients without co-existing indications for ACE inhibitor treatment the anticipated benefit of treatment (possible absolute risk reduction) should be weighed against costs and risks for side-effects, and the dose and agent used of proven efficacy for this indication" (Fox *et al* 2006b).

6.   MECHANISMS OF THE THERAPEUTIC BENEFITS OF ACE INHIBITION IN HEART FAILURE AND ISCHAEMIC HEART DISEASE

ACE inhibition has many different effects, both systemic and organ-specific (Unger *et al* 1990). The systemic effects include the reduction of circulating Ang II and aldosterone levels and the increase in kinin and AcSDKP levels. Decreased Ang II and increased kinin levels contribute to the reduction of blood pressure by ACE inhibition.

6.1.   Haemodynamic and Coronary Vascular Effects of ACE Inhibition

There is ongoing debate about the extent to which the benefits of ACE inhibition are related to blood reduction, as opposed to intrinsic benefits of ACE inhibition (Sever *et al* 2006). A major contributor to the benefits of ACE inhibition in heart failure and ischaemic heart disease may be the reduction in systemic blood pressure, and consequent reduction in heart work. ACE inhibition may improve cardiac function by reducing coronary vascular resistance in patients with heart failure, thereby augmenting cardiac blood flow (Dietz *et al* 1993).

6.2. Effects of ACE Inhibition on Ang II Levels

ACE inhibition reduces circulating and tissue levels of Ang II in both animals and humans (Campbell *et al* 1994; Duncan *et al* 1996; Campbell *et al* 1999; Zeitz *et al* 2003). ACE inhibition produced a modest reduction in Ang II levels in EUROPA participants (Ceconi *et al* 2007). However, the effects of ACE inhibition on Ang II levels can be variable, and depend on the responsiveness of renin secretion (Mooser *et al* 1990). In situations where renin shows little increase in response to ACE inhibition, the levels of Ang II and its metabolites show a marked fall, with little change in the levels of Ang I and its metabolites. By contrast, a large increase in renin levels in response to ACE inhibition also increases the levels of Ang I and its metabolites. The increased Ang I levels promote Ang II formation by residual uninhibited ACE and by serine protease pathways of Ang I conversion, thereby buffering any fall in Ang II levels during ACE inhibition (Juillerat *et al* 1990).

Improved survival of heart failure patients with ACE inhibitor therapy is associated with reduction in Ang II and aldosterone levels (Swedberg *et al* 1990). The role of renin in determining the response of Ang II levels to ACE inhibition is most evident in heart failure, where many patients continue to have elevated Ang II levels despite ACE inhibitor therapy (Roig *et al* 2000; Campbell *et al* 2001). It is of note that maximally recommended doses of ACE inhibitor do not completely prevent ACE mediated formation of Ang II in heart failure (Jorde *et al* 2000). The beneficial therapeutic effects of concomitant ß-blocker therapy in heart failure may be due in part to the associated reduction in renin and Ang II levels (Campbell *et al* 2001).

The effects of ACE inhibitors on Ang II levels are dose dependent (Fig. 3). Studies in rats showed tissue-specific differences in the dose-related effects of ACE inhibition on Ang II levels (Campbell 1996). Renal Ang II levels were reduced by lower doses of ACE inhibitor than were required to reduce Ang II levels in other tissues such as the heart (Fig. 3).

6.3. Effects of ACE Inhibition on Ang-(1-7) Levels

ACE inhibition is accompanied by increased levels of Ang-(1-7). This is due in part to the increase in Ang I levels, with subsequent conversion to Ang-(1-7). Another mechanism for the increase in Ang-(1-7) levels during ACE inhibition is the inhibition of Ang-(1-7) metabolism, given that ACE is an important pathway of Ang-(1-7) metabolism (Chappell *et al* 1998; Yamada *et al* 1998). Studies in rats led to the proposal that increased Ang-(1-7) levels mediate in part the hypotensive effects of ACE inhibition (Iyer *et al* 1998a; Iyer *et al* 1998b). However, there is as yet no evidence that these mechanisms operate in patients receiving ACE inhibitor therapy.

6.4.   Effects of ACE Inhibition on Kinin Peptide Levels

There is ample evidence that kinin peptides contribute to the therapeutic effects of ACE inhibitors (Linz *et al* 1995; Bönner 1997). ACE inhibitors increase circulating and tissue levels of bradykinin in animals (Fig. 3) and humans (Campbell *et al* 1994; Duncan *et al* 1996; Zeitz *et al* 2003). The effect of ACE inhibition on kinin peptide levels in any tissue compartment depends on the contribution of ACE, relative to other kininases, to kinin peptide metabolism in that compartment. ACE inhibitor therapy did not increase either bradykinin or kallidin peptide levels in cardiac atria of patients with ischaemic heart disease, despite the reduction in Ang II levels (Campbell *et al* 1999).

The maintenance of low levels of kinin peptides by their efficient metabolism is relevant to the success of ACE inhibitor therapy. ACE inhibition has only a modest effect on kinin peptide levels because of the many other kininases that contribute to kinin metabolism. It is for this reason that ACE inhibitors are generally free of the side effects, such as angioneurotic oedema, that one might expect from increased kinin peptide levels (Nussberger *et al* 1998; Nussberger *et al* 2002).

Studies with kinin receptor antagonists indicate a role for kinins in the cardiovascular actions of ACE inhibitors in animals and humans (Linz *et al* 1995). Studies in humans indicate a role for the B_2 receptor in flow-dependent vasodilatation in normal volunteers (Hornig *et al* 1997) and in the hypotensive effects in patients with hypertension (Gainer *et al* 1998; Squire *et al* 2000). A role for the B_1 receptor is indicated in the systemic haemodynamic effects of ACE inhibition in patients with heart failure (Witherow *et al* 2001; Cruden *et al* 2004).

Cardioprotective effects of ACE inhibition that were attenuated by icatibant included the reduction of arrhythmias, reduction of lactate, lactate dehydrogenase, and creatine kinase release, and increase in myocardial contractility and myocardial levels of glycogen, adenosine triphosphate and creatine phosphate during reperfusion of the ischaemic isolated working rat heart (Linz *et al* 1992). Icatibant attenuated the ACE inhibitor-induced increase in coronary flow and nitric oxide levels in dogs with myocardial ischaemia (Kitakaze *et al* 2002). Icatibant also prevented the potentiation of ischaemic preconditioning by ACE inhibition in human atria (Morris *et al* 1997). The post-ischaemic anti-arrhythmic effect of ACE inhibition may be mediated by kinin-induced suppression of endothelin release (Brunner *et al* 1996).

Icatibant prevented the reduction in myocardial infarct size and the reduction in post-infarct remodelling by ACE inhibition in animal models (Linz *et al* 1992; Hartman *et al* 1993; Stauss *et al* 1994; McDonald *et al* 1995; Hu *et al* 1998). However, a subsequent study in an *in vivo* canine model of myocardial ischaemic injury did not show an effect of ACE inhibition on infarct size (Black *et al* 1998). Moreover, icatibant did not modify the antihypertrophic effect of ACE inhibition in rats with myocardial infarction, although it partially reversed the reduction in myocardial collagen deposition by ACE inhibitor therapy in one study (Wollert *et al* 1997).

Possible mechanisms by which kinin peptides mediate the therapeutic benefits of ACE inhibition include the promotion of endothelial production of nitric oxide and prostacylin, thereby contributing to the correction of endothelial dysfunction and reduced oxidative stress (Linz et al 1995; Bönner 1997; Münzel et al 2001). ACE inhibition induced endothelial NOS (eNOS) in vasculature of control rats, and attenuated the induction of inducible NOS (iNOS) in rats administered bacterial lipopolysaccharide (Bachetti et al 2001). Icatibant prevented the increase in nitric oxide formation in the heart and reduction in myocardial oxygen consumption that accompany ACE inhibition in dogs (Zhang et al 1997). Icatibant also prevented the antiproliferative effect of ACE inhibition in neointima formation following endothelial injury to the rat carotid artery (Linz et al 1992), and the increase in capillary density induced by chronic ACE inhibitor treatment in stroke-prone spontaneously hypertensive rats (Gohlke et al 1997). Part of the benefits of ACE inhibition may be due to the enhancement of insulin-mediated muscle glucose uptake, that is also attenuated by icatibant (Henriksen et al 1996; Henriksen et al 1999).

6.5.   ACE Inhibitor Effects on the KKS Independent of Kinin Levels

ACE inhibition also affects the KKS by mechanisms separate from prevention of kinin degradation. For example, chronic ACE inhibition in mice and rats induced both renal and vascular B_1 receptor expression without modification of B_2 receptor expression (Marin-Castano et al 2002). Moreover, enalaprilat and other ACE inhibitors in nanomolar concentrations were shown to directly activate the human B_1 receptor, in the absence of ACE and B_1 receptor ligands (Ignjatovic et al 2002).

Several studies show ACE inhibitors may potentiate the effects of bradykinin by a mechanism independent of prevention of kinin metabolism, that involves direct interaction between ACE and the B_2 receptor (Fleming 2006) and attenuation of the sequestration of the B_2 receptor (Benzing et al 1999; Chen et al 2006). Additionally, membrane ACE appears to have its own signalling cascade that is activated by binding of ACE inhibitors (Fleming 2006).

6.6.   Comparison of ACE Inhibitor and ARB Therapy

One approach to differentiation of the respective roles of the RAS and KKS in mediating the therapeutic benefits of ACE inhibition is the comparison of ACE and ARB therapy. Comparison of ACE inhibitor and ARB therapy after myocardial infarction, or in patients with heart failure, did not show any difference in outcomes (Pitt et al 2000; Dickstein et al 2002; Pfeffer et al 2003; McMurray et al 2006). These studies suggest ACE inhibitor and ARB therapy act through blockade of the RAS, but a role for bradykinin cannot be excluded because losartan was shown to increase bradykinin levels in hypertensive humans (Campbell et al 2005).

Maximally recommended doses of ACE inhibitors do not completely prevent ACE mediated formation of Ang II in heart failure (Jorde *et al* 2000). Combination of ACE inhibitor and ARB therapy produces more complete blockade of the RAS that is dependent on the dose regimens of the individual therapies (Menard *et al* 1997; Azizi *et al* 2004). This combination therapy improves outcomes in heart failure patients (Cohn *et al* 2001; McMurray *et al* 2003), but not following myocardial infarction (Pfeffer *et al* 2003; McMurray *et al* 2006).

6.7.   Effects of ACE Inhibition on AcSDKP Levels

ACE inhibition causes a several-fold increase in AcSDKP levels that may contribute to decreased cardiac inflammation and fibrosis, and to increased myocardial capillary density after myocardial infarction (Wang *et al* 2004; Yang *et al* 2004). Elevated AcSDKP levels during ACE inhibitor therapy may also contribute to the anaemia experienced by heart failure patients receiving ACE inhibitor therapy (van der Meer *et al* 2005).

6.8.   Effects of ACE Inhibition on Aldosterone Levels

Heart failure patients have increased plasma aldosterone levels consequent to stimulation of aldosterone secretion by increased Ang II levels (Weber 2001). Evidence that reduced aldosterone levels may contribute to the therapeutic benefits of ACE inhibition is the reduced hypokalaemia in patients receiving ramipril therapy in the HOPE study (Mann *et al* 2005). In addition to promotion of sodium retention and oedema formation, aldosterone may promote cardiac fibrosis and deterioration in cardiac function (Brilla *et al* 1993). The possible clinical importance of this mechanism is shown by the benefits of aldosterone receptor antagonists in patients with heart failure, and in patients with LV dysfunction after myocardial infarction (Pitt *et al* 1999; Pitt *et al* 2003).

6.9.   Effects of ACE Inhibition on Sympathetic Nervous System Activity

Many authors have suggested the reduction in sympathetic activity that may accompany ACE inhibition is due to a reduction in the stimulation of sympathetic activity by Ang II. However, although ACE inhibitor therapy leads to reduction in sympathetic nervous system activity in heart failure, this is thought to be mainly secondary to the improvement of cardiovascular haemodynamics, rather than the specific consequence of reduced stimulation of the sympathetic nervous system by Ang II (Esler *et al* 2001).

6.10.   Effects of ACE Inhibition on Cardiac Remodelling

Cardiac hypertrophy is well recognised as a risk factor for death and cardiovascular events (Levy *et al* 1990). ACE inhibitors reduce cardiac hypertrophy in hypertensive patients (Dahlof *et al* 1992) and also reduce progressive LV remodelling after myocardial infarction (Ferrari 2006). Ventricular remodelling has a dominant role in the pathogenesis of heart failure, and the prevention of remodelling is considered to be an important mechanism of the benefit of ACE inhibitor therapy in heart failure and after myocardial infarction (Cohn 1995; Abdulla *et al* 2007).

6.11.   Effects of ACE Inhibition on Atherosclerosis

Reduction of myocardial infarction and other ischaemic events by ACE inhibition raises the possibility that these drugs inhibit atherosclerosis. ACE inhibitors correct endothelial dysfunction in patients with heart failure and ischaemic heart disease (Drexler *et al* 1995; Mancini *et al* 1996; Ceconi *et al* 2007). These effects of ACE inhibition may be due to the reduction of oxidative stress, vascular remodelling and inflammation by reduced Ang II levels and increased kinin levels. However, current evidence does not allow these data to be extrapolated to a reduction in atherogenesis by ACE inhibition in humans. Despite the prevention of atherosclerosis in animal models, ACE inhibitor therapy was not able to reduce atherogenesis in patients. ACE inhibition with cilazapril did not prevent restenosis after angioplasty (MERCATOR), (MERCATOR Study Group 1992; Faxon 1995). Similarly, Quinapril did not reduce restenosis after coronary stenting; in fact, late loss in minimum lumen diameter was significantly higher in the quinapril group than in controls (Meurice *et al* 2001). Additionally, ACE inhibition with enalapril failed to reduce progression of coronary atherosclerosis, as assessed by intravascular ultrasound, in patients with coronary artery disease (Nissen *et al* 2004).

A meta-analysis of randomised controlled studies of the effect of antihypertensive therapies in progression of carotid intima-media thickness showed only a weak, non-significant reduction in progression of carotid intima-media thickness by ACE inhibitor therapy, with significant heterogeneity between studies (Wang *et al* 2006). Some studies showed a reduction in progression of intima-media thickness by ACE inhibition and some did not. Of note, calcium channel blockers were significantly more effective than ACE inhibitors in their reduction of progression of intima-media thickness (Wang *et al* 2006).

6.12.   Effects of ACE Inhibition on Thrombosis

Reduced rates of myocardial infarction with ACE inhibitor therapy may also be due to an effect of this therapy on the mechanisms of thrombosis and fibrinolysis. ACE inhibition reduced plasma levels of PAI-1 antigen and activity in normal subjects on low salt diet and in subjects following myocardial infarction (Wright *et al* 1994; Moriyama *et al* 1997; Oshima *et al* 1997; Vaughan *et al* 1997; Brown *et al* 1998; Brown *et al* 1999), although this effect of ACE inhibition was not confirmed in other studies of patients with previous myocardial infarction (Zehetgruber *et al* 1996; Pedersen *et al* 1997). ACE inhibition also reduced PAI-1 antigen, but not PAI-1 activity, in subjects with congestive cardiac failure (Goodfield *et al* 1999).

6.13.   Effects of ACE Inhibition on Incidence of Type 2 Diabetes

Diabetes is well recognised to accelerate the processes of cardiovascular disease, and reduction of diabetes incidence may contribute to the therapeutic benefits of ACE inhibition. Many large clinical trials, including the HOPE, PEACE, and SOLVD studies, showed a reduced incidence of type 2 diabetes with ACE inhibitor therapy (Abuissa et al 2005). However, the Diabetes Reduction Assessment with Ramipril and Rosiglitazone Medication (DREAM) study found ramipril did not reduce diabetes incidence among persons with impaired fasting glucose levels or impaired glucose tolerance, although it significantly increased regression to normoglycaemia (The DREAM Trial Investigators 2006). This improvement in insulin resistance may be due in part to the enhancement of insulin-mediated muscle glucose uptake by ACE inhibition (Henriksen et al 1996; Henriksen et al 1999).

6.14.   Effects of ACE Inhibition on Arterial Stiffness

Aortic compliance is an important determinant of coronary blood flow (O'Rourke et al 1999). A recent meta-analysis showed ACE inhibitors decrease arterial stiffness (Mallareddy et al 2006). ACE inhibitors, by increasing aortic compliance, may reduce central systolic blood pressure and maintain diastolic blood pressure, thereby reducing heart work without compromising myocardial perfusion. Decrease in arterial stiffness by ACE inhibition may be due to reduced collagen deposition, as suggested by studies in spontaneously hypertensive rats (Benetos et al 1997). Reduction of aortic collagen deposition by ACE inhibition was not affected by icatibant, suggesting that this effect of ACE inhibition was not mediated by kinins (Benetos et al 1997).

6.15.   Effects of ACE Inhibition on Atrial Fibrillation

Atrial fibrillation is an important contributor to poor prognosis in heart failure (Wang et al 2003), and prevention of atrial fibrillation by ACE inhibition may contribute to the therapeutic benefits of this therapy (Vermes et al 2003).

6.16.   Interaction Between ACE Inhibitor and Aspirin Therapy

Given that kinin peptides mediate in part the therapeutic benefits of ACE inhibition, and that some of the actions of kinins are mediated by prostaglandins, the question arises whether a drug that inhibits prostaglandin synthesis may attenuate the effects of ACE inhibition. This question was addressed in a systematic review of the interaction between aspirin and ACE inhibitor therapy (Teo et al 2002). The SOLVD study found aspirin prevented the reduction of death by ACE inhibition, but this interaction between aspirin and ACE inhibitor therapy was not significant in the other trials examined. However, both SOLVD and the other trials showed aspirin attenuated the prevention of myocardial infarction or reinfarction by ACE inhibition.

By contrast, there was no evidence that aspirin attenuated the prevention of stroke, hospital admission for heart failure, or revascularisation by ACE inhibitor therapy. When the composite of major vascular events including death, myocardial infarction or reinfarction, hospital admission for heart failure, stroke, and revascularisation was examined, aspirin did not significantly attenuate the benefits of ACE inhibitor therapy. This analysis shows, therefore, that aspirin does interact with ACE inhibitor therapy, at least in the case of myocardial infarction. However, in the absence of clear contraindications, concomitant use of aspirin and ACE inhibitors should be considered in all patients at high risk of major vascular events (Teo *et al* 2002).

7.   CONCLUSIONS

ACE inhibitors have a major role in the treatment and prevention of heart failure and ischaemic heart disease. Reduction in Ang II levels, and increase in kinin and AcSDKP levels, are implicated in the mechanisms of the therapeutic effects of ACE inhibitors. Much of the detail of these mechanisms, however, remains to be discovered.

ACKNOWLEDGEMENTS

This work was supported by a Senior Research Fellowship from the National Health and Medical Research Council of Australia (ID 395508), and by the National Heart Foundation of Australia (ID G 06M 2654).

REFERENCES

Abbas, A., Gorelik, G., Carbini, L.A., and Scicli, A.G., 1997, Angiotensin-(1-7) induces bradykinin-mediated hypotensive responses in anesthetized rats. *Hypertension*, **30**: 217–221.

Abdulla, J., Abildstrom, S.Z., Christensen, E., Kober, L., and Torp-Pedersen, C., 2004, A meta-analysis of the effect of angiotensin-converting enzyme inhibitors on functional capacity in patients with symptomatic left ventricular systolic dysfunction. *Eur J Heart Fail*, **6**: 927–935.

Abdulla, J., Barlera, S., Latini, R., Kjoller-Hansen, L., Sogaard, P., Christensen, E., Kober, L., and Torp-Pedersen, C., 2007, A systematic review: Effect of angiotensin converting enzyme inhibition on left ventricular volumes and ejection fraction in patients with a myocardial infarction and in patients with left ventricular dysfunction. *Eur J Heart Fail*: (in press).

Abuissa, H., Jones, P.G., Marso, S.P., and O'Keefe, J.H., Jr., 2005, Angiotensin-converting enzyme inhibitors or angiotensin receptor blockers for prevention of type 2 diabetes: a meta-analysis of randomized clinical trials. *J Am Coll Cardiol*, **46**: 821–826.

Ader, R., Chatterjee, K., Ports, T., Brundage, B., Hiramatsu, B., and Parmley, W., 1980, Immediate and sustained hemodynamic and clinical improvement in chronic heart failure by an oral angiotensin-converting enzyme inhibitor. *Circulation*, **61**: 931–937.

Al-Mallah, M.H., Tleyjeh, I.M., Abdel-Latif, A.A., and Weaver, W.D., 2006, Angiotensin-converting enzyme inhibitors in coronary artery disease and preserved left ventricular systolic function: a systematic review and meta-analysis of randomized controlled trials. *J Am Coll Cardiol*, **47**: 1576–1583.

Azizi, M., Ezan, E., Nicolet, L., Grognet, J.M., and Ménard, J., 1997, High plasma level of *N*-acetyl-seryl-aspartyl-lysyl-proline - A new marker of chronic angiotensin-converting enzyme inhibition. *Hypertension*, **30**: 1015–1019.

Azizi, M., and Menard, J., 2004, Combined blockade of the renin-angiotensin system with angiotensin-converting enzyme inhibitors and angiotensin II type 1 receptor antagonists. *Circulation*, **109**: 2492–2499.

Bachetti, T., Comini, L., Pasini, E., Cargnoni, A., Curello, S., and Ferrari, R., 2001, Ace-inhibition with quinapril modulates the nitric oxide pathway in normotensive rats. *J Mol Cell Cardiol*, **33**: 395–403.

Baxter, G.F., and Ebrahim, Z., 2002, Role of bradykinin in preconditioning and protection of the ischaemic myocardium. *Br J Pharmacol*, **135**: 843–854.

Benetos, A., Levy, B.I., Lacolley, P., Taillard, F., Duriez, M., and Safar, M.E., 1997, Role of angiotensin II and bradykinin on aortic collagen following converting enzyme inhibition in spontaneously hypertensive rats. *Arterioscler Thromb Vasc Biol*, **17**: 3196–3201.

Benter, I.F., Diz, D.I., and Ferrario, C.M., 1993, Cardiovascular actions of angiotensin(1-7). *Peptides*, **14**: 679–684.

Benter, I.F., Ferrario, C.M., Morris, M., and Diz, D.I., 1995, Antihypertensive actions of angiotensin-(1-7) in spontaneously hypertensive rats. *Am J Physiol*, **269**: H313–H319.

Benzing, T., Fleming, I., Blaukat, A., Muller-Esterl, W., and Busse, R., 1999, Angiotensin-converting enzyme inhibitor ramiprilat interferes with the sequestration of the B2 kinin receptor within the plasma membrane of native endothelial cells. *Circulation*, **99**: 2034–2040.

Bhoola, K.D., Figueroa, C.D., and Worthy, K., 1992, Bioregulation of kinins: kallikreins, kininogens, and kininases. *Pharmacol Rev*, **44**: 1–80.

Black, S.C., Driscoll, E.M., and Lucchesi, B.R., 1998, Effect of ramiprilat or captopril on myocardial infarct size: assessment in canine models of ischemia alone and ischemia with reperfusion. *Pharmacology*, **57**: 35–46.

Bönner, G., 1997, The role of kinins in the antihypertensive and cardioprotective effects of ACE inhibitors. *Drugs*, **54(Suppl. 5)**: 23–30.

Bonnet, D., Lemoine, F.M., Pontvert-Delucq, S., Baillou, C., Najman, A., and Guigon, M., 1993, Direct and reversible inhibitory effect of the tetrapeptide acetyl-N-Ser-Asp-Lys-Pro (Seraspenide) on the growth of human CD34+ subpopulations in response to growth factors. *Blood*, **82**: 3307–3314.

Brilla, C.G., Matsubara, L.S., and Weber, K.T., 1993, Anti-aldosterone treatment and the prevention of myocardial fibrosis in primary and secondary hyperaldosteronism. *J Mol Cell Cardiol*, **25**: 563–575.

Brosnihan, K.B., Li, P., and Ferrario, C.M., 1996, Angiotensin-(1-7) dilates canine coronary arteries through kinins and nitric oxide. *Hypertension*, **27**: 523–528.

Brown, N.J., Agirbasli, M., and Vaughan, D.E., 1999, Comparative effect of angiotensin-converting enzyme inhibition and angiotensin II type I receptor antagonism on plasma fibrinolytic balance in humans. *Hypertension*, **34**: 285–290.

Brown, N.J., Agirbasli, M.A., Williams, G.H., Litchfield, W.R., and Vaughan, D.E., 1998, Effect of activation and inhibition of the renin-angiotensin system on plasma PAI-1. *Hypertension*, **32**: 965–971.

Brunner, F., and Kukovetz, W.R., 1996, Postischemic antiarrhythmic effects of angiotensin-converting enzyme inhibitors: role of suppression of endogenous endothelin secretion. *Circulation*, **94**: 1752–1761.

Burrell, L.M., Risvanis, J., Kubota, E., Dean, R.G., MacDonald, P.S., Lu, S., Tikellis, C., Grant, S.L., Lew, R.A., Smith, A.I., Cooper, M.E., and Johnston, C.I., 2005, Myocardial infarction increases ACE2 expression in rat and humans. *Eur Heart J*, **26**: 369-375; discussion 322–364.

Campbell, D.J., 1996, Endogenous angiotensin II levels and the mechanism of action of angiotensin-converting enzyme inhibitors and angiotensin receptor type 1 antagonists. *Clin Exp Pharmacol Physiol*, **Suppl. 3**: S125–S131.

Campbell, D.J., 2003, The renin-angiotensin and the kallikrein-kinin systems. *Int J Biochem Cell Biol*, **35**: 784–791.

Campbell, D.J., 2006, The biology of angiotensin II (formation, metabolism, fragments, measurement). In *Molecular Mechanisms in Hypertension* (R.N. Re, D.J. DiPette, E.L. Schiffrin and J.R. Sowers, eds.), Taylor & Francis, New York, USA: 61–68.

Campbell, D.J., Aggarwal, A., Esler, M., and Kaye, D., 2001, ß-blockers, angiotensin II, and ACE inhibitors in patients with heart failure. *Lancet*, **358**: 1609–1610.

Campbell, D.J., Alexiou, T., Xiao, H.D., Fuchs, S., McKinley, M.J., Corvol, P., and Bernstein, K.E., 2004a, Effect of reduced angiotensin-converting enzyme gene expression and angiotensin-converting enzyme inhibition on angiotensin and bradykinin peptide levels in mice. *Hypertension*, **43**: 854–859.

Campbell, D.J., Duncan, A.-M., and Kladis, A., 1999, Angiotensin converting enzyme inhibition modifies angiotensin, but not kinin peptide levels in human atrial tissue. *Hypertension*, **34**: 171–175.

Campbell, D.J., Kladis, A., and Duncan, A.-M., 1993, Nephrectomy, converting enzyme inhibition and angiotensin peptides. *Hypertension*, **22**: 513–522.

Campbell, D.J., Kladis, A., and Duncan, A.-M., 1994, Effects of converting enzyme inhibitors on angiotensin and bradykinin peptides. *Hypertension*, **23**: 439–449.

Campbell, D.J., Krum, H., and Esler, M.D., 2005, Losartan increases bradykinin levels in hypertensive humans. *Circulation*, **111**: 315–320.

Campbell, D.J., Zeitz, C.J., Esler, M.D., and Horowitz, J.D., 2004b, Evidence against a major role for angiotensin converting enzyme-related carboxypeptidase (ACE2) in angiotensin peptide metabolism in the human coronary circulation. *J Hypertens*, **22**: 1971–1976.

Carey, R.M., Jin, X.H., and Siragy, H.M., 2001, Role of the angiotensin AT2 receptor in blood pressure regulation and therapeutic implications. *Am J Hypertens*, **14**: 98S–102S.

Cavasin, M.A., Rhaleb, N.E., Yang, X.P., and Carretero, O.A., 2004, Prolyl oligopeptidase is involved in release of the antifibrotic peptide Ac-SDKP. *Hypertension*, **43**: 1140–1145.

Ceconi, C., Fox, K.M., Remme, W.J., Simoons, M.L., Bertrand, M., Parrinello, G., Kluft, C., Blann, A., Cokkinos, D., and Ferrari, R., 2007, ACE inhibition with perindopril and endothelial function. Results of a substudy of the EUROPA study: PERTINENT. *Cardiovasc Res*, **73**: 237–246.

Chao, J.L., Schmaier, A., Chen, L.M., Yang, Z.R., and Chao, L., 1996, Kallistatin, a novel human tissue kallikrein inhibitor: Levels in body fluids, blood cells, and tissues in health and disease. *J Lab Clin Med*, **127**: 612–620.

Chappell, M.C., Pirro, N.T., Sykes, A., and Ferrario, C.M., 1998, Metabolism of angiotension-(1-7) by angiotensin-converting enzyme. *Hypertension*, **31**: 362–367.

Chen, Z., Deddish, P.A., Minshall, R.D., Becker, R.P., Erdos, E.G., and Tan, F., 2006, Human ACE and bradykinin B2 receptors form a complex at the plasma membrane. *FASEB J*, **20**: 2261–2270.

Cohn, J.N., 1995, Structural basis for heart failure. Ventricular remodeling and its pharmacological inhibition. *Circulation*, **91**: 2504–2507.

Cohn, J.N., Johnson, G., Ziesche, S., Cobb, F., Francis, G., Tristani, F., Smith, R., Dunkman, W.B., Loeb, H., Wong, M., Bhat, G., Goldman, S., Fletcher, R.D., Doherty, J., Hughes, C.V., Carson, P., Cintron, G., Shabetai, R., and Haakenson, C., 1991, A comparison of enalapril with hydralazine-isosorbide dinitrate in the treatment of chronic congestive heart failure. *N Engl J Med*, **325**: 303–310.

Cohn, J.N., Tognoni, G., and for the Valsartan Heart Failure Trial Investigators, 2001, A randomized trial of the angiotensin-receptor blocker valsartan in chronic heart failure. *N Engl J Med*, **345**: 1667–1675.

Crackower, M.A., Sarao, R., Oudit, G.Y., Yagil, C., Kozieradzki, I., Scanga, S.E., Oliveira-dos-Santos, A.J., da Costa, J., Zhang, L., Pei, Y., Scholey, J., Ferrario, C.M., Manoukian, A.S., Chappell, M.C., Backx, P.H., Yagil, Y., and Penninger, J.M., 2002, Angiotensin-converting enzyme 2 is an essential regulator of heart function. *Nature*, **417**: 822–828.

Cruden, N.L., Witherow, F.N., Webb, D.J., Fox, K.A., and Newby, D.E., 2004, Bradykinin contributes to the systemic hemodynamic effects of chronic angiotensin-converting enzyme inhibition in patients with heart failure. *Arterioscler Thromb Vasc Biol*, **24**: 1043–1048.

Dagenais, G.R., Pogue, J., Fox, K., Simoons, M.L., and Yusuf, S., 2006, Angiotensin-converting-enzyme inhibitors in stable vascular disease without left ventricular systolic dysfunction or heart failure: a combined analysis of three trials. *Lancet*, **368**: 581–588.

Dahlof, B., Pennert, K., and Hansson, L., 1992, Reversal of left ventricular hypertrophy in hypertensive patients. A metaanalysis of 109 treatment studies. *Am J Hypertens*, **5**: 95–110.

Danser, A.H.J., Van Kats, J.P., Admiraal, P.J.J., Derkx, F.H.M., Lamers, J.M.J., Verdouw, P.D., Saxena, P.R., and Schalekamp, M.A.D.H., 1994, Cardiac renin and angiotensins: Uptake from plasma versus in situ synthesis. *Hypertension*, **24**: 37–48.

De Mello, W.C., and Danser, A.H., 2000, Angiotensin II and the heart : on the intracrine renin-angiotensin system. *Hypertension*, **35**: 1183–1188.

Deddish, P.A., Marcic, B., Jackman, H.L., Wang, H.Z., Skidgel, R.A., and Erdös, E.G., 1998, N-domain-specific substrate and C-domain inhibitors of angiotensin-converting enzyme angiotensin-(1-7) and Keto-ACE. *Hypertension*, **31**: 912–917.

Dell'Italia, L.J., and Husain, A., 2002, Dissecting the role of chymase in angiotensin II formation and heart and blood vessel diseases. *Curr Opin Cardiol*, **17**: 374–379.

Dickstein, K., and Kjekshus, J., 2002, Effects of losartan and captopril on mortality and morbidity in high-risk patients after acute myocardial infarction: the OPTIMAAL randomised trial. Optimal Trial in Myocardial Infarction with Angiotensin II Antagonist Losartan. *Lancet*, **360**: 752–760.

Dielis, A.W., Smid, M., Spronk, H.M., Hamulyak, K., Kroon, A.A., ten Cate, H., and de Leeuw, P.W., 2005, The prothrombotic paradox of hypertension: role of the renin-angiotensin and kallikrein-kinin systems. *Hypertension*, **46**: 1236–1242.

Dietz, R., Waas, W., Süsselbeck, T., Willenbrock, R., and Osterziel, K.J., 1993, Improvement of cardiac function by angiotensin converting enzyme inhibition: Sites of action. *Circulation*, **87(Suppl. 4)**: IV-108-IV-116.

Donoghue, M., Hsieh, F., Baronas, E., Godbout, K., Gosselin, M., Stagliano, N., Donovan, M., Woolf, B., Robison, K., Jeyaseelan, R., Breitbart, R.E., and Acton, S., 2000, A novel angiotensin-converting enzyme-related carboxypeptidase (ACE2) converts angiotensin I to angiotensin 1-9. *Circ Res*, **87**: E1–9.

Dostal, D.E., and Baker, K.M., 1999, The cardiac renin-angiotensin system: conceptual, or a regulator of cardiac function? *Circ Res*, **85**: 643–650.

Drexler, H., Kurz, S., Jeserich, M., Münzel, T., and Hornig, B., 1995, Effect of chronic angiotensin-converting enzyme inhibition on endothelial function in patients with chronic heart failure. *Am J Cardiol*, **76**: 13E–18E.

Duncan, A.-M., Burrell, L.M., Kladis, A., and Campbell, D.J., 1996, Effects of angiotensin converting enzyme inhibition on angiotensin and bradykinin peptides in rats with myocardial infarction. *J Cardiovasc Pharmacol*, **28**: 746–754.

Duncan, A.-M., Kladis, A., Jennings, G.L., Dart, A.M., Esler, M., and Campbell, D.J., 2000, Kinins in humans. *Am J Physiol*, **278**: R897–R904.

Duncan, A.M., Burrell, L.M., Kladis, A., and Campbell, D.J., 1997, Angiotensin and bradykinin peptides in rats with myocardial infarction. *J Card Fail*, **3**: 41–52.

Duncan, A.M., James, G.M., Anastasopoulos, F., Kladis, A., Briscoe, T.A., and Campbell, D.J., 1999, Interaction between neutral endopeptidase and angiotensin converting enzyme inhibition in rats with myocardial infarction: effects on cardiac hypertrophy and angiotensin and bradykinin peptide levels. *J Pharmacol Exp Ther*, **289**: 295–303.

Duprez, D.A., 2006, Role of the renin-angiotensin-aldosterone system in vascular remodeling and inflammation: a clinical review. *J Hypertens*, **24**: 983–991.

Dzau, V.J., 2001, Tissue angiotensin and pathobiology of vascular disease: a unifying hypothesis. *Hypertension*, **37**: 1047–1052.

Ehlers, M.R.W., and Riordan, J.F., 1990, Angiotensin-converting enzyme: biochemistry and molecular biology. In *Hypertension: Pathophysiology, Diagnosis, and Management* (J.H. Laragh and B.M. Brenner, ed.∧eds.), Raven Press, New York: 1217–1231.

Emanueli, C., Bonaria Salis, M., Stacca, T., Pintus, G., Kirchmair, R., Isner, J.M., Pinna, A., Gaspa, L., Regoli, D., Cayla, C., Pesquero, J.B., Bader, M., and Madeddu, P., 2002, Targeting kinin B_1 receptor for therapeutic neovascularization. *Circulation*, **105**: 360–366.

Erdos, E.G., 1990, Angiotensin I converting enzyme and the changes in our concepts through the years. *Hypertension*, **16**: 363–370.

Esler, M., and Brunner-La Rocca, H.P., 2001, Does the renin-angiotensin system exert an important stimulatory influence on the sympathetic nervous system? In *Angiotensin II Receptor Antagonists* (M. Epstein and H.R. Brunner, ed.∧eds.), Hanley & Belfus, Inc., Philadelphia: 119–128.

Faxon, D.P., 1995, Effect of high dose angiotensin-converting enzyme inhibition on restenosis: Final results of the MARCATOR study, a multicenter, double-blind, placebo-controlled trial of cilazapril. *J Am Coll Cardiol*, **25**: 362–369.

Feener, E.P., Northrup, J.M., Aiello, L.P., and King, G.L., 1995, Angiotensin II induces plasminogen activator inhibitor-1 and -2 expression in vascular endothelial and smooth muscle cells. *J Clin Invest*, **95**: 1353–1362.

Ferrari, R., 2006, Effects of angiotensin-converting enzyme inhibition with perindopril on left ventricular remodeling and clinical outcome: results of the randomized Perindopril and Remodeling in Elderly with Acute Myocardial Infarction (PREAMI) Study. *Arch Intern Med*, **166**: 659–666.

Ferrario, C.M., Brosnihan, K.B., Diz, D.I., Jaiswal, N., Khosla, M.C., Milsted, A., and Tallant, E.A., 1991, Angiotensin-(1-7): A new hormone of the angiotensin system. *Hypertension*, **18(Suppl. 3)**: III-126-III-133.

Flather, M.D., Yusuf, S., Kober, L., Pfeffer, M., Hall, A., Murray, G., Torp-Pedersen, C., Ball, S., Pogue, J., Moye, L., and Braunwald, E., 2000, Long-term ACE-inhibitor therapy in patients with heart failure or left-ventricular dysfunction: a systematic overview of data from individual patients. *Lancet*, **355**: 1575–1581.

Fleming, I., 2006, Signaling by the angiotensin-converting enzyme. *Circ Res*, **98**: 887–896.

Foult, J.-M., Tavolaro, O., Antony, I., and Nitenberg, A., 1988, Direct myocardial and coronary effects of enalaprilat in patients with dilated cardiomyopathy: assessment by a bilateral intracoronary infusion technique. *Circulation*, **77**: 337–344.

Fox, K., Ferrari, R., Yusuf, S., and Borer, J.S., 2006a, Should angiotensin-converting enzyme-inhibitors be used to improve outcome in patients with coronary artery disease and 'preserved' left ventricular function? *Eur Heart J*, **27**: 2154–2157.

Fox, K., Garcia, M.A., Ardissino, D., Buszman, P., Camici, P.G., Crea, F., Daly, C., De Backer, G., Hjemdahl, P., Lopez-Sendon, J., Marco, J., Morais, J., Pepper, J., Sechtem, U., Simoons, M., Thygesen, K., Priori, S.G., Blanc, J.J., Budaj, A., Camm, J., Dean, V., Deckers, J., Dickstein, K., Lekakis, J., McGregor, K., Metra, M., Osterspey, A., Tamargo, J., and Zamorano, J.L., 2006b, Guidelines on the management of stable angina pectoris: executive summary: the Task Force on the Management of Stable Angina Pectoris of the European Society of Cardiology. *Eur Heart J*, **27**: 1341–1381.

Francis, G.S., Cohn, J.N., Johnson, G., Rector, T.S., Goldman, S., Simon, A., and Group, f.t.V.-H.V.C.S., 1993, Plasma norepinephrine, plasma renin activity, and congestive heart failure: relations to survival and the effects of therapy in V-HeFT II. *Circulation*, **87(Suppl. VI)**: VI-40-VI-48.

Friedrich, S.P., Lorell, B.H., Rousseau, M.F., Hayashida, W., Hess, O.M., Douglas, P.S., Gordon, S., Keighley, C.S., Benedict, C., Krayenbuehl, H.P., Grossman, W., and Pouleur, H., 1994, Intracardiac angiotensin-converting enzyme inhibition improves diastolic function in patients with left ventricular hypertrophy due to aortic stenosis. *Circulation*, **90**: 2761–2771.

Gainer, J.V., Morrow, J.D., Lovelend, A., King, D.J., and Brown, N.J., 1998, Effect of bradykinin-receptor blockade on the response to angiotensin-converting-enzyme inhibitor in normotensive and hypertensive subjects. *N Engl J Med*, **339**: 1285–1292.

Gallagher, A.M., Yu, H., and Printz, M.P., 1998, Bradykinin-induced reductions in collagen gene expression involve prostacyclin. *Hypertension*, **32**: 84–88.

Gavras, H., Faxon, D.P., Berkoben, J., Brunner, H.R., and Ryan, T.J., 1978, Angiotensin converting enzyme inhibition in patients with congestive heart failure. *Circulation*, **58**: 770–776.

GISSI-3 Gruppo, 1994, GISSI-3: Effects of lisinopril and transdermal glyceryl trinitrate singly and together on 6-week mortality and ventricular function after acute myocardial infarction. *Lancet*, **343**: 1115–1122.

Gohlke, P., Kuwer, I., Schnell, A., Amann, K., Mall, G., and Unger, T., 1997, Blockade of bradykinin B$_2$ receptors prevents the increase in capillary density induced by chronic angiotensin-converting enzyme inhibitor treatment in stroke-prone spontaneously hypertensive rats. *Hypertension*, **29**: 478–482.

Goodfield, N.E., Newby, D.E., Ludlam, C.A., and Flapan, A.D., 1999, Effects of acute angiotensin II type 1 receptor antagonism and angiotensin converting enzyme inhibition on plasma fibrinolytic parameters in patients with heart failure. *Circulation*, **99**: 2983–2985.

Gorelik, G., Carbini, L.A., and Scicli, A.G., 1998, Angiotensin 1-7 induces bradykinin-mediated relaxation in porcine coronary artery. *J Pharmacol Exp Ther*, **286**: 403–410.

Griol-Charhbili, V., Messadi-Laribi, E., Bascands, J.L., Heudes, D., Meneton, P., Giudicelli, J.F., Alhenc-Gelas, F., and Richer, C., 2005, Role of tissue kallikrein in the cardioprotective effects of ischemic and pharmacological preconditioning in myocardial ischemia. *FASEB J*, **19**: 1172–1174.

Groves, P., Kurz, S., Just, H., and Drexler, H., 1995, Role of endogenous bradykinin in human coronary vasomotor control. *Circulation*, **92**: 3424–3430.

Gurley, S.B., Allred, A., Le, T.H., Griffiths, R., Mao, L., Philip, N., Haystead, T.A., Donoghue, M., Breitbart, R.E., Acton, S.L., Rockman, H.A., and Coffman, T.M., 2006, Altered blood pressure responses and normal cardiac phenotype in ACE2-null mice. *J Clin Invest*, **116**: 2218–2225.

Haber, H.L., Powers, E.R., Gimple, L.W., Wu, C.C., Subbiah, K., Johnson, W.H., and Feldman, M.D., 1994, Intracoronary angiotensin-converting enzyme inhibition improves diastolic function in patients with hypertensive left ventricular hypertrophy. *Circulation*, **89**: 2616–2625.

Hamming, I., Timens, W., Bulthuis, M.L., Lely, A.T., Navis, G.J., and van Goor, H., 2004, Tissue distribution of ACE2 protein, the functional receptor for SARS coronavirus. A first step in understanding SARS pathogenesis. *J Pathol*, **203**: 631–637.

Harmer, D., Gilbert, M., Borman, R., and Clark, K.L., 2002, Quantitative mRNA expression profiling of ACE 2, a novel homologue of angiotensin converting enzyme. *FEBS Lett*, **532**: 107–110.

Hartman, J.C., Wall, T.M., Hullinger, T.G., and Shebuski, R.J., 1993, Reduction of myocardial infarct size in rabbits by ramiprilat: reversal by the bradykinin antagonist HOE 140. *J Cardiovasc Pharmacol*, **21**: 996–1003.

Hecquet, C., Tan, F., Marcic, B.M., and Erdos, E.G., 2000, Human bradykinin B(2) receptor is activated by kallikrein and other serine proteases. *Mol Pharmacol*, **58**: 828–836.

Henriksen, E.J., Jacob, S., Augustin, H.J., and Dietze, G.J., 1996, Glucose transport activity in insulin-resistant rat muscle: effects of angiotensin-converting enzyme inhibitors and bradykinin antagonism. *Diabetes*, **45(Suppl. 1)**: S125–S128.

Henriksen, E.J., Jacob, S., Kinnick, T.R., Youngblood, E.B., Schmit, M.B., and Dietze, G.J., 1999, ACE inhibition and glucose transport in insulinresistant muscle: roles of bradykinin and nitric oxide. *Am J Physiol*, **277**: R332–R336.

Herizi, A., Jover, B., Bouriquet, N., and Mimran, A., 1998, Prevention of the cardiovascular and renal effects of angiotensin II by endothelin blockade. *Hypertension*, **31**: 10–14.

Hirsch, A.T., Talsness, C.E., Schunkert, H., Paul, M., and Dzau, V.J., 1991, Tissue-specific activation of cardiac angiotensin converting enzyme in experimental heart failure. *Circ Res*, **69**: 475–482.

Hooper, N.M., 1991, Angiotensin converting enzyme: implications from molecular biology for its physiological functions. *Int J Biochem*, **23**: 641–647.

Hornig, B., Kohler, C., and Drexler, H., 1997, Role of bradykinin in mediating vascular effects of angiotensin-converting enzyme inhibitors in humans. *Circulation*, **95**: 1115–1118.

Hu, K., Gaudron, P., Anders, H.J., Weidemann, F., Turschner, O., Nahrendorf, M., and Ertl, G., 1998, Chronic effects of early started angiotensin converting enzyme inhibition and angiotensin AT_1-receptor subtype blockade in rats with myocardial infarction: role of bradykinin. *Cardiovasc Res*, **39**: 401–412.

Hunt, S.A., Baker, D.W., Chin, M.H., Cinquegrani, M.P., Feldman, A.M., Francis, G.S., Ganiats, T.G., Goldstein, S., Gregoratos, G., Jessup, M.L., Noble, R.J., Packer, M., Silver, M.A., Stevenson, L.W., Gibbons, R.J., Antman, E.M., Alpert, J.S., Faxon, D.P., Fuster, V., Jacobs, A.K., Hiratzka, L.F., Russell, R.O., and Smith, S.C., Jr., 2001, ACC/AHA guidelines for the evaluation and management of chronic heart failure in the adult: executive summary. A report of the American College of Cardiology/American Heart Association Task Force on Practice Guidelines (Committee to revise the 1995 Guidelines for the Evaluation and Management of Heart Failure). *J Am Coll Cardiol*, **38**: 2101–2113.

Ignjatovic, T., Tan, F., Brovkovych, V., Skidgel, R.A., and Erdos, E.G., 2002, Novel mode of action of angiotensin I converting enzyme inhibitors: direct activation of bradykinin B1 receptor. *J Biol Chem*, **277**: 16847–16852.

ISIS-4 Collaborative Group, 1995, ISIS-4: A randomised factorial trial assessing early oral captopril, oral mononitrate, and intravenous magnesium sulphate in 58 050 patients with suspected acute myocardial infarction. *Lancet*, **345**: 669–685.

Iyer, S.N., Chappell, M.C., Averill, D.B., Diz, D.I., and Ferrario, C.M., 1998a, Vasodepressor actions of angiotensin-(1-7) unmasked during combined treatment with lisinopril and losartan. *Hypertension*, **31**: 699–705.

Iyer, S.N., Ferrario, C.M., and Chappell, M.C., 1998b, Angiotensin-(1-7) contributes to the antihypertensive effects of blockade of the renin-angiotensin system. *Hypertension*, **31**: 356–361.

Jaspard, E., Wei, L., and Alhenc-Gelas, F., 1993, Differences in the properties and enzymatic specificities of the two active sites of angiotensin I-converting enzyme (kininase II). Studies with bradykinin and other natural peptides. *J Biol Chem*, **268**: 9496–9503.

Johnson, D.B., Foster, R.E., Barilla, F., Blackwell, G.G., Roney, M., Stanley, A.W.H., Jr., Kirk, K., Orr, R.A., Van der Geest, R.J., Reiber, J.H.C., and Dell'Italia, L.J., 1997, Angiotensin-converting enzyme inhibitor therapy affects left ventricular mass in patients with ejection fraction >40% after acute myocardial infarction. *J Am Coll Cardiol*, **29**: 49–54.

Jorde, U.P., Ennezat, P.V., Lisker, J., Suryadevara, V., Infeld, J., Cukon, S., Hammer, A., Sonnenblick, E.H., and Le Jemtel, T.H., 2000, Maximally recommended doses of angiotensin-converting enzyme (ACE) inhibitors do not completely prevent ACE-mediated formation of angiotensin II in chronic heart failure. *Circulation*, **101**: 844–846.

Ju, H., Venema, V.J., Marrero, M.B., and Venema, R.C., 1998, Inhibitory interactions of the bradykinin B2 receptor with endothelial nitric-oxide synthase. *J Biol Chem*, **273**: 24025–24029.

Juillerat, L., Nussberger, J., Ménard, J., Mooser, V., Christen, Y., Waeber, B., Graf, P., and Brunner, H.R., 1990, Determinants of angiotensin II generation during converting enzyme inhibition. *Hypertension*, **16**: 564–572.

Kerins, D.M., Hao, Q., and Vaughan, D.E., 1995, Angiotensin induction of PAI-1 expression in endothelial cells is mediated by the hexapeptide angiotensin IV. *J Clin Invest*, **96**: 2515–2520.

Keuper, W., and Verheugt, F.W., 2005, Hotline sessions of the 27th European congress of cardiology. *Eur Heart J*, **26**: 2596–2599.

Kitakaze, M., Asanuma, H., Funaya, H., Node, K., Takashima, S., Sanada, S., Asakura, M., Ogita, H., Kim, J., and Hori, M., 2002, Angiotensin-converting enzyme inhibitors and angiotensin II receptor blockers synergistically increase coronary blood flow in canine ischemic myocardium: role of bradykinin. *J Am Coll Cardiol*, **40**: 162–166.

Kober, L., Torp-Pedersen, C., Carlsen, J.E., Bagger, H., Eliasen, P., Lyngborg, K., Videbek, J., Cole, D.S., Auclert, L., Pauly, N.C., Aliot, E., Persson, S., and Camm, A.J., 1995, A clinical trial of the angiotensin-converting-enzyme inhibitor trandolapril in patients with left ventricular dysfunction after myocardial infarction. *N Engl J Med*, **333**: 1670–1676.

Koch, M., Spillmann, F., Dendorfer, A., Westermann, D., Altmann, C., Sahabi, M., Linthout, S.V., Bader, M., Walther, T., Schultheiss, H.P., and Tschope, C., 2006, Cardiac function and remodeling is attenuated in transgenic rats expressing the human kallikrein-1 gene after myocardial infarction. *Eur J Pharmacol*, **550**: 143–148.

Kohno, M., Horio, T., Ikeda, M., Yokokawa, K., Fukui, T., Yasunari, K., Kurihara, N., and Takeda, T., 1992, Angiotensin II stimulates endothelin-1 secretion in cultured rat mesangial cells. *Kidney Int*, **42**: 860–866.

Kozik, A., Moore, R.B., Potempa, J., Imamura, T., Rapala-Kozik, M., and Travis, J., 1998, A novel mechanism for bradykinin production at inflammatory sites. Diverse effects of a mixture of neutrophil elastase and mast cell tryptase *versus* tissue and plasma kallikreins on native and oxidized kininogens. *J Biol Chem*, **273**: 33224–33229.

Lamontagne, D., König, A., Bassenge, E., and Busse, R., 1992, Prostacyclin and nitric oxide contribute to the vasodilator action of acetylcholine and bradykinin in the intact rabbit coronary bed. *J Cardiovasc Pharmacol*, **20**: 652–657.

Lawrence, A.C., Evin, G., Kladis, A., and Campbell, D.J., 1990, An alternative strategy for the radioimmunoassay of angiotensin peptides using amino-terminal-directed antisera: measurement of eight angiotensin peptides in human plasma. *J Hypertens*, **8**: 715–724.

Le Tran, Y., and Forster, C., 1997, Angiotensin-(1-7) and the rat aorta: Modulation by the endothelium. *J Cardiovasc Pharmacol*, **30**: 676–682.

Lenfant, M., Wdzieczak-Bakala, J., Guittet, E., Prome, J.C., Sotty, D., and Frindel, E., 1989, Inhibitor of hematopoietic pluripotent stem cell proliferation: purification and determination of its structure. *Proc Natl Acad Sci USA*, **86**: 779–782.

Lenzen, M.J., Boersma, E., Reimer, W.J., Balk, A.H., Komajda, M., Swedberg, K., Follath, F., Jimenez-Navarro, M., Simoons, M.L., and Cleland, J.G., 2005, Under-utilization of evidence-based drug treatment in patients with heart failure is only partially explained by dissimilarity to patients enrolled in landmark trials: a report from the Euro Heart Survey on Heart Failure. *Eur Heart J*, **26**: 2706–2713.

Levy, D., Garrison, R.J., Savage, D.D., Kannel, W.B., and Castelli, W.P., 1990, Prognostic implications of echocardiographically determined left ventricular mass in the Framingham study. *N Engl J Med*, **322**: 1561–1566.

Li, J.M., and Shah, A.M., 2004, Endothelial cell superoxide generation: regulation and relevance for cardiovascular pathophysiology. *Am J Physiol Regul Integr Comp Physiol*, **287**: R1014–R1030.

Li, P., Chappell, M.C., Ferrario, C.M., and Brosnihan, K.B., 1997, Angiotensin-(1-7) augments bradykinin-induced vasodilation by competing with ACE and releasing nitric oxide. *Hypertension*, **29**: 394–400.

Lima, C.V., Paula, R.D., Resende, F.L., Khosla, M.C., and Santos, R.A.S., 1997, Potentiation of the hypotensive effect of bradykinin by short-term infusion of angiotensin-(1-7) in normotensive and hypertensive rats. *Hypertension*, **30**: 542–548.

Linz, W., and Schölkens, B.A., 1992, Role of bradykinin in the cardiac effects of angiotensin-converting enzyme inhibitors. *J Cardiovasc Pharmacol*, **20(Suppl. 9)**: S83–S90.

Linz, W., Wiemer, G., Gohlke, P., Unger, T., and Schölkens, B.A., 1995, Contribution of kinins to the cardiovascular actions of angiotensin-converting enzyme inhibitors. *Pharmacol Rev*, **47**: 25–49.

Lonn, E.M., Yusuf, S., Jha, P., Montague, T.J., Teo, K.K., Benedict, C.R., and Pitt, B., 1994, Emerging role of angiotensin-converting enzyme inhibitors in cardiac and vascular protection. *Circulation*, **90**: 2056–2069.

Mallareddy, M., Parikh, C.R., and Peixoto, A.J., 2006, Effect of angiotensin-converting enzyme inhibitors on arterial stiffness in hypertension: systematic review and meta-analysis. *J Clin Hypertens (Greenwich)*, **8**: 398–403.

Mancini, G.B.J., Henry, G.C., Macaya, C., O'Neill, B.J., Pucillo, A.L., Carere, R.G., Wargovich, T.J., Mudra, H., Luscher, T.F., Klibaner, M.I., Haber, H.E., Uprichard, A.C.G., Pepine, C.J., and Pitt, B., 1996, Angiotensin-converting enzyme inhibition with quinapril improves endothelial vasomotor dysfunction in patients with coronary artery disease – The TREND (Trial on Reversing ENdothelial Dysfunction) study. *Circulation*, **94**: 258–265.

Mann, J.F., Yi, Q.L., Sleight, P., Dagenais, G.R., Gerstein, H.C., Lonn, E.M., and Bosch, J., 2005, Serum potassium, cardiovascular risk, and effects of an ACE inhibitor: results of the HOPE study. *Clin Nephrol*, **63**: 181–187.

Marcic, B., Deddish, P.A., Jackman, H.L., and Erdos, E.G., 1999, Enhancement of bradykinin and resensitization of its B2 receptor. *Hypertension*, **33**: 835–843.

Marin-Castano, M.E., Schanstra, J.P., Neau, E., Praddaude, F., Pecher, C., Ader, J.L., Girolami, J.P., and Bascands, J.L., 2002, Induction of functional bradykinin b(1)-receptors in normotensive rats and mice under chronic Angiotensin-converting enzyme inhibitor treatment. *Circulation*, **105**: 627–632.

McDonald, K.M., Mock, J., D'Aloia, A., Parrish, T., Hauer, K., Francis, G., Stillman, A., and Cohn, J.N., 1995, Bradykinin antagonism inhibits the antigrowth effect of converting enzyme inhibition in the dog myocardium after discrete transmural myocardial necrosis. *Circulation*, **91**: 2043–2048.

McMurray, J., Solomon, S., Pieper, K., Reed, S., Rouleau, J., Velazquez, E., White, H., Howlett, J., Swedberg, K., Maggioni, A., Kober, L., Van de Werf, F., Califf, R., and Pfeffer, M., 2006, The effect of valsartan, captopril, or both on atherosclerotic events after acute myocardial infarction: an analysis of the Valsartan in Acute Myocardial Infarction Trial (VALIANT). *J Am Coll Cardiol*, **47**: 726–733.

McMurray, J.J., Ostergren, J., Swedberg, K., Granger, C.B., Held, P., Michelson, E.L., Olofsson, B., Yusuf, S., and Pfeffer, M.A., 2003, Effects of candesartan in patients with chronic heart failure and reduced left-ventricular systolic function taking angiotensin-converting-enzyme inhibitors: the CHARM-Added trial. *Lancet*, **362**: 767–771.

Mehta, P.K., and Griendling, K.K., 2007, Angiotensin II Cell Signaling: Physiological and Pathological Effects in the Cardiovascular System. *Am J Physiol Cell Physiol*: in press.

Menard, J., Campbell, D.J., Azizi, M., and Gonzales, M.F., 1997, Synergistic effects of ACE inhibition and Ang II antagonism on blood pressure, cardiac weight, and renin in spontaneously hypertensive rats. *Circulation*, **96**: 3072–3078.

MERCATOR Study Group, 1992, Does the new angiotensin converting enzyme inhibitor cilazapril prevent restenosis after percutaneous transluminal coronary angioplasty? Results of the MERCATOR study: A multicenter, randomized, double-blind placebo-controlled trial. *Circulation*, **86**: 100–110.

Meurice, T., Bauters, C., Hermant, X., Codron, V., VanBelle, E., Mc Fadden, E.P., Lablanche, J., Bertrand, M.E., and Amouyel, P., 2001, Effect of ACE inhibitors on angiographic restenosis after coronary stenting (PARIS): a randomised, double-blind, placebo-controlled trial. *Lancet*, **357**: 1321–1324.

Mooser, V., Nussberger, J., Juillerat, L., Burnier, M., Waeber, B., Bidiville, J., Pauly, N., and Brunner, H.R., 1990, Reactive hyperreninemia is a major determinant of plasma angiotensin II during ACE inhibition. *J Cardiovasc Pharmacol*, **15**: 276–282.

Moreau, P., D'Uscio, L.V., Shaw, S., Takase, H., Barton, M., and Lüscher, T.F., 1997, Angiotensin II increases tissue endothelin and induces vascular hypertrophy - Reversal by ET_A-receptor antagonist. *Circulation*, **96**: 1593–1597.

Moriyama, Y., Ogawa, H., Oshima, S., Takazoe, K., Honda, Y., Hirashima, O., Arai, H., Sakamoto, T., Sumida, H., Suefuji, H., Kaikita, K., and Yasue, H., 1997, Captopril reduced plasminogen activator inhibitor activity in patients with acute myocardial infarction. *Jpn Circ J*, **61**: 308–314.

Morris, S.D., and Yellon, D.M., 1997, Angiotensin-converting enzyme inhibitors potentiate preconditioning through bradykinin B_2 receptor activation in human heart. *J Am Coll Cardiol*, **29**: 1599–1606.

Münzel, T., and Keaney, J.F., Jr., 2001, Are ACE inhibitors a "magic bullet" against oxidative stress? *Circulation*, **104**: 1571–1574.

Nakamoto, H., Ferrario, C.M., Fuller, S.B., Robaczewski, D.L., Winicov, E., and Dean, R.H., 1995, Angiotensin-(1-7) and nitric oxide interaction in renovascular hypertension. *Hypertension*, **25**: 796–802.

Nissen, S.E., Tuzcu, E.M., Libby, P., Thompson, P.D., Ghali, M., Garza, D., Berman, L., Shi, H., Buedendorf, E., and Topol, E.J., 2004, Effect of antihypertensive agents on cardiovascular events in patients with coronary disease and normal blood pressure: the CAMELOT study: a randomized controlled trial. *JAMA*, **292**: 2217–2225.

Nolly, H., Carbini, L.A., Scicli, G., Carretero, O.A., and Scicli, A.G., 1994, A local kallikrein-kinin system is present in rat hearts. *Hypertension*, **23**: 919–923.

Nolly, H.L., Saed, G., Scicli, G., Carretero, O.A., and Scicli, A.G., 1992, The kallikrein-kinin system in cardiac tissue. In *Recent Progress on Kinins Pharmacological and Clinical Aspects of the Kallikrein-Kinin System Part II* (G. Bönner, H. Fritz, B. Schoelkens, G. Dietze and K. Luppertz, ed.∧eds.), Birkhèuser Verlag, Basel: 62–72.

Nussberger, J., Cugno, M., Amstutz, C., Cicardi, M., Pellacani, A., and Agostoni, A., 1998, Plasma bradykinin in angio-oedema. *Lancet*, **351**: 1693–1697.

Nussberger, J., Cugno, M., and Cicardi, M., 2002, Bradykinin-mediated angioedema. *N Engl J Med*, **347**: 621–622.

O'Rourke, M.F., and Mancia, G., 1999, Arterial stiffness. *J Hypertens*, **17**: 1–4.

Oettgen, P., 2006, Regulation of vascular inflammation and remodeling by ETS factors. *Circ Res*, **99**: 1159–1166.

Ohkubo, N., Matsubara, H., Nozawa, Y., Mori, Y., Murasawa, S., Kijima, K., Maruyama, K., Masaki, H., Tsutumi, Y., Shibazaki, Y., Iwasaka, T., and Inada, M., 1997, Angiotensin type 2 receptors are reexpressed by cardiac fibroblasts from failing myopathic hamster hearts and inhibit cell growth and fibrillar collagen metabolism. *Circulation*, **96**: 3954–3962.

Oshima, S., Ogawa, H., Mizuno, Y., Yamashita, S., Noda, K., Saito, T., Sumida, H., Suefuji, H., Kaikita, K., Soejima, H., and Yasue, H., 1997, The effects of the angiotensin-converting enzyme inhibitor imidapril on plasma plasminogen activator inhibitor activity in patients with acute myocardial infarction. *Am Heart J*, **134**: 961–966.

Oza, N.B., Schwartz, J.H., Goud, H.D., and Levinsky, N.G., 1990, Rat aortic smooth muscle cells in culture express kallikrein, kininogen, and bradykininase activity. *J Clin Invest*, **85**: 597–600.

Park, S.S., Zhao, H., Mueller, R.A., and Xu, Z., 2006, Bradykinin prevents reperfusion injury by targeting mitochondrial permeability transition pore through glycogen synthase kinase 3beta. *J Mol Cell Cardiol*, **40**: 708–716.

Paul, M., Poyan Mehr, A., and Kreutz, R., 2006, Physiology of local renin-angiotensin systems. *Physiol Rev*, **86**: 747–803.

Paula, R.D., Lima, C.V., Khosla, M.C., and Santos, R.A.S., 1995, Angiotensin-(1-7) potentiates the hypotensive effect of bradykinin in conscious rats. *Hypertension*, **26**: 1154–1159.

Pedersen, O.D., Gram, J., Jeunemaitre, X., Billaud, E., and Jespersen, J., 1997, Does long-term angiotensin converting enzyme inhibition affect the concentration of tissue-type plasminogen activator plasminogen activator inhibitor-1 in the blood of patients with a previous myocardial infarction. *Coronary Artery Dis*, **8**: 283–291.

Pelc, L.R., Gross, G.J., and Warltier, D.C., 1991, Mechanism of coronary vasodilation produced by bradykinin. *Circulation*, **83**: 2048–2056.

Pfeffer, J.M., Pfeffer, M.A., and Braunwald, E., 1985a, Influence of chronic captopril therapy on the infarcted left ventricle of the rat. *Circ Res*, **57**: 84–95.

Pfeffer, M.A., Braunwald, E., Moyé, L.A., Basta, L., Brown, E.J., Jr., Cuddy, T.E., Davis, B.R., Geltman, E.M., Goldman, S., Flaker, G.C., Klein, M., Lamas, G.A., Packer, M., Rouleau, J., Rouleau, J.L., Rutherford, J., Wertheimer, J.H., Hawkins, C.M., and on behalf of the SAVE Investigators, 1992, Effect of captopril on mortality and morbidity in patients with left ventricular dysfunction after myocardial infarction. Results of the survival and ventricular enlargement trial. *N Engl J Med*, **327**: 669–677.

Pfeffer, M.A., Lamas, G.A., Vaughan, D.E., Parisi, A.F., and Braunwald, E., 1988, Effect of captopril on progressive ventricular dilatation after anterior myocardial infarction. *N Engl J Med*, **319**: 80–86.

Pfeffer, M.A., McMurray, J.J., Velazquez, E.J., Rouleau, J.L., Kober, L., Maggioni, A.P., Solomon, S.D., Swedberg, K., Van De Werf, F., White, H., Leimberger, J.D., Henis, M., Edwards, S., Zelenkofske, S., Sellers, M.A., and Califf, R.M., 2003, Valsartan, captopril, or both in myocardial infarction complicated by heart failure, left ventricular dysfunction, or both. *N Engl J Med*, **349**: 1893–1906.

Pfeffer, M.A., Pfeffer, J.M., Steinberg, C., and Finn, P., 1985b, Survival after an experimental myocardial infarction: beneficial effects of long-term therapy with captopril. *Circulation*, **72**: 406–412.

Pitt, B., 2004, ACE inhibitors for patients with vascular disease without left ventricular dysfunction–may they rest in PEACE? *N Engl J Med*, **351**: 2115–2117.

Pitt, B., Poole-Wilson, P.A., Segal, R., Martinez, F.A., Dickstein, K., Camm, A.J., Konstam, M.A., Riegger, G., Klinger, G.H., Neaton, J., Sharma, D., and Thiyagarajan, B., 2000, Effect of losartan compared with captopril on mortality in patients with symptomatic heart failure: randomised trial – the Losartan Heart Failure Survival Study ELITE II. *Lancet*, **355**: 1582–1587.

Pitt, B., Remme, W., Zannad, F., Neaton, J., Martinez, F., Roniker, B., Bittman, R., Hurley, S., Kleiman, J., and Gatlin, M., 2003, Eplerenone, a selective aldosterone blocker, in patients with left ventricular dysfunction after myocardial infarction. *N Engl J Med*, **348**: 1309–1321.

Pitt, B., Zannad, F., Remme, W.J., Cody, R., Castaigne, A., Perez, A., Palensky, J., and Wittes, J., 1999, The effect of spironolactone on morbidity and mortality in patients with severe heart failure. Randomized Aldactone Evaluation Study Investigators. *N Engl J Med*, **341**: 709–717.

Pörsti, I., Bara, A.T., Busse, R., and Hecker, M., 1994, Release of nitric oxide by angiotensin-(1-7) from porcine coronary endothelium: Implications for a novel angiotensin receptor. *Br J Pharmacol*, **111**: 652–654.

Pradelles, P., Frobert, Y., Creminon, C., Liozon, E., Masse, A., and Frindel, E., 1990, Negative regulator of pluripotent hematopoietic stem cell proliferation in human white blood cells and plasma as analysed by enzyme immunoassay. *Biochem Biophys Res Commun*, **170**: 986–993.

Rajagopalan, S., Laursen, J.B., Borthayre, A., Kurz, S., Keiser, J., Haleen, S., Giaid, A., and Harrison, D.G., 1997, Role for endothelin-1 in angiotensin II-mediated hypertension. *Hypertension*, **30**: 29–34.

Regitz-Zagrosek, V., Fielitz, J., and Fleck, E., 1998, Myocardial angiotensin receptors in human hearts. *Basic Res Cardiol*, **93(Suppl. 2)**: 37–42.

Rhaleb, N.E., Peng, H., Harding, P., Tayeh, M., LaPointe, M.C., and Carretero, O.A., 2001, Effect of N-acetyl-seryl-aspartyl-lysyl-proline on DNA and collagen synthesis in rat cardiac fibroblasts. *Hypertension*, **37**: 827–832.

Rieger, K.-J., Saez-Servent, N., Papet, M.-P., Wdzieczak-Bakala, J., Morgat, J.-L., Thierry, J., Voelter, W., and Lenfant, M., 1993, Involvement of human plasma angiotensin I-converting enzyme in the degradation of the haemoregulatory peptide N-acetyl-seryl-aspartyl-lysyl-proline. *Biochem J*, **296**: 373–378.

Ritchie, R.H., Marsh, J.D., Lancaster, W.D., Diglio, C.A., and Schiebinger, R.J., 1998, Bradykinin blocks angiotensin II-induced hypertrophy in the presence of endothelial cells. *Hypertension*, **31**: 39–44.

Roig, E., Perez-Villa, F., Morales, M., Jimenez, W., Orus, J., Heras, M., and Sanz, G., 2000, Clinical implications of increased plasma angiotensin II despite ACE inhibitor therapy in patients with congestive heart failure. *Eur Heart J*, **21**: 53–57.

Rousseau, A., Michaud, A., Chauvet, M.-T., Lenfant, M., and Corvol, P., 1995, The hemoregulatory peptide N-acetyl-Ser-Asp-Lys-Pro is a natural and specific substrate of the N-terminal active site of human angiotensin-converting enzyme. *J Biol Chem*, **270**: 3656–3661.

Sato, F., and Nagasawa, S., 1988, Mechanism of kinin release from human low-molecular-mass-kininogen by the synergistic action of human plasma kallikrein and leukocyte elastase. *Biol Chem Hoppe Seyler*, **369**: 1009–1017.

Sever, P.S., Poulter, N.R., Elliott, W.J., Jonsson, M.C., and Black, H.R., 2006, Blood pressure reduction is not the only determinant of outcome. *Circulation*, **113**: 2754–2772; discussion 2773–2754.

Sharpe, N., Smith, H., Murphy, J., Greaves, S., Hart, H., and Gamble, G., 1991, Early prevention of left ventricular dysfunction after myocardial infarction with angiotensin-converting-enzyme inhibition. *Lancet*, **337**: 872–876.

Shigematsu, S., Ishida, S., Gute, D.C., and Korthuis, R.J., 1999, Bradykinin prevents postischemic leukocyte adhesion and emigration and attenuates microvascular barrier disruption. *Am J Physiol*, **277**: H161–H171.

Smart, N., Risebro, C.A., Melville, A.A., Moses, K., Schwartz, R.J., Chien, K.R., and Riley, P.R., 2007, Thymosin beta4 induces adult epicardial progenitor mobilization and neovascularization. *Nature*: (in press).

Sogaard, P., Gotzsche, C.-O., Ravkilde, J., and Thygesen, K., 1993, Effects of captopril on ischemia and dysfunction of the left ventricle after myocardial infarction. *Circulation*, **87**: 1093–1099.

Spillmann, F., Van Linthout, S., Schultheiss, H.P., and Tschope, C., 2006, Cardioprotective mechanisms of the kallikrein-kinin system in diabetic cardiopathy. *Curr Opin Nephrol Hypertens*, **15**: 22–29.

Squire, I.B., O'Kane, K.P., Anderson, N., and Reid, J.L., 2000, Bradykinin B(2) receptor antagonism attenuates blood pressure response to acute angiotensin-converting enzyme inhibition in normal men. *Hypertension*, **36**: 132–136.

Stauss, H.M., Zhu, Y.-C., Redlich, T., Adamiak, D., Mott, A., Kregel, K.C., and Unger, T., 1994, Angiotensin-converting enzyme inhibition in infarct-induced heart failure in rats: bradykinin versus angiotensin II. *J Cardiovasc Risk*, **1**: 255–262.

Struthers, A.D., MacFadyen, R., Fraser, C., Robson, J., Morton, J.J., Junot, C., and Ezan, E., 1999, Nonadherence with angiotensin-converting enzyme inhibitor therapy: a comparison of different ways of measuring it in patients with chronic heart failure. *J Am Coll Cardiol*, **34**: 2072–2077.

Studer, R., Reinecke, H., Müller, B., Holtz, J., Just, H., and Drexler, H., 1994, Increased angiotensin-I converting enzyme gene expression in the failing human heart. Quantification by competitive RNA polymerase chain reaction. *J Clin Invest*, **94**: 301–310.

Sun, Y., Zhang, J., Zhang, J.Q., and Weber, K.T., 2001, Renin expression at sites of repair in the infarcted rat heart. *J Mol Cell Cardiol*, **33**: 995–1003.

Swedberg, K., Cleland, J., Dargie, H., Drexler, H., Follath, F., Komajda, M., Tavazzi, L., Smiseth, O.A., Gavazzi, A., Haverich, A., Hoes, A., Jaarsma, T., Korewicki, J., Levy, S., Linde, C., Lopez-Sendon, J.L., Nieminen, M.S., Pierard, L., and Remme, W.J., 2005, Guidelines for the diagnosis and treatment of chronic heart failure: executive summary (update 2005): The Task Force for the Diagnosis and Treatment of Chronic Heart Failure of the European Society of Cardiology. *Eur Heart J*, **26**: 1115–1140.

Swedberg, K., Eneroth, P., Kjekshus, J., Wilhelmsen, L., and Group, f.t.C.T.S., 1990, Hormones regulating cardiovascular function in patients with severe congestive heart failure and their relation to mortality. *Circulation*, **82**: 1730–1736.

Swedberg, K., Held, P., Kjekshus, J., Rasmussen, K., Rydén, L., and Wedel, H., 1992, Effects of the early administration of enalapril on mortality in patients with acute myocardial infarction–Results of the Cooperative New Scandinavian Enalapril Survival Study II (CONSENSUS II). *N Engl J Med*, **327**: 678–684.

Takano, M., Horie, M., Narahara, M., Miyake, M., and Okamoto, H., 1999, Expression of kininogen mRNAs and plasma kallikrein mRNA by cultured neurons, astrocytes and meningeal cells in the rat brain. *Immunopharmacology*, **45**: 121–126.

Teo, K.K., Yusuf, S., Pfeffer, M., Torp-Pedersen, C., Kober, L., Hall, A., Pogue, J., Latini, R., and Collins, R., 2002, Effects of long-term treatment with angiotensin-converting-enzyme inhibitors in the presence or absence of aspirin: a systematic review. *Lancet*, **360**: 1037–1043.

The Acute Infarction Ramipril Efficacy (AIRE) Study Investigators, 1993, Effect of ramipril on mortality and morbidity of survivors of acute myocardial infarction with clinical evidence of heart failure. *Lancet*, **342**: 821–828.

The CONSENSUS Trial Study Group, 1987, Effects of enalapril on mortality in severe congestive heart failure: results of the Cooperative North Scandinavian Enalapril Survival Study (CONSENSUS). *N Engl J Med*, **316**: 1429–1435.

The DREAM Trial Investigators, 2006, Effect of ramipril on the incidence of diabetes. *N Engl J Med*, **355**: 1551–1562.

The European Trial on Reduction of Cardiac Events with Perindopril in Stable Coronary Artery Disease Investigators, 2003, Efficacy of perindopril in reduction of cardiovascular events among patients with stable coronary artery disease: randomised, double-blind, placebo-controlled, multicentre trial (the EUROPA study). *Lancet*, **362**: 782–788.

The Heart Outcomes Prevention Evaluation Study Investigators, 2000, Effects of an angiotensin-converting-enzyme inhibitor, ramipril, on cardiovascular events in high-risk patients. *N Engl J Med*, **342**: 145–153.

The PEACE Trial Investigators, 2004, Angiotensin-converting-enzyme inhibition in stable coronary artery disease. *N Engl J Med*, **351**: 2058–2068.

The SOLVD Investigators, 1991, Effect of enalapril on survival in patients with reduced left ventricular ejection fractions and congestive heart failure. *N Engl J Med*, **325**: 293–302.

The SOLVD Investigators, 1992, Effect of enalapril on mortality and the development of heart failure in asymptomatic patients with reduced left ventricular ejection fractions. *N Engl J Med*, **327**: 685–691.

Tipnis, S.R., Hooper, N.M., Hyde, R., Karran, E., Christie, G., and Turner, A.J., 2000, A human homolog of angiotensin-converting enzyme. Cloning and functional expression as a captopril-insensitive carboxypeptidase. *J Biol Chem*, **275**: 33238–33243.

Unger, T., Gohlke, P., and Gruber, M.-G., 1990, Converting enzyme inhibitors. In *Pharmacology of Antihypertensive Therapeutics Handbook of Experimental Pharmacology, Vol 93* (D. Ganten and P.J. Mulrow, ed.∧eds.), Springer-Verlag, Berlin: 377–481.

Urata, H., Kinoshita, A., Misono, K.S., Bumpus, F.M., and Husain, A., 1990, Identification of a highly specific chymase as the major angiotensin II-forming enzyme in the human heart. *J Biol Chem*, **265**: 22348–22357.

van der Meer, P., Lipsic, E., Westenbrink, B.D., van de Wal, R.M., Schoemaker, R.G., Vellenga, E., van Veldhuisen, D.J., Voors, A.A., and van Gilst, W.H., 2005, Levels of hematopoiesis inhibitor N-acetyl-seryl-aspartyl-lysyl-proline partially explain the occurrence of anemia in heart failure. *Circulation*, **112**: 1743–1747.

Van Leeuwen, R.T.J., Kol, A., Andreotti, F., Kluft, C., Maseri, A., and Sperti, G., 1994, Angiotensin II increases plasminogen activator inhibitor type 1 and tissue-type plasminogen activator messenger RNA in cultured rat aortic smooth muscle cells. *Circulation*, **90**: 362–368.

Vaughan, D.E., Rouleau, J.L., Ridker, P.M., Arnold, J.M.O., Menapace, F.J., and Pfeffer, M.A., 1997, Effects of ramipril on plasma fibrinolytic balance in patients with acute anterior myocardial infarction. *Circulation*, **96**: 442–447.

Vermes, E., Tardif, J.C., Bourassa, M.G., Racine, N., Levesque, S., White, M., Guerra, P.G., and Ducharme, A., 2003, Enalapril decreases the incidence of atrial fibrillation in patients with left ventricular dysfunction: insight from the Studies Of Left Ventricular Dysfunction (SOLVD) trials. *Circulation*, **107**: 2926–2931.

Vickers, C., Hales, P., Kaushik, V., Dick, L., Gavin, J., Tang, J., Godbout, K., Parsons, T., Baronas, E., Hsieh, F., Acton, S., Patane, M., Nichols, A., and Tummino, P., 2002, Hydrolysis of biological peptides by human angiotensin-converting enzyme-related carboxypeptidase. *J Biol Chem*, **277**: 14838–14843.

Voros, S., Yang, Z., Bove, C.M., Gilson, W.D., Epstein, F.H., French, B.A., Berr, S.S., Bishop, S.P., Conaway, M.R., Matsubara, H., Carey, R.M., and Kramer, C.M., 2006, Interaction between AT1 and AT2 receptors during postinfarction left ventricular remodeling. *Am J Physiol Heart Circ Physiol*, **290**: H1004–H1010.

Wang, D., Carretero, O.A., Yang, X.Y., Rhaleb, N.E., Liu, Y.H., Liao, T.D., and Yang, X.P., 2004, N-acetyl-seryl-aspartyl-lysyl-proline stimulates angiogenesis in vitro and in vivo. *Am J Physiol Heart Circ Physiol*, **287**: H2099–H2105.

Wang, J.G., Staessen, J.A., Li, Y., Van Bortel, L.M., Nawrot, T., Fagard, R., Messerli, F.H., and Safar, M., 2006, Carotid intima-media thickness and antihypertensive treatment: a meta-analysis of randomized controlled trials. *Stroke*, **37**: 1933–1940.

Wang, T.J., Larson, M.G., Levy, D., Vasan, R.S., Leip, E.P., Wolf, P.A., D'Agostino, R.B., Murabito, J.M., Kannel, W.B., and Benjamin, E.J., 2003, Temporal relations of atrial fibrillation and congestive heart failure and their joint influence on mortality: the Framingham Heart Study. *Circulation*, **107**: 2920–2925.

Webb, M.L., Dickinson, K.E.J., Delaney, C.L., Liu, E.C.-K., Serafino, R., Cohen, R.B., Monshizadegan, H., and Moreland, S., 1992, The endothelin receptor antagonist, BQ-123, inhibits angiotensin II-induced contractions in rabbit aorta. *Biochem Biophys Res Commun*, **185**: 887–892.

Weber, K.T., 2001, Aldosterone in congestive heart failure. *N Engl J Med*, **345**: 1689–1697.

Wei, L., Alhenc-Gelas, F., Corvol, P., and Clauser, E., 1991, The two homologous domains of human angiotensin I-converting enzyme are both catalytically active. *J Biol Chem*, **266**: 9002–9008.

Wei, L., Clauser, E., Alhenc-Gelas, F., and Corvol, P., 1992, The two homologous domains of human angiotensin I-converting enzyme interact differently with competitive inhibitors. *J Biol Chem*, **267**: 13398–13405.

Witherow, F.N., Helmy, A., Webb, D.J., Fox, K.A., and Newby, D.E., 2001, Bradykinin contributes to the vasodilator effects of chronic angiotensin-converting enzyme inhibition in patients with heart failure. *Circulation*, **104**: 2177–2181.

Wollert, K.C., Studer, R., Doerfer, K., Schieffer, E., Holubarsch, C., Just, H., and Drexler, H., 1997, Differential effects of kinins on cardiomyocyte hypertrophy and interstitial collagen matrix in the surviving myocardium after myocardial infarction in the rat. *Circulation*, **95**: 1910–1917.

Wright, R.A., Flapan, A.D., Alberti, K.G.M.M., Ludlam, C.A., and Fox, K.A.A., 1994, Effects of captopril therapy on endogenous fibrinolysis in men with recent, uncomplicated myocardial infarction. *J Am Coll Cardiol*, **24**: 67–73.

Xiong, W., Chen, L.-M., Woodley-Miller, C., Simson, J.A., and Chao, J., 1990, Identification, purification, and localization of tissue kallikrein in rat heart. *Biochem J*, **267**: 639–646.

Yamada, K., Iyer, S.N., Chappell, M.C., Ganten, D., and Ferrario, C.M., 1998, Converting enzyme determines plasma clearance of angiotensin-(1-7). *Hypertension*, **32**: 496–502.

Yamamoto, K., Chappell, M.C., Brosnihan, K.B., and Ferrario, C.M., 1992, In vivo metabolism of angiotensin I by neutral endopeptidase (EC 3.4.24.11) in spontaneously hypertensive rats. *Hypertension*, **19**: 692–696.

Yang, F., Yang, X.P., Liu, Y.H., Xu, J., Cingolani, O., Rhaleb, N.E., and Carretero, O.A., 2004, Ac-SDKP reverses inflammation and fibrosis in rats with heart failure after myocardial infarction. *Hypertension*, **43**: 229–236.

Yousef, G.M., and Diamandis, E.P., 2001, The new human tissue kallikrein gene family: structure, function, and association to disease. *Endocr Rev*, **22**: 184–204.

Yusuf, S., Pepine, C.J., Garces, C., Pouleur, H., Salem, D., Kostis, J., Benedict, C., Rousseau, M., Bourassa, M., and Pitt, B., 1992, Effect of enalapril on myocardial infarction and unstable angina in patients with low ejection fractions. *Lancet*, **340**: 1173–1178.

Zehetgruber, M., Beckmann, R., Gabriel, H., Christ, G., Binder, B.R., and Huber, K., 1996, The ACE-inhibitor lisinopril affects plasma insulin levels but not fibrinolytic parameters. *Thromb Res*, **83**: 143–152.

Zeitz, C.J., Campbell, D.J., and Horowitz, J.D., 2003, Myocardial uptake and biochemical and hemody-namic effects of ACE inhibitors in humans. *Hypertension*, **41**: 482–487.

Zhang, X., Xie, Y.W., Nasjletti, A., Xu, X., Wolin, M.S., and Hintze, T.H., 1997, ACE inhibitors promote nitric oxide accumulation to modulate myocardial oxygen consumption. *Circulation*, **95**: 176–182.

Zisman, L.S., Keller, R.S., Weaver, B., Lin, Q., Speth, R., Bristow, M.R., and Canver, C.C., 2003, Increased angiotensin-(1-7)-forming activity in failing human heart ventricles: evidence for upregu-lation of the angiotensin-converting enzyme homologue ACE2. *Circulation*, **108**: 1707–1712.

CHAPTER 3

PROTEASES OF THE RENIN-ANGIOTENSIN SYSTEM IN HUMAN ACUTE PANCREATITIS

R. PEZZILLI AND L. FANTINI

Department of Internal Medicine and Gastroenterology, Sant'Orsola-Malpighi Hospital, Bologna, Italy

1.   INTRODUCTION

It is well-known that acute pancreatitis originates in the acinar cells and then involves all body structures; in other words, acute pancreatitis evolves from an organ disease to a systemic disease. Thus, it is important to understand why this happens; the basic mechanisms of acute pancreatitis are strictly linked to the anatomy and the physiology of the pancreatic acinar cells and their products, even if most of the data on this process come from basic research and not from human studies. In this chapter, we will review the advance in understanding the origin and development of acute pancreatitis in humans with particular regard to the participation of the renin-angiotensin system in the setting of acute pancreatic inflammation.

2.   PANCREAS DEVELOPMENT

It has been suggested that there is a common pancreatic progenitor of both acinar and islet cells (Fishman and Melton 2002); pancreatic acinar cells appear during the third month of intrauterine life as small clusters of cells along the lateral walls and at the distal ends of the ducts. Glycogen presence can be demonstrated at the end of the third month; in the following month, the basophilia of the acinar cells increases and small granules with non-specific esterase activity can be found in the basal cytoplasm and the pancreatic acinar cells then become capable of secretion during prenatal life (Laitio *et al* 1974). It is worth noting that pancreatic cells may transdifferentiate into ductal cells during the course of acute and chronic disease, mainly pancreatitis and pancreatic cancer (Bockman 1997). However, we have no information as to the role of the renin-angiotensin system in the differentiation development.

55

Po Sing Leung (ed.), Frontiers in Research of the Renin-Angiotensin System on Human Disease, 55–71.
© 2007 *Springer.*

3.   PHYSIOLOGY

The exocrine part of the pancreatic gland secretes about 3 litres of fluid and a clear secretion rich in enzymes and bicarbonates (Gullo *et al* 1987). The water and bicarbonates are mainly secreted by the pancreatic ductal epithelium whereas acinar cells synthesize, store and secrete digestive enzymes in order to catalyze the hydrolysis of food constituents into absorbable forms. Pancreatic acinar cell secretion contains three major categories of enzymes: amylolytic, lipolytic and proteolytic enzymes which are able to digest carbohydrates, fats and proteins, respectively. Synthesis of the digestive enzymes begins at the ribosomes located in the cytosol of the acinar cell. To permit regulated exocytosis, these enzymes must be sorted from the constitutively secreted proteins and stored in secretory granules. The sorting and packing of these enzymes involves protein selection at the level of the trans-Golgi network and the removal of residual lysosomal enzymes, as well as secreted proteins during the post-Golgi maturation of secretory granules. Pancreatic proteases are secreted as inactive precursors into the duodenum where enterokinase, an enzyme located along the brush border of duodenal enterocytes, initiates their activation. Acinar cell secretion is primarily induced by the ingestion of food, which initiates multiple endocrine, neurocrine and paracrine pathways regulating the release of appropriate amounts of acinar digestive enzymes. There are several neurohormonal regulators released in response to the ingestion of food mainly represented by cholecystokinin, secretin, vasoactive intestinal polypeptide, acetylcholine, or angiotensin II. Upon binding of these secretagogues to their respective receptors on the basolateral membrane of pancreatic acinar cells, various types of signal transduction pathways are evoked. Both cholecystokinin and acetylcholine activate inositol triphosphate/diacyl glycerol signaling pathways which raise cytosolic Ca^{2+} concentration with the concurrent activation of protein kinase C and the consequent triggering of Ca^{2+}-dependent exocytosis. In contrast, the signaling pathway initiated by secretin and vasoactive intestinal peptides is mediated by the increase of the cAMP level and the subsequent activation of protein kinase A. On the other hand, local RAS seems to play an important role in the physiology of pancreatic acinar cells (Leung and Carlsson 2001); in fact, angiotensin II could stimulate a dose-dependent release of digestive enzymes from the pancreatic acinar cells, probably via the mediation of intracellular calcium.

4.   ACUTE PANCREATITIS

4.1.   Definition

Acute pancreatitis is an inflammatory disease characterized by pancreatic tissue edema, acinar cell necrosis, hemorrhage and inflammation of the damaged gland. Clinically the pancreatitis is characterized in more than 95% of the cases by abdominal pain associated with an increase of pancreatic enzymes in serum and/or urine. The major etiologic factors of acute pancreatitis are gallstones and alcoholism, which are present in more than 80% of the cases whereas the remaining pancreatitis cases are for the most part idiopathic (Pezzilli *et al* 1998). From a clinical point of view, we can distinguish the pancreatitis according to the clinical evolution of the disease (Bradley 1993): mild acute pancreatitis characterized by an uneventful course with mortality near 0% and severe pancreatitis which is characterized by local and distant organ involvement with mortality varying from 30 to 50%. We can also identify various phases in the development of severe acute pancreatitis (Fig. 1): the initial phase characterized mainly altered intra-acinar protein traffic and by the accumulation of trypsinogen in the interstitial space (as in the mild form of the disease), an early-middle phase characterized by the activation of various protease cascades which determine formation of necrosis of the pancreatic tissue, and the late phase characterized by the infection of pancreatic necrotic tissue due to translocation of bacteria from the gastrointestinal tract.

It is clear that the early identification of severely ill patients is helpful in ensuring rapid appropriate treatment; in fact, endoscopic sphincterotomy has became more widely used for the management of severe gallstone-induced acute pancreatitis and other specific therapies are also available (e.g. antibiotic prophylaxis, enteral nutrition, etc.).

4.2.   Pathophysiology

In 1896, the concept that the cause of the pathophysiological changes in acute pancreatitis lay in the autodigestion of the pancreas mediated by the pancreatic enzymes was proposed for the first time (Chiari 1896). Numerous studies published so far indicate that the activation of trypsin in acinar cells is an important early mechanism in this disease; in animal models of acute pancreatitis, several processes have been observed in acinar cells leading to the inhibition of secretion and subsequent autodigestion. These mechanisms include premature activation of trypsin (Whitcomb 1999), colocalization of zymogens and lysosomes with the subsequent redistribution of lysosomal enzymes (Fig. 2), a sustained rise in intracellular calcium (Raraty *et al* 2000; Parekh 2000), breakdown of apical F-actin (Jungermann *et al*

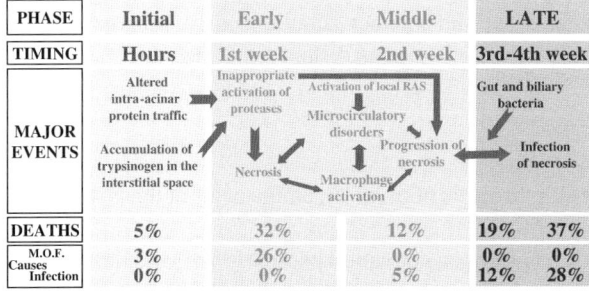

Figure 1. Physiopathological and clinical phases of acute pancreatitis (from Pezzilli, 2004, modified). RAS: renin-angiotensin system

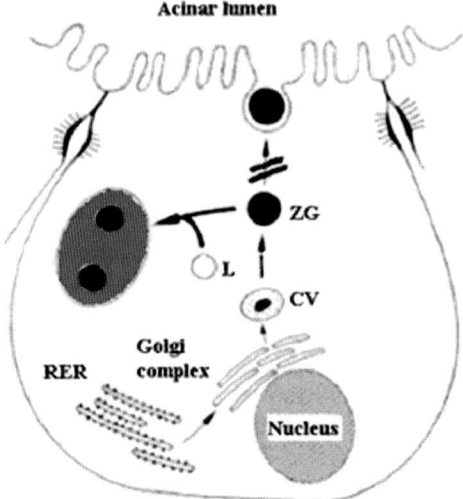

Figure 2. Mechanism of acute pancreatitis. The initial event is blockage of the secretion, leading to the accumulation of zymogen granules within the acinar cells. After this event, there is a fusion of lysosomes and zymogens within large vacuoles and, finally, there is the activation of enzymes and acute intracellular injury. L=lysosome; ZG=zymogens; CV=condensing vacuole; RER=rough endoplamatic reticulum

1995; Fallon *et al* 1995) and the activation of the transcription of nuclear factor-*k*B (NF-*k*B) (Steinle *et al* 1999).

Even if many causes have been postulated to be associated with the development of acute pancreatitis, such as biliary tract disease, alcohol etc., the exact event capable of initiating the intracellular activation of trypsin is under investigation. In fact, even if the basic mechanism of the activation of trypsin is now partially known, the factor capable of initiating these events is still unknown. After the initiation of acute pancreatitis, other mechanisms are involved in the progression of the disease such as the chemokine cascade, the kallikrein-kinin system, the complement activation system, the coagulation system and the renin-angiotensin system (RAS). All these systems act and interact simultaneously, thus explaining the effects of acute pancreatitis in various organs distant from the pancreas.

4.3.   Trypsin

Trypsinogen is activated by the hydrolysis of up to ten amino acids at the N-terminus (Fig. 3).

The cleaved region is called trypsinogen activation peptide (TAP) and the removal of this peptide from the pro-enzyme renders the trypsinogen active (trypsin) by inducing conformational changes. To better understand the activation of trypsin, we must remember that the co-localization theory postulates that trypsin activation

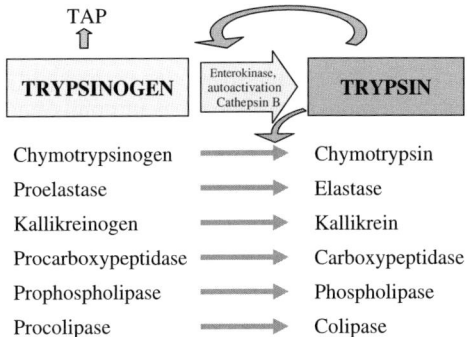

Chymotrypsinogen ⟹ Chymotrypsin

Proelastase ⟹ Elastase

Kallikreinogen ⟹ Kallikrein

Procarboxypeptidase ⟹ Carboxypeptidase

Prophospholipase ⟹ Phospholipase

Procolipase ⟹ Colipase

Figure 3. Activation of trypsinogen: trypsinogen could be activated into active trypsin either by the brush border enzyme enterokinase in the small intestine or by cathepsin-B, a lysosomal enzyme present in acinar cells. Another mechanism consists of trypsinogen autoactivation. Once trypsin is activated, it can catalyze the other digestive pro enzymes. TAP: Trypsinogen activating peptide

occurs within cytosolic vacuoles containing both digestive enzymes and lysosomal enzymes, such as cathepsin B. Some authors (Otani *et al* 1998; Hofbauer 1998) have detected immunoreactivity against TAP in vacuoles positive for lysosomal markers and cathepsin B. Cathepsin B is capable of removing the TAP region from the trypsinogen; thus, it seems to be able to transform trypsinogen into trypsin in cellular compartments. However, the inhibition of trypsin activation in knockout mice is not complete; thus, other mechanisms or premature activation by other lysosomal proteases should be hypothesized. Another possible mechanism in the activation of trypsinogen involves intracellular calcium; it has been demonstrated (Kruger *et al* 2000) that premature trypsin activation takes place in the apical cell in response to supramaximal cholecystokinin stimulation and that this activation is dependent on the spatial and temporal distribution of Ca^{2+} release within the same subcellular compartment. Whereas in resting acinar cells, trypsinogen is stored within zymogen granules located in the apical part of the cells, after stimulation with physiological doses of cholecystokinin, the granules are exocytosed in a calcium-dependent manner. However, using supramaximal doses of cholecystokinin, trypsin activation begins in a defined region in apical acinar cells and a sustained rise in calcium triggers vacuole formation in response to supramaximal cerulein stimulation. Both trypsin activation and vacuole formation can be inhibited by the interruption of Ca^{2+} signals (Raraty *et al* 2000). Thus, these studies provide a demonstration that a sustained rise in calcium is an important cofactor of acute pancreatitis.

4.4. Chemokines

The destruction of the pancreatic parenchyma during acute pancreatitis quickly induces an inflammatory reaction at the site of injury. The initial cellular response involves the infiltration of polymorphonuclear leukocytes into the perivascular regions of the pancreas. Within a few hours, macrophages and lymphocytes accumulate and phagocyte-derived oxygen radicals participate in a primary injury to the pancreatic capillary endothelial cells. Increased microvascular permeability facilitates margination and extravascular migration of additional neutrophils and monocytes amplifying the inflammatory process. Following an experimental insult, there is rapid expression of tumor necrosis factor-alpha (TNF-alpha), interleukin-1 (IL-1) and other chemokines such as interleukin-6 (IL-6) and interleukin-8 (IL-8) by pancreatic acinar cells and/or transmigrated leukocytes (Norman 1998). IL-1 and TNF-alpha are the primary inducers of IL-6 and IL-8 production and they are known to initiate and propagate many metabolic consequences of sepsis including fever, hypotension, acidosis and acute respiratory distress syndrome (Lowry 1993; Dinarello 1996a; Dinarello 1996b) (Fig. 4).

The cellular mechanisms underlying cytokine production are not entirely known. The transcription factor NF-kB is important for the activation of many inflammatory mediators and cytokines such as IL-1 and IL-6 (Mercurio and Manning 1999). Initially, NF-kB is sequestered in the cytoplasm bound to its inhibitory element named IKB. On stimulation, IKB is phosphorylated and degraded by proteosomes and the degradation of IkB releases NF-kB, allowing it to translocate into the nucleus; in the nucleus, NF-kB binds to its consensus sequence within the promoter region of a number of proinflammatory genes (Thanos and Maniatis 1995). Early induction of NF-kB binding activity and decreased IkB expression were shown in cerulein-induced pancreatitis (Tando *et al* 1999; Steinle *et al* 1999, Han and Logsdon 2000), and NF-kB activity seems to be dependent on Ca^{2+} influx and protein kinase C activation (Han and Logsdon 2000; Tando *et al* 1999; Ethridge *et al* 2002). Increased NF-kB activity seems to play an important role in the induction of

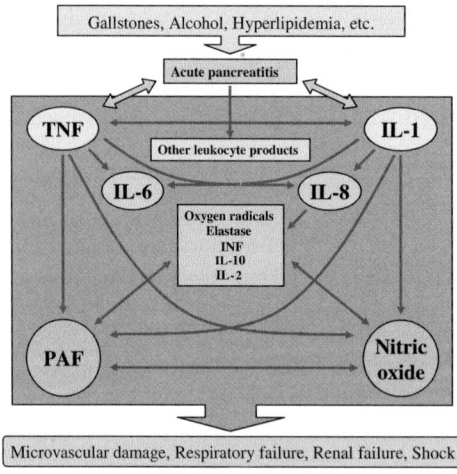

Figure 4. Pathogenesis of acute pancreatitis according to the chemokine theory. TNF: tumor necrosis factor. IL: interleukin; INF: Interferon; PAF: Platelet activating factor

proinflammatory cytokines. Furthermore, in the severe forms of acute pancreatitis, there is also a low production of anti-inflammatory cytokines, such as interleukin-10 (IL-10), capable of blocking the action of the pro-inflammatory cytokines (Pezzilli *et al* 1997).

4.5.   Kallikrein-kinin System

Kinins released during the course of inflammatory injury are one of the major cause of vascular symptoms, i.e. pancreatic oedema formation and its consequences, such as haemoconcentration, hypovolaemia and hypotension. Kinins are also involved in the accumulation of potentially cytotoxic factors in the pancreatic tissue (Griesbacher 2000). While glandular prekallikrein is synthesised in the pancreas, both kininogens and plasma prekallikrein are probably produced mainly in the liver. The kinin system also interacts with the prostaglandins, mostly through kininogens and kallikreins and not through bradykinin. While bradykinin is rapidly degraded by kinases, kallikrein is inactivated by complex formation with alpha-2 macroglobulin, with a C1 inhibitor and also with a few other inhibitors. For the most part, studies of the kinin system in acute pancreatitis have been carried out in animals and activation of this system has been found to be most pronounced in the peritoneal cavity. In humans, there are very few studies; one of these (Uehara *et al* 1989.) demonstrated that plasma prekallikrein decreased in acute pancreatitis and there was a negative correlation between plasma prekallikrein and kallikrein-like activity. Finally, this study demonstrated that both high and low molecular weight kininogens decreased in an acutely damaged pancreas.

4.6.   Complement Activation System

Complement activation has been shown to occur in patients with acute pancreatitis. In fact, the serum complement system is capable of damaging viable unaltered cell membranes (Balldin *et al* 1981.), but there are no sufficient data on the involvement of this system in human acute pancreatitis.

4.7.   Coagulation System

The importance of disseminated intravascular coagulation during the course of acute pancreatitis is well-known. Lasson and Ohlsson (Lasson and Ohlsson 1986.) analysed the activation of the coagulation and fibrinolytic systems in 27 attacks of acute human pancreatitis of differing severity. Consumptive coagulopathy was suggested by decreased platelet counts, decreased prothrombin values and the consumption of fibrinogen during the first days of severe attacks. Factor X was slightly decreased for the first 5 days of the attacks. Increased fibrinolysis was suggested by decreased plasminogen values in severe attacks. Fibrinogen degradation products were seen in the blood in 40% of patients and in the peritoneal fluid in all patients with severe attacks. Furthermore, the plasma levels of antithrombin III and alpha 2-macroglobulin were low while the levels of C1-inhibitor and alpha 2-antiplasmin were high. In conclusion, severe acute pancreatitis results in both consumptive coagulopathy and increased fibrinolysis. A local antiprotease deficiency is seen in the peritoneal cavity and high levels of protease-antiprotease complexes are also seen in the plasma. All these changes are closely correlated to the severity of the disease and probably determine the clinical outcome of the acute attack.

4.8.   Renin-Angiotensin System

Recently, characterization of the RAS in the pancreas has been reported in laboratory animals as well as in humans (Chappell *et al* 1991; Chappell *et al* 1992a; Ghiani and Masini 1995; Tahmasebi *et al* 1999.).

In the 1990s, two studies demonstrating key components which comprise an intrinsic RAS within the canine pancreas have been published (Chappell *et al* 1991; Chappell *et al* 1992a). These studies documented the expression of the bioactive peptides angiotensin II, angiotensin III, and angiotensin-(1-7), the mRNA levels of the precursor angiotensinogen as well as the distribution of the AT_2 and AT_1 receptor subtypes. Subsequent studies confirmed these findings in the rat, the mouse and, most importantly, in the human pancreas (Leung *et al* 1997; Leung *et al* 1999; Tahmasebi *et al* 1999) (Fig. 5).

Indeed, in one of the few reports aimed at studying the *in vivo* regulation of pancreatic angiotensin II receptors, an increase in angiotensin II binding sites in the pancreas of normotensive rats maintained on a high-salt diet has been demonstrated (Ghiani and Masini 1995).

Although angiotensin II receptors were distributed throughout the pancreas, the highest density of sites comprised the AT_2 receptor subtype and they are localized, at least in the dog and the monkey, to acinar cells and the ductal epithelium (Chappell *et al* 1992a, Chappell *et al* 1994a). The pancreas is one of the few tissues which primarily expresses the AT_2 receptor subtype and only recently has a more complete understanding of the functional role of the AT_2 receptor emerged. In vitro receptor autoradiography of angiotensin II receptors in the primate pancreas using the non-selective angiotensin ligand ^{125}I-(Sar1, Thre8)-angiotensin II, named Sarthran, revealed the distribution of sites throughout the tissue, but with the highest density in acinar cells (Chappell *et al* 1994a; Chappell MC *et al* 1994b). The majority of Sarthran binding (>80%) was attenuated by the AT_2 selective antagonist PD123319. High resolution emulsion autoradiography of this tissue revealed a very high expression of Sarthran binding surrounding the islet cells and a lower density of sites within the islet field; addition of the PD123319 compound essentially abolished binding. These findings, demonstrating the predominant expression of the AT_2 subtype in the exocrine components of the pancreas prompted further investigation of angiotensin II receptors and other components of the RAS in an acinar cell model. Angiotensin II receptor binding in the AR42J acinar cell line was characterized, and a high density of binding sites was found (Chappell *et al* 1995);

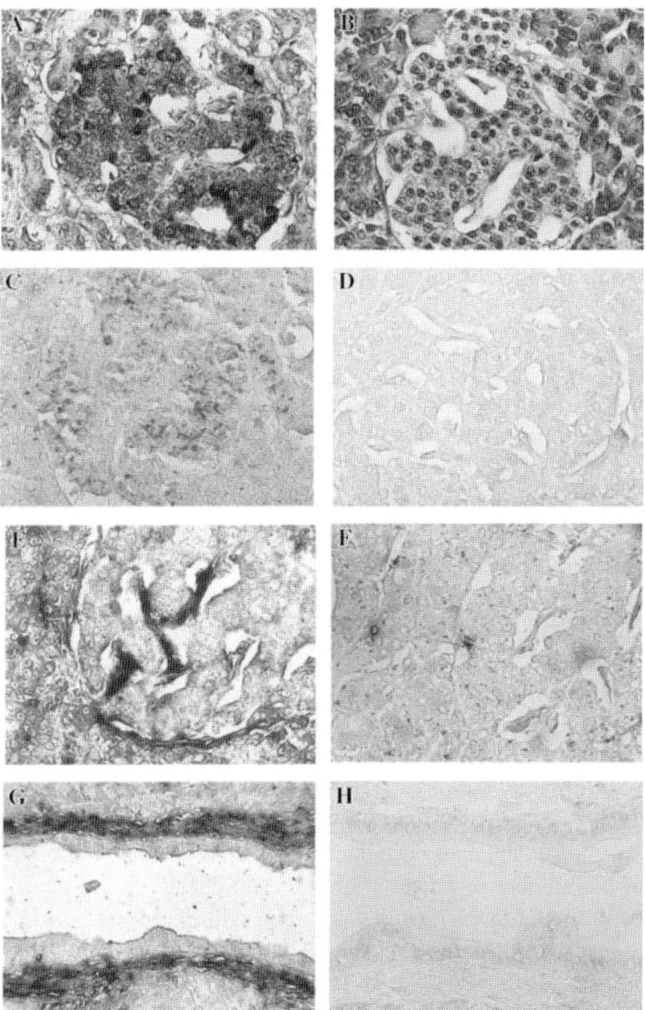

Figure 5. Immunocytochemistry shows the distribution of AT_1 receptors (brown stain) in beta cells of the islets of Langerhans in the human pancreas. It is absent from reticular fibres (A). Control sections, using antibody presaturated with peptide antigen, showed no staining (B). The distribution of renin (brown stain) is similarly confined to beta cells of the islets (C). Control sections again showed no immunoreactivity (D). In situ hybridisation shows that prorenin mRNA (dark stain) was transcribed in the reticular fibres of the islets (E) and the fibroblasts and connective tissue surrounding blood vessels (G). The negative controls, using a sense probe, showed no staining (F & H). Magnification x166 throughout. (Tahmasebi M et al, 1999)

the majority of these receptors were the AT_2 subtype with a minority of sites (<15%) for the AT_1 antagonist losartan. Although the proportion of AT_1 receptors expressed in the AR42J cell line was small, application of angiotensin II to cells loaded with fluorescent calcium dye Fura-2 resulted in an immediate and significant increase in intracellular calcium. The angiotensin II-dependent rise in calcium was abolished by the AT_1 antagonist, but was not modified by AT_2 antagonists (Chappell et al 1995). Subsequent studies also reported AT_1-dependent changes in intracellular calcium by angiotensin II (Barnhardt et al 1999). The biochemical characterization of the AT_2 binding sites utilized cross-linking of radiolabeled Sarthran and SDS/P AGE fractionation. These studies revealed an AT_2 site with a molecular mass of approximately 110 kDa which was substantially greater than the predicted mass of 40 kDa based on the protein sequence of the AT_2 receptor. Analysis of the AT_2 sequence indicated a high number of glycosylation sites which likely influences the larger molecular mass observed in these cells (Servant et al 1994). However, internalization of the AT_2 receptor (another characteristic quite distinct from the rapid down-regulation of the AT_1 receptor subtype following agonist binding (De Gasparo et al 2000)) has not been demonstrated until now. Regarding the functional aspects of the AT_2 receptor, a link to the activation of tyrosine phosphatase has been reported (Takahasi et al 1994; Bottari et al 1992). In the AR42J cells, activation of somatostatin receptors increased tyrosine phosphatase activity and inhibited cell proliferation (Tahiri-Jouti et al 1992). Chappell et al found that, in the presence of an AT_1 blockade, angiotensin II increased vanadate-inhibitable tyrosine phosphatase activity as measured with para-nitrophenol phosphate (Chappell et al 2001). In the presence of both AT_2 and AT_1 antagonists, angiotensin II did not change phosphatase activity. Regarding the regulation of the AT_2 receptor subtype, it has been found that treatment with the glucocorticoid agonist dexamethasone resulted in a significant decline in PD123319-sensitive binding within six hours and a maximal decrease in binding within 24 hours (Chappell et al 1992b). The addition of cortisol also substantially reduced binding, but other steroid agents including estrogen, and aldosterone had little or no effect.

Saturation analysis of the dexamethasone-induced inhibition of the AT_2 binding reflected a decrease in the number of receptor sites and no change in the relative affinity of the receptor to the Sarthran ligand. Consistent with the decrease in the number of receptors, the assessment of AT_2 mRNA levels by RT-PCR revealed an almost complete inhibition of mRNA expression by dexamethasone in these cells. In contrast, estrogen treatment had no effect on angiotensin II binding or AT_2 mRNA expression. Further studies are necessary to determine whether this reduction in AT_2 mRNA results from an attenuation in transcriptional activity or decreased mRNA stability. In view of the contrasting actions of AT_1 and AT_2 receptors, glucocorticoids are known to increase AT_1 binding and AT_1 mRNA, as well as ACE activity (Fishel et al 1995; Guo et al 1995). Thus, glucocorticoid-induced hypertension may comprise a shift in the balance of effects between the AT_1 and AT_2 receptors in the presence of elevated levels of angiotensin II. Glucocorticoid down-regulation of the AT_2 receptors may also be relevant to the recent findings that endogenous glucocorticoids suppress apoptosis in an induced-pancreatitis model (Kimura et al 1998). An up-regulation of the pancreatic RAS including increased expression of AT_2 mRNA in a chronic model of hypoxia, as well as augmented angiotensinogen in induced pancreatitis have been demonstrated

(Chan *et al* 2000; Leung *et al* 2000). Thus, the activation of pancreatic RAS, particularly the AT_2 receptor, may promote cellular apoptosis and influence pancreatitis. Furthermore, the expression of additional components of the pancreatic RAS in AR42J cells is under investigation (Chappell *et al* 2001) and preliminary studies using RT-PCR revealed that the AR42J cells express mRNA for both AT_{1a} and AT_{1b} isotypes as well as those for renin, angiotensinogen and ACE. Although the expression of these components may result from the transformed phenotype, the AR42J cells constitute a unique cell model capable of exploring the processing of angiotensin II and angiotensin I. Indeed, these cells may more closely model an autocrine system in which the local production of angiotensin II or other active metabolites acting through different receptor subtypes may influence its tissue of origin be means of a feedback mechanism. This may be of particular relevance in hypertensive patients as AT_1 receptor blockers may supplant ACE inhibitors and other anti-hypertensive treatments. AT_1 receptor blocker treatment not only blocks AT_1 receptors, but significantly increases angiotensin II levels which may result in greater activation of the AT_2 and other receptor subtypes. Furthermore, the acinar cell model may be of relevance to study more novel components of the RAS such as the AT_4 receptor and the biologically active ligands, angiotensin-(3-8) and angiotensin-(3-7); these endogenous peptides exhibit high affinity for the AT_4 binding site (De Gasparo *et al* 2000; Harding *et al* 1994). Although a high density of AT_4 sites are found in a number of tissues such as the heart, adrenal glands, and the vascular endothelium, whether this site is expressed on the exocrine or endocrine elements of the pancreas is not known at this time. In addition, numerous studies demonstrate a functional role for angiotensin-(1-7) in the vasculature, brain and kidneys which is mediated by a non-AT_1,-AT_2 receptor (Chappell *et al* 1998; Chappell *et al* 2000). Indeed, elevated levels of angiotensin-(1-7) contribute to the anti-hypertensive actions of ACE inhibitors and AT_1 receptor antagonists (Iyer *et al* 1998; Iyer *et al* 2000). Although Chappell *et al* originally measured significant angiotensin-(1-7) levels in the dog pancreas, whether this peptide influences pancreatic function is also unknown (Chappell *et al* 2001). All knowledge accumulated up to now has stimulated further investigation into defining the importance of RAS in various pancreatic disease; specifically, a lot of papers have focused their interest on acute pancreatitis. In fact, angiotensinogen and angiotensin receptors may play an important role in the induction of inflammation and microcirculatory regulation in the pancreas, and this, in turn, may contribute to pancreatic tissue injury in acute pancreatitis. Indeed, pancreatic microcirculatory changes such as vasoconstriction, capillary stasis, decreased oxygen tension and progressive ischemia have been shown to occur early in the course of acute pancreatitis (Knoefel *et al* 1994). It would be logical to ask if local RAS could control or determine the extension of inflammatory activation in the pancreas and it may be involved in the regulation of vascular injuries (Janiak *et al* 1992). Data on the effects of blocking local RAS activation in human acute pancreatitis are lacking. Molecules in the families of reactive oxygen metabolites and reactive nitrogen species have been shown to be mediated by RAS in the circulatory system (Fernandez-Alfonso and Gonzalez,

1999; Berry *et al* 2000). Nitric oxide is known to increase pancreatic secretion as well as improve pancreatic perfusion (Patel *et al* 1995) while reactive oxygen metabolites are important mediators in ischaemic-reperfusion injury (Granger *et al* 1994). Obviously, their roles in acute pancreatitis in relation to the local RAS remain to be investigated.

Activation of plasma RAS, as shown by an elevation of plasma renin, has been demonstrated in patients with acute pancreatitis (Greenstein *et al* 1987). We recently re-assessed these data (Pezzilli *et al* 2006) and we studied 21 patients with acute pancreatitis (13 males, 8 females, mean age 57.9 years, range 20-84 years) within 24 hours of pain onset. None of the patients had arterial hypertension or other known diseases and none were taking drugs capable of modifying the RAS. According to the Atlanta criteria, 14 patients (67%) had mild acute pancreatitis and seven (33%) had the severe form of the disease. In all patients, plasma renin activity (reference range: 0.2-2.8 ng/mL/h), plasma angiotensin I converting enzyme activity (reference range: 65.8-114.4 U/L) and plasma aldosterone concentration (reference range: 33-489 pg/mL) were determined immediately after hospital admission using commercially available kits. Serum amylase and lipase activities were also determined. The results of our experience are reported in Fig. 6.

In brief, considering all patients with acute pancreatitis, mean±SD plasma renin activity, angiotensin I converting enzyme activity and aldosterone concentration were 0.73±0.84 ng/mL/h, 56.8±30.4 U/L, and 92.2±112.8 pg/mL, respectively. In particular, the plasma renin activity was above the reference range in one patient with severe pancreatitis (5%); the plasma angiotensin I converting enzyme activity was above the reference range in one patient (5%) with mild acute pancreatitis and below the reference range in 15 patients (71%) (ten with mild acute pancreatitis and five with the severe form of the disease); plasma aldosteron concentration was below the reference range in five patients (24%) (three with mild acute pancreatitis and two with the severe pancreatitis). In addition, no significant relationship was found between serum amylase or lipase activities and plasma renin activity, plasma angiotensin I converting enzyme activity or aldosteron concentration. Furthermore, no significant relationship was found between plasma renin activity, angiotensin

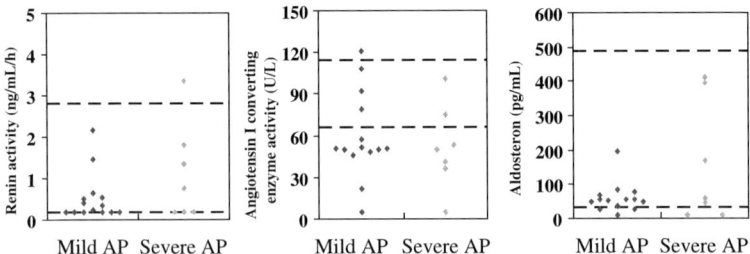

Figure 6. Individual values of plasma renin, angiotensin I converting enzyme activity and aldosterone in acute pancreatitis (AP) patients divided according to the mild or the severe course of the disease. Dotted lines represent the reference ranges

I converting enzyme activity and aldosteron concentration and the severity of the disease. Thus, the RAS appears to be impaired in patients with acute pancreatitis even if the impairment does not seem to be related to the severity of the disease. Although circulatory hypovolaemia was thought to be the main cause of the activation of plasma RAS, it may be hypothesized that activation of local RAS may be related to plasma RAS, either directly or through other inflammatory mediators.

5. THERAPEUTIC POSSIBILITIES FOR MANIPULATING THE RENIN-ANGIOTENSIN SYSTEM

Recent studies have explored the differential effects of RAS blockers and their potential use in the treatment of pancreatic inflammation. Prophylactic administration of saralasin, a non-specific renin-angiotensin blocker, was shown to improve acute pancreatitis-induced injury in the pancreas, while ramiprilat, an angiotensin-converting enzyme inhibitor, did not (Tsang *et al* 2003). The protective mechanism of saralasin may be related to the alleviation of the increased oxidative stress caused by the upregulation of AT_1 receptors during acute pancreatitis (Ip *et al* 2003). In addition, prophylactic and therapeutic administration of AT_1-R (losartan) and AT_2-R (PD1233 19) antagonists reveal a distinctive action against pancreatitis-induced oxidative stress (Tsang *et al* 2004). This beneficial effect may be due, in part, to inhibition of the AT_1-R-mediated NADPH oxidase-dependent production of free radicals and in part to the impaired pancreatic microcirculation seen in acute pancreatitis. Another study has demonstrated that the angiotensin-converting enzyme inhibitor does attenuate chronic pancreatitis-induced injury and pancreatic fibrosis, possibly by means of the prevention of pancreatic stellate cell activation (Kuno *et al* 2003). Despite the fact that these studies demonstrate the involvement of the RAS blockade in acute pancreatitis, it should be stressed that these results are based on an animal model of mild edematous pancreatitis and they might not mimic the clinical situation which usually occurs in humans (Foitzik *et al* 2000). Moreover, all available data support the potential value of a RAS blockade in treating pancreatic inflammation in the future, even if few reports indicate that angiotensin-converting enzyme inhibitor induces acute pancreatitis in some patients (Kanbay *et al* 2004; Anagnostopoulos *et al* 2003; Cheng *et al* 2003). This may be due to the fact that angiotensin-converting enzyme inhibitor prevents the breakdown of bradykinins. Nevertheless, the accumulated data on the effects of a RAS blockade in pancreatic inflammation and injury, the selective use of a specific renin-angiotensin blocker and/or a combination therapy of a renin-angiotensin blocker plus angiotensin-converting enzyme inhibitors may provide indications for synergistic action in the treatment of pancreatic inflammation. Another possibility of modulating the RAS in acute pancreatitis has come from the use of Rhodiola, a type of Chinese herb, which may protect hypoxia-induced pancreatic injury in two ways. It prevents hypoxia-induced biological changes by increasing intracellular oxygen diffusion and efficiency of oxygen utilization; alternatively, it reduces hypoxia-induced oxidative damage by its antioxidant activities (Ip *et al* 2001) There is the need to design and carry out clinical trials in order to investigate RAS blocker therapy in patients with pancreatitis.

6.   CONCLUSIONS

Local RAS is present in pancreatic acinar cells and it is activated during the course of acute pancreatitis. This fact represents a new and important finding in recent research and development, not only regarding the knowledge of the pathophysiology of the acute pancreatic inflammation but also regarding the possible therapeutic applications. However, the differential actions of AT_1 and AT_2 receptors in mediating the acinar secretion of digestive enzymes have yet to be better defined. Application of selective angiotensin II receptor inhibitors, such as the AT_1 receptor antagonist, could be an effective approach in inhibiting the oversecretion of digestive enzymes and in attenuating pancreatic injury.

REFERENCES

Anagnostopoulos GK, Kostopoulos P, Tsiakos S, Margantinis G, Arvanitidis D., 2003, Fulminant pancreatitis associated with ramipril therapy. *Pancreas.* **27**: 278–279.

Balldin G, Eddeland A, Ohlsson K., 1981, Studies on the role of the plasma protease inhibitors on in vitro C3 activation and in acute pancreatitis. *Scand J Gastroenterol.* **16**: 603–609.

Barnhardt DC, Sarosi GA, Romanchuk G Jr, Mulholland MW., 1999, Calcium signaling induced by angiotensin II in the pancreatic acinar cell line AR42J. *Pancreas.* **18**: 189–196.

Berry C, Hamilton CA, Brosnan J, Magill FG, Berg GA, McMurray JJV, Dominiczak AF., 2000, Investigation into the sources of superoxide in human blood vessels: angiotensin II increases superoxide production in human internal mammary arteries. *Circulation.* **101**: 2206–2212.

Bockman DE., 1997, Morphology of the exocrine pancreas related to pancreatitis. *Microsc Res Tech.* **37**: 509–519.

Bottari SP, King IN, Reichlin S, Dahlstrom I, Lydon N, De Gasparo M., 1992, The AT2 receptor stimulates protein tyrosine phosphatase activity and mediates inhibition of particulate guanylate cyclase. *Biochem Biophys Res Commun.* **183**: 206–211.

Bradley EL 3rd., 1993, A clinically based classification system for acute pancreatitis. Summary of the International Symposium on Acute Pancreatitis, Atlanta, Ga, September 11 through 13, 1992. *Arch Surg.* **128**: 586–590.

Chan WP, Fung ML, Nobiling R, Leung PS, 2000, Activation of local renin-angiotensin system by chronic hypoxia in rat pancreas. *Mol Cell Endocrinol.* **160**: 107–114.

Chappell MC, Milsted A, Diz DI, Brosnihan KB, Ferrario CM., 1991, Evidence for an intrinsic angiotensin system in the canine pancreas. *J Hypertens.* **9**: 751–759.

Chappell MC, Diz DI, Jacobsen DW., 1992a, Pharmacological characterization of angiotensin II binding sites in the canine pancreas. *Peptides.* **13**: 311–318.

Chappell MC, Jacobsen DW, Tallant EA., 1992b, Glucocorticoid regulation of angiotensin II receptors in pancreatic acinar AR42J cells. *Growth Factors, Peptides, Receptors.* **7**: 66.

Chappell MC, Bosch SM, Hansen BC, Ferrario CM, Diz DI., 1994a, Differential expression of AT2 angiotensin II receptors in the primate and rat pancreas. *J Hypertens.* **12**: S181.

Chappell MC, Bosch SM, Hansen BC, Ferrario CM, Diz DI., 1994b, Angiotensin II receptor subtype expression in the primate pancreas. *Am J Hypertens.* **7**: 94A.

Chappell MC, Jacobsen DW, Tallant EA., 1995, Characterization of angiotensin II receptor subtypes in pancreatic acinar AR42J cells. *Peptides.* **16**: 741–747.

Chappell MC, Iyer SN, Diz DI, Ferrario CM., 1998, Antihypertensive effects of angiotensin-(1-7). *Braz J Med Biol Res*. **31**: 1205–1212.

Chappell MC, Tallant EA, Diz DI, Ferrario CM., 2000, The renin-angiotensin system and cardiovascular homeostasis. In *Drugs, Enzymes and Receptors of the Renin-Angiotensin System: Celebrating a Century of Discovery*. (A. Husain, and R.M. Graham, eds.), Harwood Academic Publishers, Amsterdam, pp 3–22.

Chappell MC, Diz DI, Gallagher PE, 2001, The renin-angiotensin system and the exocrine pancreas. *JOP*. **2**: 33–39.

Cheng RM, Mamdani M, Jackevicius CA, Tu K., 2003, Association between ACE inhibitors and acute pancreatitis in the elderly. *Ann Pharmacother*. **37**: 994–998.

Chiari H., 1896, Uber die Selbstverdauung des menschlichen Pankreas. *Z Heilk*. **17**: 69–96.

De Gasparo M, Catt KJ, Inagami T, Wright JW, Unger TH., 2000, The angiotensin II receptors. *Pharmacol Rev*. **52**: 415–472.

Dinarello CA., 1996a, Biologic basis for interleukin-1 in disease. *Blood*. **87**: 2095–2147.

Dinarello CA., 1996b, Cytokines as mediators in the pathogenesis of septic shock. *Curr Top Microbiol Immunol*. **216**: 133–165.

Ethridge RT, Hashimoto K, Chung DH, Ehlers RA, Rajaraman S, Evers BM., 2002, Selective inhibition of NF-kappaB attenuates the severity of cerulein- induced acute pancreatitis. *J Am Coll Surg*. **195**: 497–505.

Fallon MB, Gorelick FS, Anderson JM, Mennone A, Saluja A, Steer ML., 1995, Effect of cerulein hyperstimulation on the paracellular barrier of rat exocrine pancreas. *Gastroenterology*. **108**: 1863–1872.

Fernandez-Alfonso MS, Gonzalez C., 1999, Nitric oxide and the renin-angiotensin system: is there a physiological interplay between the system? *J Hypertens*. **17**: 1355–1361.

Fishel RS, Eisenberg S, Shai SY, Redden RA, Bernstein KE, Berk BC., 1995, Glucocorticoids induce angiotensin-converting enzyme expression in vascular smooth muscle. *Hypertension*. **25**: 343–349.

Fishman MP, Melton DA., 2002, Pancreatic lineage analysis using a retroviral vector in embryonic mice demonstrates a common progenitor for endocrine and exocrine cells. *Int J Dev Biol*. **46**: 201–207.

Foitzik T, Hotz HG, Eibl G, Buhr HJ., 2000, Experimental models of acute pancreatitis: are they suitable for evaluating therapy? *Int J Colorectal Dis*. **15**: 127–135.

Ghiani BU, Masini MA., 1995, Angiotensin II binding sites in the rat pancreas and their modulation after sodium loading and depletion. *Comp Biochem Physiol A Physiol*. **111**: 439–444.

Granger D, Grisham M, Kvietys P., 1994, Mechanisms of microvascular injury. In: *Physiology of the Gastrointestinal Tract* (L.R. John, ed.), Raven Press, New York, pp 1693–722.

Greenstein RJ, Krakoff LR, Felton K., 1987, Activation of the renin system in acute pancreatitis. *Am J Med*. **82**: 401–404.

Griesbacher T., 2000, Kallikrein-kinin system in acute pancreatitis: potential of B(2)-bradykinin antagonists and kallikrein inhibitors. *Pharmacology*. **60**: 113–120.

Gullo L, Pezzilli R, Priori P, Baldoni F, Paparo F, Mattioli G., 1987, Pure pancreatic juice collection over 24 consecutive hours. *Pancreas*. **2**: 620–623.

Guo DF, Uno S, Ishihata A, Nakamura N, Inagami T., 1995, Identification of a cis-acting glucocorticoid responsive element in the rat angiotensin II type 1A promoter. *Circ Res*. **77**: 249–257.

Han B, Logsdon CD., 2000, CCK stimulates mob-1 expression and NF-kappaB activation via protein kinase C and intracellular Ca(2).*Am J Physiol Cell Physiol*. **278**: C344–C351.

Harding JW, Wright JW, Swanson GN, Hanesworth JM, Krebs LT., 1994, AT4 receptors: specificity and distribution. *Kidney Int*. **46**: 1510–1512.

Hofbauer B, Saluja AK, Lerch MM, Bhagat L, Bhatia M, Lee HS, Frossard JL, Adler G, Steer ML., 1998, Intra-acinar cell activation of trypsinogen during caerulein-induced pancreatitis in rats. *Am J Physiol*. **275**: G352–G362.

Ip SP, Che CT, Leung PS., 2001, Association of free radicals and the tissue renin-angiotensin system: prospective effects of Rhodiola, a genus of Chinese herb, on hypoxia-induced pancreatic injury. *JOP*. **2**: 16–25.

Ip SP, Tsang SW, Wong TP, Che CT, Leung PS., 2003, Saralasin, a nonspecific angiotensin II receptor antagonist, attenuates oxidative stress and tissue injury in cerulein-induced acute pancreatitis. *Pancreas.* **26**: 224–229.

Iyer SN, Ferrario CM, Chappell MC., 1998, Angiotensin-(1-7) contributes to the antihypertensive effects of blockade of the renin-angiotensin system. *Hypertension.* **31**: 356–361.

Iyer SN, Yamada K, Diz DI, Ferrario CM, Chappell MC., 2000, Evidence that prostaglandins mediate the antihypertensive actions of angiotensin-(1-7) during chronic blockade of the renin-angiotensin system. *J Cardiovasc Pharmacol.* **36**: 109–117.

Janiak P, Pillon A, Prost JF, Vilaine JP., 1992, Role of angiotensin subtype 2 receptor in neointima formation after vascular injury. *Hypertension.* **20**: 737–745.

Jungermann J, Lerch MM, Weidenbach H, Lutz MP, Kruger B, Adler G., 1995, Disassembly of rat pancreatic acinar cell cytoskeleton during supramaximal secretagogue stimulation. *Am J Physiol.* **268**: G328–G338.

Kanbay M, Korkmaz M, Yilmaz U, Gur G, Boyacioglu S., 2004, Acute pancreatitis due to ramipril therapy. *Postgrad Med J.* **80**: 617–618.

Kimura K, Shimosegawa T, Sasano H, Abe R, Satoh A, Masamune A, Koizumi M, Nagura H, Toyota T., 1998, Endogenous glucocorticoids decrease the acinar cell sensitivity to apoptosis during cerulein pancreatitis in rats. *Gastroenterology.* **114**: 372–381.

Knoefel WT, Kollias N, Warshaw AL, Waldner H, Nishioka NS, Rattner DW., 1994, Pancreatic microcirculatory changes in experimental pancreatitis of graded severity in rat. *Surgery.* **116**: 904–913.

Kruger B, Albrecht E, Lerch MM., 2000, The role of intracellular calcium signaling in premature protease activation and the onset of pancreatitis. *Am J Pathol.* **157**: 43–50.

Kuno A, Yamada T, Masuda K, Ogawa K, Sogawa M, Nakamura S, Nakazawa T, Ohara H, Nomura T, Joh T, Shirai T, Itoh M., 2003, Angiotensin-converting enzyme inhibitor attenuates pancreatic inflammation and fibrosis in male Wistar Bonn/Kobori rats. *Gastroenterology.* **124**: 1010–1019.

Laitio M, Lev R, Orlic D., 1974, The developing human fetal pancreas: an ultrastructural and histochemical study with special reference to exocrine cells. *J Anat.* **117**: 619–634.

Lasson A, Ohlsson K., 1986, Consumptive coagulopathy, fibrinolysis and protease-antiprotease interactions during acute human pancreatitis. *Thromb Res.* **41**: 167–183.

Leung PS, Chan HC, Fu LXM, Wong PYD., 1997, Localization of angiotensin II receptor subtypes AT1 and AT2 in the pancreas of rodents. *J Endocrinol.* **153**: 269–274.

Leung PS, Chan WP, Wong TP, Sernia C., 1999, Expression and localization of the renin-angiotensin system in the rat pancreas. *J Endocrinol.* **160**: 13–19.

Leung PS, Chan WP, Nobiling R., 2000, Regulated expression of pancreatic renin-angiotensin system in experimental pancreatitis. *Mol Cell Endocrinol.* **166**: 121–128.

Leung PS, Carlsson PO., 2001, Tissue renin-angiotensin system: its expression, localization, regulation and potential role in the pancreas. *J Mol Endocrinol.* **26**: 155–164.

Lowry SF., 1993, Cytokine mediators of immunity and inflammation. Arch Surg. **128**: 1235–1241.

Mercurio F, Manning AM., 1999, NF-kappaB as a primary regulator of the stress response. *Oncogene.* **18**: 6163–6171.

Norman J., 1998, The role of cytokines in the pathogenesis of acute pancreatitis. *Am J Surg.* **175**: 76–83.

Otani T, Chepilko SM, Grendell JH, Gorelick FS., 1998, Codistribution of TAP and the granule membrane protein GRAMP-92 in rat caerulein-induced pancreatitis. *Am J Physiol.* **275**: G999–G1009.

Parekh AB., 2000, Calcium signaling and acute pancreatitis: specific response to a promiscuous messenger. *Proc Natl Acad Sci USA.* **97**: 12933–12934.

Patel AG, Toyama MT, Nguyen TN, Cohen GA, Ignarro LJ, Reber HA, Ashley SW., 1995, Role of nitric oxide in the relationship of pancreatic blood flow and exocrine secretion in cats. Gastroenterology. **108**: 1215–1220.

Pezzilli R, Billi P, Miniero R, Barakat B., 1997, Serum interleukin-10 in human acute pancreatitis. *Dig Dis Sci.* **42**: 1469–1472.

Pezzilli R, Billi P, Morselli-Labate AM., 1998, Severity of acute pancreatitis: relationship with etiology, sex and age. *Hepatogastroenterology.* **45**: 1859–1864.

Pezzilli R, Ceciliari R, Corinaldesi R., 2004, The pathogenesis of acute pancreatitis: from the basic research to the bedside. *Osp Ital Chir.* **10**: 314–323.

Pezzilli R, Barakat B, Fantini L, Timpano A, Morselli Labate AM, Corinaldesi R., 2006, The plasma renin-angiotensin system in human acute pancreatitis. *Dig Liv Dis.* **38**: S88.

Raraty M, Ward J, Erdemli G, Vaillant C, Neoptolemos JP, Sutton R, Petersen OH., 2000, Calcium-dependent enzyme activation and vacuole formation in the apical granular region of pancreatic acinar cells. *Proc Natl Acad Sci USA.* **97**: 13126–13131.

Servant G, Dudley DT, Escher E, Guillemette G., 1994, The marked disparity between the sizes of angiotensin type 2 receptors from different tissues is related to different degrees of N-glycosylation. *Mol Pharmacol.* **45**: 1112–1118.

Steinle AU, Weidenbach H, Wagner M, Adler G, Schmid RM., 1999, NF-kappaB/Rel activation in cerulein pancreatitis. *Gastroenterology.* **116**: 420–430.

Tahiri-Jouti N, Cambillau C, Viguerie N, Vidal C, Buscail L, Laurent NS, Vaysse N, Susini C., 1992, Characterization of a membrane tyrosine phosphatase in AR42J cells: regulation by somatostatin. *Am J Physiol.* **262**: G1007–G1014.

Tahmasebi M, Puddefoot JR, Inwang ER, Vinson GP., 1999, The tissue renin-angiotensin system in human pancreas. *J Endocrinol.* **161**: 317–322.

Takahasi K, Bardhan S, Kambayashi Y, Shirai H, Inagami T., 1994, Protein tyrosine phosphatase inhibition by angiotensin II in rat pheochromocytoma cells through type 2 receptor, AT2. *Biochem Biophys Res Commun.* **198**: 60–66.

Tando Y, Algul H, Wagner M, Weidenbach H, Adler G, Schmid RM., 1999, Caerulein-induced NF-kappaB/Rel activation requires both Ca2 and protein kinase C as messengers. *Am J Physiol.* **277**: G678–G686.

Thanos D, Maniatis T., 1995, NF-kappa B: A lesson in family values. *Cell.* **80**: 529–532.

Tsang SW, Ip SP, Wong TP, Che CT, Leung PS., 2003, Differential effects of saralasin and ramiprilat, the inhibitors of renin-angiotensin system, on cerulein-induced acute pancreatitis. *Regul Pept.* **111**: 47–53.

Tsang SW, Ip SP, Leung PS., 2004, Prophylactic and therapeutic treatments with AT 1 and AT 2 receptor antagonists and their effects on changes in the severity of pancreatitis. *Int J Biochem Cell Biol.* **36**: 330–339.

Uehara S, Honjyo K, Furukawa S, Hirayama A, Sakamoto W., 1989, Role of the kallikrein-kinin system in human pancreatitis. *Adv Exp Med Biol.* **247B**: 643–648.

Whitcomb DC., 1999, Early trypsinogen activation in acute pancreatitis. *Gastroenterology.* **116**: 770–772.

CHAPTER 4

THE RENIN-ANGIOTENSIN SYSTEM IN PANCREATIC STELLATE CELLS: IMPLICATIONS IN THE DEVELOPMENT AND PROGRESSION OF TYPE 2 DIABETES MELLITUS

SEUNG-HYUN KO, YU-BAI AHN, KI-HO SONG, AND KUN-HO YOON

Division of Endocrinology & Metabolism, Department of Internal Medicine, The Catholic University of Korea, Seoul, Korea

1. INTRODUCTION

The number of people with type 2 diabetes mellitus (T2DM) has increased explosively throughout the world (Yoon *et al* 2006). The World Health Organization estimates that more than 180 million people worldwide have diabetes. This number is likely to more than double by 2030 (WHO. http://www.who.int/mediacentre/factsheets). Because the economic burden of diabetes and its related complications is enormous, early diagnosis and prompt prevention of diabetes are important and a promising health issue. Only strict glycaemic control can prevent or delay diabetic complications. However, in practice, less than 40% of people with T2DM have a glycaeted haemoglobin level within the target range. At present, regular physical exercise and suitable diet therapy are considered the "gold standard" in preventing T2DM in high-risk patients (Lindstrom *et al* 2006).

Recent clinical trials have shown that lifestyle modification cannot prevent diabetes mellitus completely in high-risk patients with impaired glucose tolerance (Lindstrom *et al* 2006). When these patients are clinically diagnosed with diabetes mellitus, their beta cell function is remarkably low (Fukushima *et al* 2004), indicating that beta cell function is already impaired in the glucose-intolerant state and that early intervention may be too late to prevent the development of diabetes mellitus. These results prompted our interest in the use of drugs such as metformin, acarbose, troglitazone, and orlistat (Liberopoulos *et al* 2006) in individuals at high risk of diabetes mellitus.

Po Sing Leung (ed.), Frontiers in Research of the Renin-Angiotensin System on Human Disease, 73–86.
© 2007 *Springer.*

In the recent Heart Outcomes Prevention Evaluation (HOPE) study, the angiotensin converting enzyme inhibitor (ACEI) ramipril reduced the rates of death, myocardial infarction, stroke, and heart failure, the risk of complications related to diabetes, and the number of new cases of diabetes (Yusuf *et al* 2000; Yusuf *et al* 2001). Similar results have been reported by the recent Captopril Prevention Project (CAPPP) study, the Losartan Intervention for Endpoint reduction in hypertension study (LIFE) study (Hansson *et al* 1999; Lindholm *et al* 2002), the VALUE study (Kjeldsen *et al* 2006), and the CHARM study (Yusuf *et al* 2005). These large-scale clinical studies suggest that ACEIs and angiotension receptor blockers (ARBs) can reduce the rate of diabetes onset, regardless of the mechanisms involved. In addition, some studies have described the presence of angiotensin II (Ang II) receptors on the surface of pancreatic islet beta cells, and the effects of the local renin–angiotensin system (RAS) on isolated beta cells or islets (Leung *et al* 1999; Leung *et al* 2001; Leung *et al* 2003). In the human pancreas, the angiotensin I receptor has been identified in islets (Leung *et al* 2005), especially on beta cells and endothelial cells, although this requires additional clarification. Thus, ACEIs may directly influence pancreatic islets in animal models or in patients with T2DM.

In terms of the morphological changes of islets in T2DM, several common findings have been noted, including islet hyalinization or islet amyloid polypeptide deposition in islets (Ken *et al* 1979; Gept and Lecompte, 1981; Kloppel *et al* 1985), islet fibrosis, decreased beta cell mass (Stefan *et al* 1982; Clark *et al* 1988; Sakuraba *et al* 2002; Yoon *et al* 2003), and increased proportion (relative volume) of alpha cells (Yoon *et al* 2003). Recent data from our laboratory and others indicate that pancreatic stellate cells (PSCs) are involved in pancreatic islets fibrosis in an animal model of T2DM, RAS activation, and even in the islets of patients with T2DM (unpublished data). Understanding the role of PSCs and local RAS in islet fibrosis and the development of T2DM would be helpful in developing alternative strategies to prevent or treat T2DM.

2.   PSCS AND ISLET FIBROSIS

2.1.   PSCs

PSCs were first described in the pancreas in 1982 (Watari *et al* 1982). Since their isolation in 1998, PSCs have been identified as the major source of the extracellular matrix proteins found in chronic pancreatitis or pancreatic fibrosis in both experimental animals and humans (Apte *et al* 1999). Stellate-shaped cells comprise about 4% of all pancreatic cells and have a periacinar distribution (Apte *et al* 1998). In the quiescent state, PSCs contain numerous vitamin A-storing lipid droplets in their cytoplasm and stain for desmin and glial fibrillary acidic protein (Fig. 1) (Apte *et al* 1998; Bachem *et al* 1998). PSCs are activated by various cytokines and growth factors, such as platelet-derived growth factor (PDGF), transforming growth factor β (TGF-β), activin A, TGF-α, basic fibroblast growth factor, tumour necrosis factor α (TNF-α), interleukin 1 (IL-1), and IL-6 (Powell *et al* 1999; Jaster

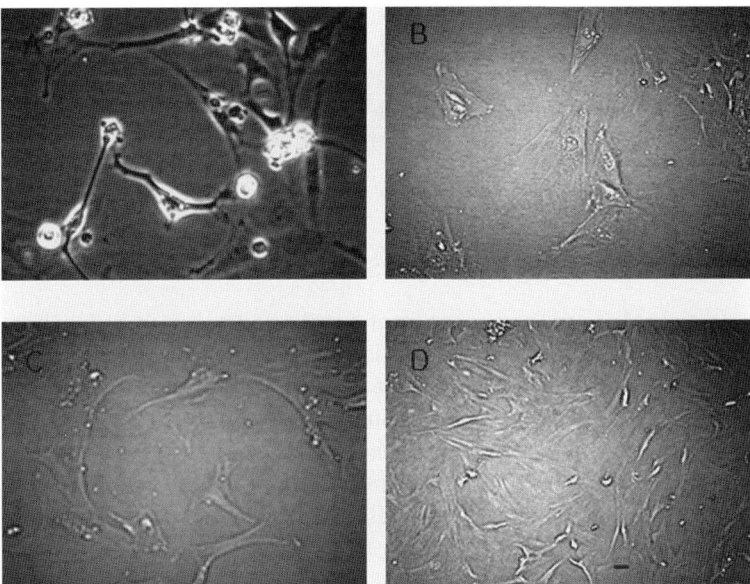

Figure 1. Phase-contrast microscopy of cultured PSCs isolated from rat pancreas. (A) PSCs showing perinuclear fat droplets three days after seeding. (B) PSCs showing fewer fat droplets and long cytoplasmic extensions after seven days in primary culture

et al 2002; Jaster *et al* 2004). Of these, PDGF and TGF-β exert potent proliferative effects on PSCs (Kruse *et al* 2000; Jaster *et al* 2002). PSCs can also synthesize and secret cytokines, such as TNF-α, IL-1, PDGF, and TGF-β, suggesting that PSCs have an autocrine action once activated by pancreatic inflammation (Powell *et al* 1999). PSCs transform into myofibroblast cells and stain positively for alpha-smooth muscle actin (α-SMA) (Fig. 2) (Apte *et al* 1999). PSCs characteristically display prominent cytoplasmic actin filaments, and they are connected to each other

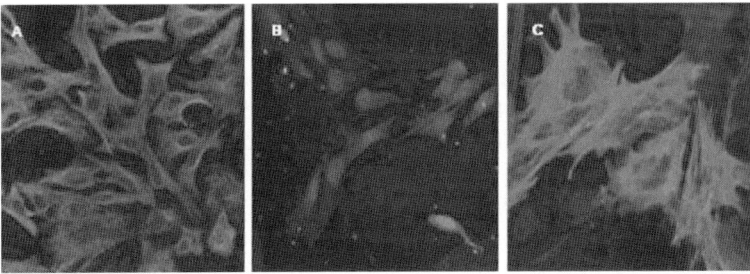

Figure 2. Immunofluorescence staining for vimentin (green colour, A), desmin (green colour, B), α-SMA (green colour, C) in cultured PSCs isolated from rat pancreas (original magnification 400×). Blue, nuclei of PSCs stained with DAPI

by gap junctions. Activated PSCs show markedly increased synthesis of extracel-lular matrix protein, such as collagen type I and type III, fibronectin, and laminin, in response to various stimuli (Haber *et al* 1999; Yokota *et al* 2002). Many recent reports provide evidence that activated PSCs are involved in pancreatic fibrogenesis, including chronic pancreatitis and pancreatic fibrosis (Haber *et al* 1999; Yokota *et al* 2002).

2.2.   Pancreatic Fibrosis and Pancreatic Stellate Cells (PSCs)

PSCs play a crucial role in the pathogenesis of pancreatic fibrosis in both experi-mental animals and humans. Pancreatic fibrosis is caused by alcohol abuse (Suda *et al* 1994), pancreatic duct obstruction (Suda *et al* 1990), biliary disease (Suda and Miyano 1985), and acute pancreatitis (Suda and Tsukahara 1992). Chronic alcohol abuse is the most common cause of pancreatic fibrosis and chronic pancre-atitis (Singh and Sinsek 1990). Fibrosis is accompanied by the appearance of cells with anti-α-SMA immunoreactivity (Suda 2000). An increased number of α-SMA-positive cells have been observed in cerulein-induced acute pancreatitis (Yokota *et al* 2002), TNBS-induced chronic pancreatitis (Haber *et al* 1999), and pancreatic sections from human alcoholic pancreatitis. In such conditions, the α-SMA-positive cells surround the pancreatic acini, and extracellular matrix protein is then deposited. These studies suggest that PSCs are activated in these experimental and human pancreatic fibrosis models and that the activated PSCs are the main cellular source of collagen in acute and chronic pancreatitis.

2.3.   Islet Fibrosis and PSCs

In our previous report, the ACEI ramipril significantly attenuated islet fibrosis in Otsuka Long Evans Tokushima fatty (OLETF) rats, an animal model of T2DM (Ko *et al* 2004]. Interestingly, the proliferation of α-SMA-positive PSCs, fibrosis of the pancreatic islets, and extracellular matrix production in the pancreas increased significantly in OLETF rats, and this effect was attenuated by ramipril treatment (Fig. 3). We found prominent islet fibrosis with destroyed islet architecture, which was accompanied by α-SMA-positive cells in advanced a T2DM animal model without evidence of pancreatitis. This differed somewhat from the results of previous studies, which described the role of PSCs in pancreatic exocrine fibrosis.

   In general, the pathological manifestation of pancreatic islets in patients with T2DM includes reduced beta cell mass, amyloid deposition, and eventually islet fibrosis similar to the islet fibrosis observed in OLETF rats (Yoon *et al* 2003; Cooper *et al* 2006). OLETF rats with diabetic progression display severe islet destruction as a result of fibrosis, which is accompanied by increased pancreatic expression of α-SMA, a specific marker of PSCs, especially surrounding the destroyed islets (Yoshikawa *et al* 2002; Ko *et al* 2004). These data suggest that PSCs have a role in both pancreatic exocrine fibrosis and islet fibrosis in models of T2DM, although

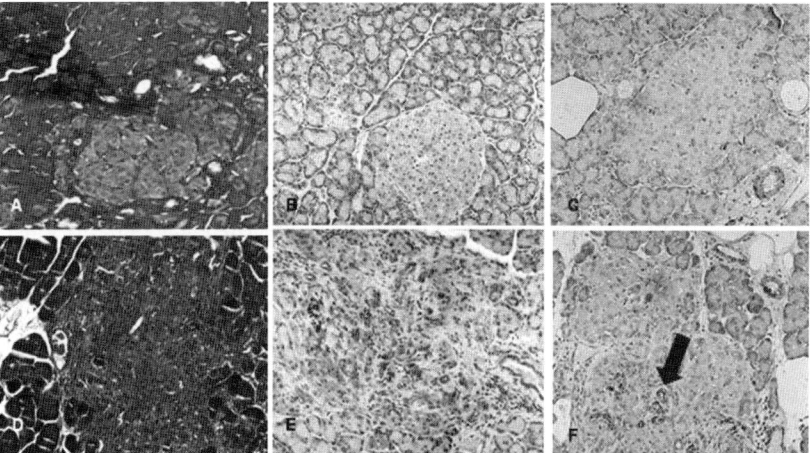

Figure 3. Immunohistochemical staining with trichrome (A, D), TGF-β (B, E) and α-SMA (C, F) in the pancreatic tissue of OLETF rats. In ramipril-treated OLETF rats (A–C), TGF-β expression (brown colour) was relatively confined to the islets and some exocrine tissues (B). However, in OLETF controls, more extensive TGF-β staining was detected in the whole pancreas (E) compared with the ramipril-treated animals (B), and was accompanied by destroyed islet structure and profound islet fibrosis (D). Expression of α-SMA showed a similar pattern. Compared with ramipril-treated OLETF rats (C), more intense brown-coloured α-SMA immunostaining (arrow) was observed in small ring-shaped vessels in the enlarged and disorganized pancreatic islets of the control OLETF rats (F). Reproduced with permission from BBRC

this needs to be clarified. There are no reports on whether PSCs are involved in the pathogenesis of T2DM in any model of pancreatic inflammation.

We have also reported that ACEIs attenuate islet destruction by fibrosis and have some beneficial effects on extracellular matrix protein expression; these effects are accompanied by the suppression of α-SMA expression in an animal model of T2DM. These findings imply that islet fibrosis and PSC proliferation are related to the renin–angiotensin system.

3. RAS AND PSCS

3.1. Expression of RAS in PSCs

Classically, the systemic RAS plays a crucial role in maintaining blood pressure and electrolyte balance through its action on vascular smooth muscle cells and aldosterone secretion. Ang II is a vasoactive agent that participates in haemodynamic regulation. The RAS system works both systemically and locally; the local RAS exists in the kidney, adrenal gland, pituitary gland, brain, adipose tissue, and pancreas (Vinson *et al* 1998; McKinley *et al* 2003; Crandall *et al* 1994). Ang II also plays an important role in tissue inflammation beyond its haemodynamic effects (Ruiz-Ortega *et al* 2000; Suzuki *et al* 2003), and this effect is mediated mainly through the local RAS. Ang II receptor subtypes are present in the rodent pancreas, predominantly in the epithelia of pancreatic ducts and vessels and in pancreatic acinar cells (Leung *et al* 1999; Leung and Carlsson 2001).

Locally produced Ang II promotes the recruitment of inflammatory cells, induces the expression and secretion of extracellular matrix proteins, and inhibits collagen degradation (Wolf and Neilson 1993; Ruiz-Ortega and Egido 1997; Suzuki *et al* 2003). Ang II modulates cell growth by inducing hyperplasia or hypertrophy, depending on the cell type (Ruiz-Ortega *et al* 2000) and participates in tissue repair and fibrogenesis of extra-cardiovascular organs during inflammation (Nagashio *et al* 2004). Ang II also promotes pulmonary fibrosis accompanying lung injury (Marshall *et al* 2004), and mediates hepatic fibrosis after chemically induced chronic liver injury (Yoshiji *et al* 2001). In addition, in renal fibrosis, Ang II activates mesangial cells, tubular cells, and interstitial fibroblasts; activation increases the expression and synthesis of extracellular matrix proteins mediated by the release of growth factors (Wolf and Neilson, 1990; Wolf *et al* 1993).

The RAS is believed to play a key role in tissue remodelling and fibrogenesis in the kidney, heart, and liver, suggesting that Ang II plays some part in pancreatic inflammation. Experimentally induced acute and chronic pancreatitis or chemically induced pancreatic injury increase Ang II receptors and angiotensinogen in the pancreas (Yoshiji *et al* 2001; Nagashio *et al* 2004), and ACEIs attenuate pancreatic fibrosis an in vivo model (Kuno *et al* 2003). More recent studies have shown that blocking the RAS attenuates pancreatic inflammation and fibrosis (Kuno *et al* 2003) and liver fibrosis (Yoshiji *et al* 2001). Blockade of RAS activity by ACEIs or ARB in animal models of chronic liver disease attenuates the progression of liver fibrosis. Therefore, the RAS is believed to play a role in tissue remodelling and fibrogenesis in the kidney, heart, and blood vessels (Campbell and Katwa 1997; Marshall *et al* 2004), liver (Yoshiji *et al* 2001), and pancreas.

We have previously observed increased expression of mRNA for components of the tissue RAS, such as angiotensin 1a (Ang 1a), angiotensin 1b (Ang 1b), angiotensinogen, and Ang II in PSC cultures, suggesting that the RAS is involved in PSC proliferation or activation (Reinehr *et al* 2004; Ko *et al* 2006). Most known actions of Ang II are mediated by angiotensin I, including vasoconstriction and the deposition of matrix proteins (Leehey *et al* 2000; Bataller *et al* 2003). In our study, Ang 1a receptor was upregulated significantly in response to high glucose concentration, whereas Ang 1b and Ang 2 mRNA expression was unchanged. Ang 1a protein expression was upregulated significantly by high glucose concentration, suggesting that the effect of Ang II on PSCs is also mediated by Ang 1a (Ko *et al* 2006). Combined with data obtained in our in vivo model, these data suggest that PSCs and the RAS are, at least partially, involved in the pathogenesis of T2DM.

3.2.   Effect of Glucose on the Expression of RAS in PSCs

We have shown that PSCs are activated by high glucose concentrations and that PSC proliferation following high-glucose stimulation is accompanied by

Ang II production. Moreover, extracellular matrix protein and TGF-β expression increased in the culture medium containing high glucose concentration after the increase in Ang II. In addition, high-glucose concentration-induced Ang II production was virtually abolished by preincubation of the PSCs with an ACEI. This decrease was greater in ramipril-treated PSCs than in candesartan-treated PSCs (Fig. 4).

The mechanism underlying the Ang II increase in response to glucose has not been clarified. In the proximal tubule cells of the kidney, a glucose response element has been identified in the angiotensinogen gene promoter, and high glucose stimulates angiotensinogen synthesis in a concentration-dependent manner (Zhang *et al* 1999; Hsieh *et al* 2002; Giacchetti *et al* 2005). In mesangial cells, high glucose concentration increases Ang II generation due to an increase in intracellular renin activity mediated by three or more factors: the time-dependent stimulation of (pro)renin gene transcription, reduction in prorenin enzyme secretion, and an increased rate of conversion of prorenin to active renin, probably mediated by cathepsin B (Vidott *et al* 2004). Further studies are required to clarify the exact

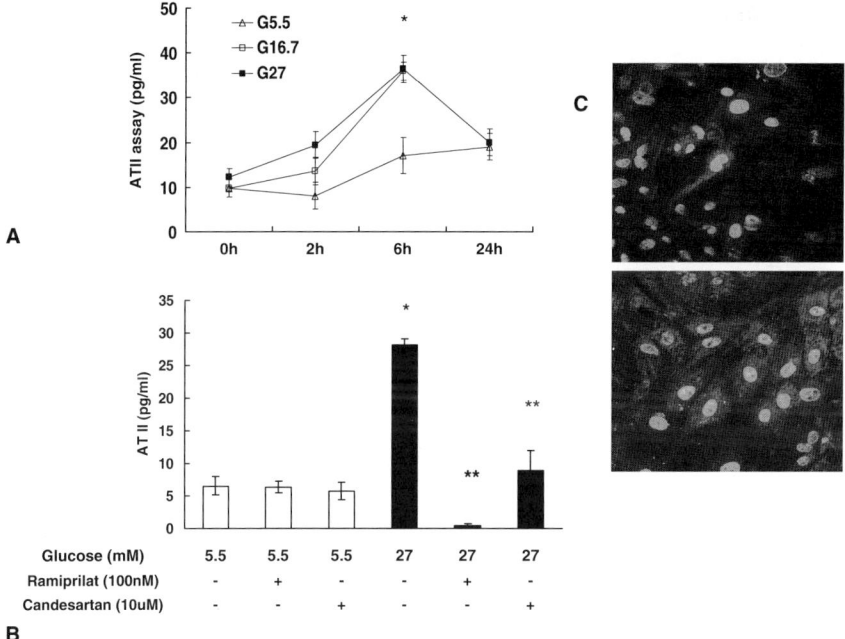

Figure 4. Effect of glucose on Ang II concentration in PSCs. (A) Ang II concentration increased significantly under high-glucose conditions. (B) PSCs treated with ramipril or candesartan showed significantly attenuated increases in Ang II concentration under high-glucose conditions. (C) The number of immunostained Ang II-positive cells increased significantly in the high glucose concentration. Reprinted with permission from J Cell Biochem

mechanism responsible for the effect of high glucose concentration on Ang II production in PSCs.

4.   TYPE 2 DIABETES AND ISLET FIBROTIC DESTRUCTION INDUCED BY PSC ACTIVATION

In contrast to acute or chronic pancreatitis, in which fibrosis involves mainly the whole exocrine pancreatic tissue, pancreatic fibrosis in people with T2DM is confined mainly to the endocrine pancreatic islet tissue, even though entire pancreatic tissue is exposed to hyperglycaemia. We propose that pancreatic fibrosis

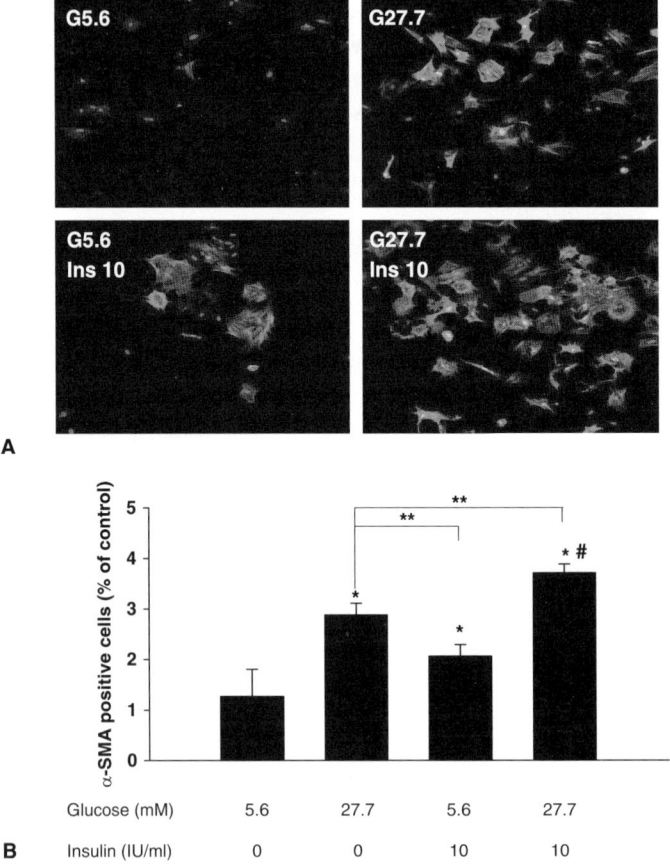

Figure 5. Effect of high glucose and insulin concentrations on the activation of quiescent PSCs assessed by immunostaining (A) and western blotting (B) with anti-α-SMA antibody. Combined stimulation by glucose (27.7 mM) and insulin (10 IU/ml) markedly increased the expression of α-SMA, a specific marker of PSCs. * p < 0.05 vs. 5.6 mM glucose; ** p < 0.05 vs. 27.7 mM glucose; # p < 0.05 5.6 mM glucose + 10 IU/ml insulin vs. 27.7 mM glucose + 10 IU/ml insulin (unpublished data)

is an important factor explaining the decreased pancreatic beta cell mass and progressive loss of beta cells in patients with T2DM. One possibility is that PSCs in the islets are exposed to both hyperglycaemia hyperinsulinaemia. Insulin or insulin-like growth factor 1 is a well-known mitogen for fibroblasts and smooth muscle cells, and PSCs in the islets might be predisposed to activate and proliferate by hyperglycaemia or hyperinsulinaemia or both.

Insulin is a potent cell growth factor and is secreted continuously at a relatively high concentration into the capillaries within the islets, although relative insulin deficiency in the whole body occurs in T2DM. We hypothesized that local hyperinsulinaemia in the islets might predispose toward PSC activation and proliferation in a hyperglycaemic environment. In a recent study, we found that hyperglycaemia alone may not be enough to activate the PSCs in the whole pancreas, and we suggested that other factors that induce activation of PSCs might exist in the islets of diabetic rats. We demonstrated that glucose is more potent and enhances PSC proliferation gradually in a dose- and time-dependent manner. Although not as effective as glucose, insulin also significantly influences PSC proliferation within the limited concentration range. PSCs treated concomitantly with glucose and insulin produced a peak concentration that was nearly six times the basal level, confirming the additive effect of glucose and insulin (Fig. 5).

The signalling pathways activating stellate cells are not fully understood, although several studies show that the ERK pathway (Hama *et al* 2004) and the p38 MAPK (mitogen-activated protein kinase) pathway (Masamune *et al* 2003) are involved. In our study, glucose and insulin induced ERK 1/2 phosphorylation in a dose-dependent manner. Moreover, connective tissue growth factor, an important downstream mediator of TGF-β activity (Paradis *et al* 2001), was significantly

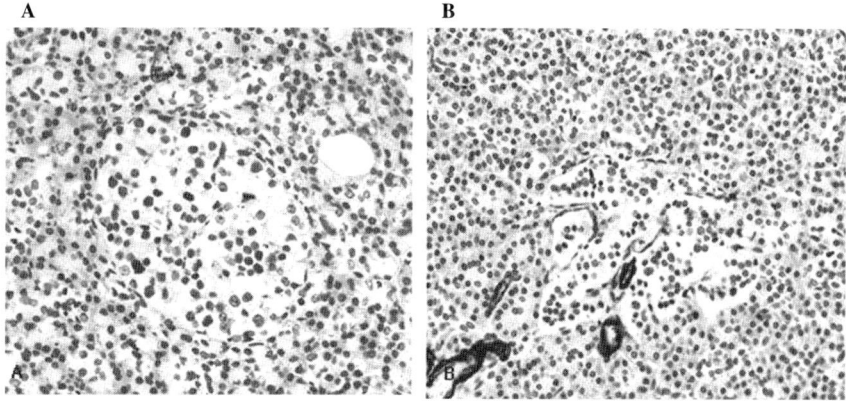

Figure 6. Immunostaining of α-SMA in a pancreatic section from a healthy human (A) and a patient with T2DM (B). Compared with the sample from the healthy person, the pancreatic islets of the diabetic patient show increased expression of α-SMA (brown colour) especially in the pancreatic islets

upregulated by high glucose and insulin concentrations and nearly completely suppressed by the MAPK inhibitor, U0126.

The clinical implication of the activated PSCs in the pathogenesis of T2DM has been investigated infrequently. We examined pancreatic sections from patients with T2DM and found prominent α-SMA immunostaining compared with staining in a sample from a healthy person (Fig. 6). The clinical significance of this finding should be further evaluated.

In summary, it appears that hyperglycaemia and hyperinsulinaemia are the two crucial mitogenic factors that induce the proliferation of PSCs; the presence of these two factors at the same time probably amplifies this effect. Therefore, rigorous control of the blood glucose concentration and improving the insulin resistance associated with diabetes may suppress fibrosis of the pancreas. Products that inhibit the fibrosis pathway, such as U0126, may be promising agents for treating diseases that induce pancreatic fibrosis, including diabetes.

5.   CONCLUSIONS

PSCs play an important role in the pathogenesis of pancreatic inflammation and fibrosis. We have found that PSCs are involved in the progression of islet fibrosis in an animal model of T2DM and, possibly, in people with T2DM. There is much evidence that the PSC activation and proliferation are associated with Ang II production in pancreatic fibrosis. High concentrations of glucose and insulin contribute to PSC proliferation, although the exact mechanisms remain to be confirmed. Both in vitro and in vivo studies indicate that ACEIs attenuate islet destruction caused by fibrosis and that these have some beneficial effects on glucose tolerance by suppressing of PSC activation and proliferation.

We suggest that PSCs are partially involved in the pathogenesis of islet-confined extracellular matrix protein deposition and fibrosis in T2DM, and we propose that ACEIs have a beneficial protective action against islet fibrosis and beta cell loss, and in preventing fibrogenesis in various tissues.

ACKNOWLEDGEMENTS

This work was supported by a grant from the Korea Health 21 Research and Development Project, ministry of Health and Welfare, Republic of Korea (Contract grant number: 0405-DB01-0104-0006) and the Research Institute of Medical Science of St. Vincent's Hospital, the Catholic University of Korea.

REFERENCES

Apte MV, Haber PS, Applegate TL, Norton ID, McCaughan GW, Korsten MA, Pirola RC, Wilson JS, 1998, Periacinar stellate shaped cells in rat pancreas: identification, isolation, and culture. *Gut.* **43**: 128–133.

Apte MV, Haber PS, Darby SJ, Rodgers SC, McCaughan GW, Korsten MA, Pirola RC, Wilson JS, 1999, Pancreatic stellate cells are activated by proinflammatory cytokines: implications for pancreatic fibrogenesis. *Gut*. **44**: 534–541.

Bachem MG, Schneider E, Gross H, Weidenbach H, Schmid RM, Menke A, Siech M, Beger H, Grunert A, Adler G, 1998, Identification, culture, and characterization of pancreatic stellate cells in rats and humans. *Gastroenterology*. **115**: 421–432.

Bataller R, Sancho-Bru P, Gines P, Lora JM, Al-Garawi A, Sole M, Colmenero J, Nicolas JM, Jimenez W, Weich N, Gutierrez-Ramos JC, Arroyo V, Rodes J. 2003. Activated human hepatic stellate cells express the renin-angiotensin system andsynthesize angiotensin II. Gastroenterology 125: 117–125.

Campbell SE, Katwa LC, 1997, Angiotensin II stimulated expression of transforming growth factor-b1 in cardiac fibroblasts and myofibroblasts. *J Mol Cell Cardiol*. **29**: 1947–1958.

Clark A, Wells CA, Buley ID, Cruickshank JK, Vanhegan RI, Matthews DR, Cooper GJ, Holman RR, Turner RC, 1988, Islet amyloid, increased A-cells, reduced B-cells and exocrine fibrosis:quantitative changes in the pancreas in type 2 diabetes. *Diabetes Res Clin Prac*. **4**: 151–159.

Cooper ME, Tikellis C, Thomas MC, 2006, Preventing diabetes in patients with hypertension: one more reason to block the renin-angiotensin system. *Journal of Hypertension*. **24**(1):S57–S63.

Crandall DL, Herzlinger HE, Saunders BD, Armellino DC, Kral JG, 1994, Distribution of angiotensin II receptors in rat and human adipocytes. *J Lipid Res*. **35**: 1378–1385.

Fukushima M, Suzuki H, Seino Y, 2004, Insulin secretion capacity in the development from normal glucose tolerance to type 2 diabetes. *Diabetes Research and Clinical Practice* **66**(Suppl1):S37–S43.

Gepts W, Lecompte PM, 1981, The pancreatic islets in diabetes. *Am J Med*. **70**:105–115.

Giacchetti G, Sechi LA, Rilli S, Carey RM, 2005, The renin-angiotensin-aldosterone system, glucose metabolism and diabetes. *Trends Endocrinol Metab*. **16**: 120–126.

Haber PS, Keogh GW, Apte MV, Moran CS, Stewart NL, Crawford DH, Pirola RC, McCaughan GW, Ramm GA, Wilson JS, 1999, Activation of pancreatic stellate cells in human and experimental pancreatic fibrosis. *Am J Pathol*. **155**: 1087–1095.

Hama K, Ohnishi H, Yasuda H, Ueda N, Mashima H, Satoh Y, Hanatsuka K, Kita H, Ohashi A, Tamada K, Sugano K, 2004, Angiotensin II stimulates DNA synthesis of rat pancreatic stellate cells by activating ERK through EGF receptor transactivation. *Biochem Biophys Res Commun*. **19**;315(4): 905–911.

Hansson L, Lindholm DH, Niskanen L, Lanke J, Hedner T, Niklason A, 1999, Effects of angiotensin-converting enzyme inhibition compared with conventional therapy on cardiovascular morbidity and mortality in hypertension: the Captopril Prevention Project (CAPP) randomized trial. *Lancet*. **353**: 611–616

Hsieh TJ, Zhang SL, Filep JG, Tang SS, Ingelfinger JR, Chan JS, 2002, High glucose stimulates angiotensinogen gene expression via reactive oxygenspecies generation in rat kidney proximal tubular cells. *Endocrinology*. **143**: 2975–2985.

Jaster R, 2004, Molecular regulation of pancreatic stellate cell function. *Mol Cancer*. **6**: 1–8.

Jaster R, Sparmann G, Emmrich J, Liebe S, 2002, Extracellular signal regulated kinases are key mediators of mitogenic signals in rat pancreatic stellate cells. *Gut*. **51**: 579–584.

Ken S, Nobuhisa Y, Tohru T, 1979, Differential volumetry of A, B and D cells in the pancreatic islets of diabetic and nondiabetic subjects. *Tohoku J Exp Med*. **129**:273–283.

Kjeldsen SE, Julius S, Mancia G, McInnes GT, Hua T, Weber MA, Coca A, Ekman S, Girerd X, Jamerson K, Larochelle P, MacDonald TM, Schmieder RE, Schork MA, Stolt P, Viskoper R, Widimsky J, Zanchetti A; VALUE Trial Investigators, 2006, Effects of valsartan compared to amlodipine on preventing type 2 diabetes in high-risk hypertensive patients: the VALUE trial. *J Hypertens*.**24**:1405–1412.

Kloppel G, Lohr M, Habich K, Oberholzer M, Heitz P, 1985, Islet pathology and pathogenesis of type 1 and type 2 diabetes mellitus revisited. *Surv Synth Path Res*. **4**:110–125.

Ko SH, Kwon HS, Kim SR, Moon SD, Ahn YB, Song KH, Son HS, Cha BY, Lee KW, Son HY, Kang SK, Park CG, Lee IK, Yoon KH, 2004, Ramipril treatment suppresses islet fibrosis in Otsuka Long-Evans Tokushima fatty rats. *Biochem Biophys Res Commun*. **26**: 114–122.

Ko SH, Hong OK, Kim JW, Ahn YB, Song KH, Cha BY, Son HY, Kim MJ, Jeong IK, Yoon KH, 2006, High glucose increases extracellular matrix production in pancreatic stellate cells by activating the renin-angiotensin system. *J Cell Biochem.* **15**:343–355.

Kruse ML, Hildebrand PB, Timke C, Folsch UR, Schmidt WE, 2000, TGF beta1 autocrine growth control in isolated pancreatic fibroblastoid cells/stellate cells in vitro. *Regul Pept.* **90**(1-3): 47–52.

Kuno A, Yamada T, Masuda K, Ogawa K, Sogawa M, Nakamura S, Nakazawa T, Ohara H, Nomura T, Joh T, Shirai T, Itoh M, 2003, Angiotensin-converting enzyme inhibitor attenuates pancreas inflammation and fibrosis in male wistar Bonn/Kobori rats. *Gastroenterology.* **124**: 1010–1019.

Leehey DJ, Singh AK, Alavi N, Singh R, 2000, Role of angiotensin II in diabetic nephropathy. *Kidney Int Suppl.* **77**: S93–98.

Leung PS, Chan WP, Wong TP, Sernia C, 1999, Expression and localization of the renin-angiotensin system in the rat pancreas. *J Endocrinol.* **160**: 13–19.

Leung PS, Carlsson PO, 2001, Tissue renin-angiotensin system: its expression, localization, regulation and potential role in the pancreas. *J Mol Endocrinol.* **26**: 155–164.

Leung PS, Chappell MC, 2003, A local pancreatic renin-angiotensin system: endocrine and exocrine roles. *Int J Biochem Cell Biol.* **35**: 838–846.

Leung PS, Carlsson PO, 2005, Pancreatic islet renin angiotensin system: its novel roles in islet function and in diabetes mellitus. *Pancreas.* **30**: 293–298.

Liberopoulos EN, Tsouli S, Mikhailidis DP, Elisaf MS, 2006, Preventing type 2 diabetes in high risk patients: an overview of lifestyle and pharmacological measures. *Curr Drug Targets.* **7**(2):211–228.

Lindholm LH, Ibsen H, Dahlof B, Devereux RB, Beevers G, de Faire U, Fyhrquist F, Julius S, Kjeldsen SE, Kristiansson K, Lederballe-Pedersen O, Nieminen MS, Omvik P, Oparil S, Wedel H, Aurup P, Edelman J, Snapinn S; LIFE Study Group, 2002, Cardiovascular morbidity and mortality in patients with diabetes in the Losartan Intervention For Endpoint reduction in hypertension study (LIFE): a randomised trial against atenolol. *Lancet.* 23: 1004–1010.

Lindstrom J, Ilanne-Parikka P, Peltonen M, Aunola S, Eriksson JG, Hemio K, Hamalainen H, Harkonen P, Keinanen-Kiukaanniemi S, Laakso M, Louheranta A, Mannelin M, Paturi M, Sundvall J, Valle TT, Uusitupa M, Tuomilehto J; Finnish Diabetes Prevention Study Groupm 2006, Sustained reduction in the incidence of type 2 diabetes by lifestyle intervention: follow-up of the Finnish Diabetes Prevention Study. *Lancet.* **368**(9548):1673–1679.

Marshall RP, Gohlke P, Chambers RC, Howell DC, Bottoms SE, Unger T, McAnulty RJ, Laurent GJ, 2004, Angiotensin II and the fibroproliferative response to acute lung injury. *Am J Physiol Lung Cell Mol Physiol.* **286**:L156-L164.

Masamune A, Satoh M, Kikuta K, Sakai Y, Satoh A, Shimosegawa T, 2003, Inhibition of p38 mitogen-activated protein kinase blocks activation of rat pancreatic stellate cells. *J Pharmacol Exp Ther.* **304**(1):8–14.

McKinley MJ, Albiston AL, Allen AM, Mathai ML, May CN, McAllen RM, Oldfield BJ, Mendelsohn FA, Chai SYI, 2003, The brain renin-angiotensin system: location and physiological roles. *Int J Biochem Cell Biol.* **35**: 901–918.

Nagashio Y, Asaumi H, Watanabe S, Nomiyama Y, Taguchi M, Tashiro M, Sugaya T, Otsuki M, 2004, Angiotensin II type 1 receptor interaction is an important regulator for the development of pancreatic fibrosis in mice. *Am J Physiol Gastrointest Liver Physiol.* **287**: G170-G177.

Paradis V, Perlemuter G, Bonvoust F, Dargere D, Parfait B, Vidaud M, Conti M, Huet S, Ba N, Buffet C, Bedossa P, 2001, High glucose and hyperinsulinemia stimulate connective tissue growth factor expression: a potential mechanism involved in progression to fibrosis in nonalcoholic steatohepatitis. *Hepatology.* **34**(4 Pt 1):738–744.

Powell DW, Mifflin RC, Valentich JD, Crowe SE, Saada JI, West AB, 1999, Myofibroblasts. I. Paracrine cells important in health and disease. *Am J Physiol.* **277**(1 Pt 1): C1-C9.

Reinehr R, Zoller S, Klonowski-Stumpe H, Kordes C, Haussinger D, 2004, Effects of angiotensin II on rat pancreatic stellate cells. *Pancreas.* **28**: 129–137.

Ruiz-Ortega M, Egido J, 1997, Angiotensin II modulates cell growth-related events and synthesis of matrix proteins in renal interstitial fibroblasts. *Kidney Int.* **52**: 1497–1510.

Ruiz-Ortega M, Lorenzo O, Ruperez M, Egido J, 2000, ACE inhibitors and AT(1) receptor antagonists-beyond the haemodynamic effect. *Nephrol Dial Transplant.* **15**: 561–565.

Sakuraba H, Mizukami H, Yagihashi N, Wada R, Hanyu C, Yagihashi S, 2002, Reduced beta-cell mass and expression of oxidative stress-related DNA damage in the islets of Japanese type II diabetic patients. *Diabetologia.* **45**:85–96.

Singh M, Sinsek H, 1990, Ethanol and the pancreas: current status. *Gastroenterology.* **98**: 1051–1062.

Stefan Y, Orci L, Malaisse-Lagae F, Perrelet A, Patel Y, Unger RH, 1982, Quantitation of endocrine cell content in the pancreas of nondiabetic and diabetic humans. *Diabetes.* **31**:694–700.

Suda K, Miyano T, 1985, Bile pancreatitis. *Arch Pathol Lab Med.* **109**: 433–436.

Suda K, Mogaki M, Oyama T, Matsumoto Y, 1990, Histopathologic and immunohistochemical studies on alcoholic pancreatitis and chronic obstructive pancreatitis: special emphasis on ductal obstruction and genesis of pancreatitis. *Am J Gastroenterol.* **85**: 271–276.

Suda K, Tsukahara M, 1992, Histopathological and immunohistochemical studies on apparently uninvolved areas of pancreas in patients with acute pancreatitis. *Arch Pathol Lab Med.* **116**: 934–937.

Suda K, SHiotsu H, Nakamura T, Akai J, Nakamura T, 1994, Pancreatic fibrosis in patients with chronic alcohol abuse: Correlation with alcoholic pancreatitis. *Am J Gastroenterol .* **89**: 2060–2062.

Suda K, 2000, Pathogenesis and progression of human pancreatic fibrosis. *Med Electron Microsc.* **33**: 200–206.

Suzuki Y, Ruiz-Ortega M, Lorenzo O, Ruperez M, Esteban V, Egido J, 2003, Inflammation and angiotensin II. *Int J Biochem Cell Biol.* **35**: 881–900.

Vidotti DB, Casarini DE, Cristovam PC, Leite CA, Schor N, Boim MA, 2004, High glucose concentration stimulates intracellular renin activity and angiotensin II generation in rat mesangial cells. *Am J Physiol Renal Physiol.* **286**: F1039–1045.

Vinson GP, Teja R, Ho MM, Hinson JP, Puddefoot JR, 1998, The role of the tissue renin-angiotensin system in the response of the rat adrenal to exogenous angiotensin II. *J Endocrinol.* **158**: 153–159.

Watari N, Hotta Y, Mabuchi Y, 1982, Morphological studies on a vitamin A-storing cell and its complex with macrophage observed in mouse pancreatic tissues following excess vitamin A administration. *Okajimas Folia Anat Jpn.* **58**: 837–858.

World Health Organization (http://www.who.int/mediacentre/factsheets. Last access 15 Dec 2006)

Wolf G, Neilson EG, 1990, Angiotensin II induces cellular hypertrophy in cultured murine proximal tubular cells. *Am J Physiol.* **259**(5 Pt 2): F768–777.

Wolf G, Neilson EG, 1993, Angiotensin II as a renal growth factor. *J Am Soc Nephrol.* **3**: 1531–1540.

Wolf G, Mueller E, Stahl RA, Ziyadeh FN, 1993, Angiotensin II-induced hypertrophy of cultured murine proximal tubular cells is mediated by endogenous transforming growth factor-beta. *J Clin Invest.* **92**: 1366–1372.

Yokota T, Denham W, Murayama K, Pelham C, Joehl R, Bell RH Jr, 2002, Pancreatic stellate cell activation and MMP production in experimental pancreatic fibrosis. *J Surg Res.* **104**: 106–111.

Yoon KH, Ko SH, Cho JH, Lee JM, Ahn YB, Song KH, Yoo SJ, Kang MI, Cha BY, Lee KW, Son HY, Kang SK, Kim HS, Lee IK, Bonner-Weir S, 2003, Selective beta-cell loss and alpha-cell expansion in patients with type 2 diabetes mellitus in Korea. *J Clin Endocrinol Metab.* **88**:2300–2308.

Yoon KH, Lee JH, Kim JW, Cho JH, Choi YH, Ko SH, Zimmet P, Son HY, 2006, Epidemic obesity and type 2 diabetes in Asia. *Lancet.* **11**:1681–1688.

Yoshiji H, Kuriyama S, Yoshii J, Ikenaka Y, Noguchi R, Nakatani T, Tsujinoue H, Fukui H, 2001, Angiotensin-II type 1 receptor interaction is a major regulator for liver fibrosis development in rats. *Hepatology.* **34**(4 Pt 1): 745–750.

Yoshikawa H, Kihara Y, Taguchi M, Yamaguchi T, Nakamura H, Otsuki M, 2002, Role of TGF-beta1 in the development of pancreatic fibrosis in Otsuka Long-Evans Tokushima Fatty rats. *Am J Physiol Gastrointest Liver Physiol.* **282**: G549–558.

Yusuf S, Sleight P, Pogue J, Bosch J, Davies R, Dagenais G, 2000, Effects of an angiotensin-converting enzyme inhibitor, ramipril, on cardiovascular events in high-risk patients. The Heart Outcomes Prevention Evaluation Study Investigators. *N Eng J Med.* **342**:145–153

Yusuf S, Gerstein H, Hoogwerf B, Pogue J, Bosch J, Wolffenbuttel BHR, Zinman B, 2001, Ramipril and the development of diabetes. *JAMA.* **286**:1882–1885

Yusuf S, Ostergren JB, Gerstein HC, Pfeffer MA, Swedberg K, Granger CB, Olofsson B, Probst-field J, McMurray JV, 2005, Candesartan in Heart Failure-Assessment of Reduction in Mortality and Morbidity Program Investigators, Effects of candesartan on the development of a new diagnosis of diabetes mellitus in patients with heart failure. *Circulation.* **5**: 48–53.

Zhang SL, Filep JG, Hohman TC, Tang SS, Ingelfinger JR, Chan JS, 1999, Molecular mechanisms of glucose action on angiotensinogen gene expression in rat proximal tubular cells. *Kidney Int.* **55**: 454–464.

CHAPTER 5

RENIN-ANGIOTENSIN SYSTEM PROTEASES AND THE CARDIOMETABOLIC SYNDROME: PATHOPHYSIOLOGICAL, CLINICAL AND THERAPEUTIC IMPLICATIONS

GUIDO LASTRA[1], CAMILA MANRIQUE[1], AND JAMES R. SOWERS[1]

[1] *Department of Internal Medicine, University of Missouri-Columbia, Columbia, MO65212, USA*

1.   INTRODUCTION

Obesity, Type 2 Diabetes Mellitus (T2DM) and Cardiovascular Disease (CVD) are worldwide leading causes of morbidity and mortality. Once considered as separate metabolic and hemodynamic/cardiovascular entities respectively, it has become nowadays clear that the relationship between these conditions is not coincidental, and has common pathophysiological features that allows considering both obesity and T2DM as part of the cardiovascular diseases spectrum. Furthermore, from a clinical standpoint it is also clear that cardiovascular risk factors seldom are isolated findings, but frequently present as a clustering of different conditions, including abnormalities in blood pressure, body weight, glucose homeostasis and albuminuria.

The tendency of CVD risk factors to cluster has been described in the medical literature since the decade of 1920s (Avogaro *et al* 1967). However, the concept of Cardiometabolic Syndrome (CMS) is still evolving, and makes reference to a group of cardiovascular /metabolic risk factors, including hypertension (HTN), dysglycemia, atherogenic dyslipidemia, albuminuria and obesity, which confer an excess high risk for CVD than its individual components.

Several names have been given to the condition, including Syndrome X, Dysmetabolic Syndrome, Insulin Resistance Syndrome, Metabolic Syndrome and more recently Cardiometabolic Syndrome. In addition, numerous worldwide organizations have described the CMS and have used different definition criteria, which take into account the current epidemiologic, clinic and pathophysiological evidence available about the condition. These include the National Cholesterol Education

Po Sing Leung (ed.), Frontiers in Research of the Renin-Angiotensin System on Human Disease, 87–111.

Program (NCEP) Adult Treatment Panel III (ATP III), the World Health Organization, the European Group for Study of Insulin Resistance (EGIR), the American Association of Clinical Endocrinologists (AACE) and the International Diabetes Federation (IDF) (Table 1). Nevertheless, despite existing debate about the different criteria required for the diagnosis of CMS and their clinical relevance, all systems do acknowledge the importance of obesity.

Obesity, largely resultant from decreased physical activity, high caloric diets rich in saturated fats and carbohydrates, appears to account for most of the steady increase in the incidence and prevalence of the CMS in the world (Manrique, et al 2005). For instance, in the U.S. general population, the prevalence of the CMS reached 22.8% in adult men and 22.6% in adult women from 1988 to 1994, according to analysis based on the Third National Health and Nutrition Survey (NHANES III) and the National Cholesterol Education Program (NCEP) (Park et al 2003). The NHANES III is considered one of the most recent surveys of a representative U.S. population. More recent analysis from the NHANES III, from 1999 to 2000, documented an increased global prevalence of 34.5% of adults. The prevalence of the CMS increases with age, and has been estimated to be approximately 43.5% in US adults over 50 years old. On the other hand, the occurrence of T2DM without CMS is uncommon, as only 13% of type 2 diabetics did not had features of CMS in a sub-analysis based on the NHANES III (Alexander et al 2003).

Furthermore, when the newer International Diabetes Federation (IDF) criteria, in which the presence of obesity is required, were used in adult US population, the estimated prevalence of the CMS further augmented to 39% (Ford, 2005). Finally, ethnicity plays also a key role in the CMS features, as is exemplified by the higher prevalence of CMS in Mexican-Americans (Ford, 2005). The ethnicity role was taken into account in the newer IDF definition criteria, as different anthropometric measurements cutoffs are used in different populations (Lorenzo et al 2006).

Data from the NHANES survey also provide concerning insights into the epidemiology of CMS in young populations. Prevalence of the condition appears to have increased from 4.2% during the period 1988–1992, to 6.4% between 1999 and 2000, reaching more than 30% of overweighed adolescents, roughly more than 2 million people (Duncan et al 2004).

As previously discussed, the dramatic increase in the incidence and prevalence of CMS appears to be largely accounted for by obesity, considered to be the epidemic of the new millennium. Indeed, both industrialized and non-industrialized countries have experienced an alarming increase in both overweight and obesity. American epidemiologic data report an increase of 110% in the prevalence of obesity during the past three decades (Stein and Colditz, 2004), while excess body weight affects roughly 65% of the general adult population (Flegal, et al 2002). These trends are not exclusive to the United States, but are closely followed by the rest of the World, according to data from the World Health Organization (WHO) (James, et al 2001).

Genetic factors certainly influence excess adiposity, but environmental factors, related to diet and exercise carry most of the responsibility in the development of

Table 1. Diagnosis of the cardiometabolic syndrome

World Health Organization 1998	European Group Insulin Resistance 1999	Adult Treatment Panel III – National Cholesterol Education Program 2001
FASTING GLYCEMIA ≥110 mg/dL or Impaired Glucose Tolerance (>140 mg/dL or insulin resistance) **AND** 2 OR MORE OF THE FOLLOWING: • HYPERLIPIDEMIA: TRIGLICERYDES ≥150 and/or HDL <35M, <40W • Blood pressure:>140/90 • MICROALBUMINURI > 20 µg/min	INSULIN RESISTANCE - HIPERINSU-LINEMIA >25% **AND** 2 OR MORE OF THE FOLLOWING: • CENTRAL OBESITY: Waist circumference ≥94 men, ≥80 women • DYSLIPIDEMIA: TG>170 or HDL<40 • HYPERTENSION: Blood pressure ≥140/90 and/or on medication • FASTING GLUCOSE ≥110 mg/dl	3 OR MORE OF THE FOLLOWING: • CENTRAL OBESITY: Waist circumference ≥102cm in men, ≥88 in women • HYPERLIPIDEMIA Triglycerides ≥150 mg/dl HDL <40 men HDL <50 women • HYPERTENSION Blood pressure: ≥135/85 or on medication • FASTING GLUCOSE > 110(100) MG/DL

International Diabetes Federation 2005

CENTRAL OBESITY PLUS 2 OTHER FACTORS
Waist Circumference ≥90 cm H, ≥80 M

DISGLYCEMIA: FASTING GLYCEMIA ≥100 mg/dl
HYPERLIPIDEMIA: Triglycerides ≥150 mg/dl OR ON MEDICATION HDL <40 MEN, <50 WOMEN mg/dl OR ON MEDICATION
HYPERTENSION: Systolic Blood Pressure ≥130 OR DBP ≥85 mm Hg OR ON MEDICATION

excess body weight. Both overweight and obesity appear to be largely related to industrialization of societies, which has produced a drastic reduction in the levels of physical activity, while simultaneously energy intake has increased, and is based mainly in highly caloric and fat-dense foods. On the other hand, distribution of adiposity appears to be also of paramount importance. In addition to obesity, it has been estimated that visceral-type adipose tissue distribution is associated with the presence of CMS in both men and women above 70 years old, even in presence of normal body weight (Goodpaster, *et al* 2005). Excess and dysfunctional visceral adipose tissue could serve as a source of increased fatty acid (FA) delivery to the portal circulation, leading to insulin resistance in the liver, as demonstrated by Bergman and coworkers in experimental conditions (Bergman, *et al* 2001).

However, other experimental evidence only partially supports the above mentioned hypothesis, as both subcutaneous adiposity and total fat body content have also been related to insulin resistance (Albu, *et al* 2000). An alternative "ectopic fat storage" hypothesis has been proposed, in which lipids are abnormally deposited in tissues such as liver, skeletal muscle and pancreatic beta cells, leading to insulin resistance and T2DM (Ravussin and Smith, 2002). Certainly, studies have reported a strong association between triglycerides accumulation in skeletal muscle, in particular intramyocellular triglyceride content, and insulin resistance *in vivo* (Krssak, *et al* 1999). Abnormalities in the development of adipose tissue, as is the case in lipodystrophic disorders, lead to ectopic lipid deposits in the liver, skeletal muscle and, and are related to insulin resistance. In fact, it has been also postulated that obesity is itself a disorder of ectopic lipid storage, as in addition to increased adipose tissue, obese patients (as well as type 2 diabetics) also exhibit excessive liver and skeletal muscle lipid deposits (Goodpaster *et al* 2000). As is widely known, adipose tissue in obese individuals is dysfunctional, both from functional and morphologic standpoints. Enlargement of adipocytes has been proven to be strongly related to insulin resistance (Schneider, 1981, Ravussin *et al* 2002). Adipocytes are derived from mesenchymal pluripotential stem cells, in a process that involves numerous transcriptional and posttranscriptional events. Disturbances in these differentiation and proliferation steps could lead to failure of adipose tissue in adaptation to excess caloric intake, dysfunctional adipose tissue characterized by enlarged adipocytes, and ectopic lipid storage, a process in which abnormalities in lipid oxidation can also participate (Ravussin *et al* 2002).

2.   ADIPOSE TISSUE AS AN ENDOCRINE ORGAN AND INSULIN RESISTANCE

It is known that adipose tissue is not an inert tissue only dedicated to lipids and energy storage. Instead, adipose tissue, which includes not only adipocytes but also vascular structures, stromal tissue and preadipocytes, is an active endocrine organ with multiple functions and is a key player in the modulation of energy homeostasis. Numerous adipokines, with endocrine, autocrine and paracrine activities are originated in adipose tissue (Fig. 1).

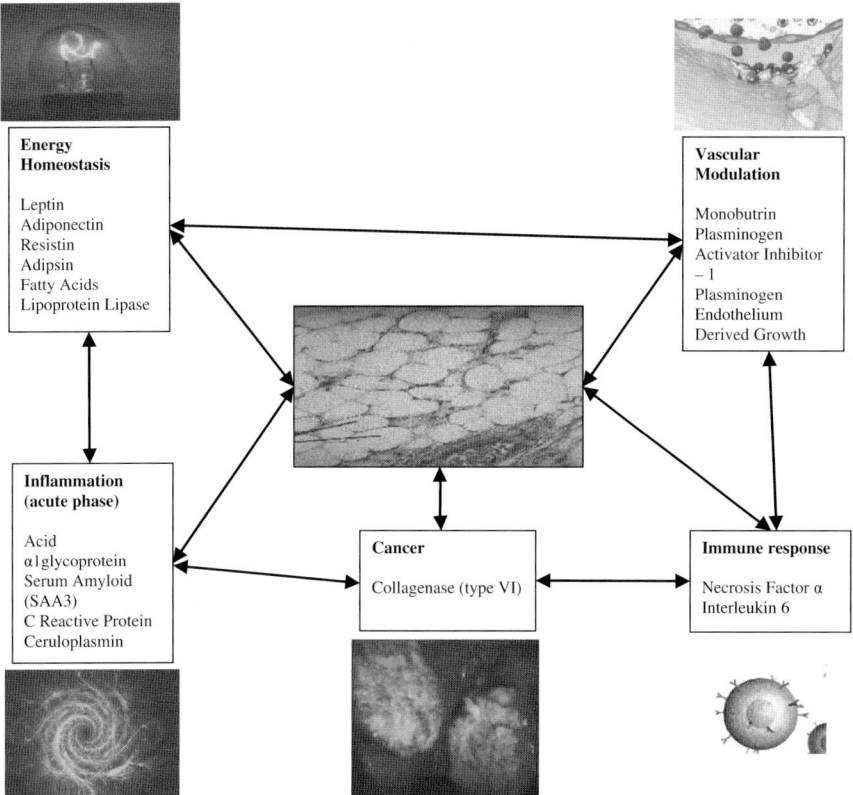

Figure 1. Adipose tissue production of adipokynes and their role in diverse biologic processes

As previously discussed, in obesity, as well as in CMS, adipose tissue is dysfunctional and contributes both to the development of a chronic low-grade inflammatory environment and to insulin resistance (Pickup, 2004).

Several substances, such as Fatty Acids (FA) are released from dysfunctional adipocytes, and have been strongly implicated in development of insulin resistance. In insulin resistance conditions, the antilipolytic effect of insulin is impaired, and persistently elevated FA levels promote hepatic gluconeogenesis (by stimulation of pyruvate carboxylase and phosphoenolpyruvate carboxykinase), interfere intracellular insulin signaling, and ultimately promote oxidative stress and insulin resistance (Bays *et al* 2004). In addition, adipokines such as resistin can also induce hepatic insulin resistance, as well as impairment of skeletal muscle glucose uptake and hepatic glucose production (Pittas *et al* 2004). Tumor Necrosis Factor α (TNF-α), one of the first cytokines implicated in inflammation has been shown to induce insulin resistance. Mainly through paracrine actions, TNF-α appears to contribute to increased FA concentrations and reduced secretion of adiponectin, an adipokyne with insulin sensitizing activity. TNF-α also induces serine phosphorylation of the first Insulin Receptor Substrate (IRS-1), hampering the tyrosine phosphorylation process required for normal insulin signaling, and activates the inflammatory Nuclear Factor κB (NF-κB) pathway, increasing the expression of adhesion molecules in endothelial cells and in vascular smooth muscle cells (VSMC) (Hotamisligil et al 1994).

As opposed to TNF-α, Interleukin-6 (IL-6) action is both endocrine and paracrine. Circulating levels of IL-6 are significantly associated with body mass index (BMI), insulin resistance and impaired glucose tolerance (Fernández-Real and Ricart, 2003). The mechanisms explaining the influence of IL-6 on insulin sensitivity are not fully uncovered, but appear to involve the expression of Suppressor of Cytokines 3 (SOCS-3), which secondarily impairs insulin transduction (Senn et al 2003), as well as an antagonistic effect on Adiponectin secretion (Kristiansen and Mandrup-Poulse, 2005).

On the other hand Adiponectin, first characterized in 1995 and previously known by multiple names including adipoQ, AcrP30 and Gelatin Ligand Protein, appears to confer a protective effect against the metabolic abnormalities that characterize the CMS (Kadowaki et al 2006). The mechanisms underlying Adiponectin actions are still to be characterized, and include increased FA oxidation in skeletal muscle, reduced hepatic glucose output, suppression of the expression of adhesion molecules, and inflammatory molecules (TNF-α), reduction of intimal vascular proliferation and stimulation of Nitric Oxide (NO) synthesis (Goldstein and Scalia, 2004, Ouchi et al 2003). Adiponectin is also able to stimulate the AMP-activated Protein Kinase (AMPK) cascade, thus promoting lipid as well as carbohydrates oxidation (Hardie, 2004).

3. THE RENIN-ANGIOTENSIN SYSTEM AND ITS PROTEASES: EVOLVING CONCEPTS

The Renin-Angiotensin System (RAS) can be conceptualized as a complex network of tightly regulated hormonal cascades that participate in the regulation of cardiovascular, renal and adrenal functions, which ultimately contribute to the control of blood pressure and electrolyte sodium/potassium balance. The RAS system has been characterized for more than 30 years (Peach, 1977) and is still an active and exciting field of research. Over the last decade, numerous advances in cellular and molecular biology have allowed to greatly expand our knowledge about the RAS, including the discovery of new proteins, novel functions of already known peptides, new receptors, interactions within the system and with other systems, and the existence of local RAS systems.

Classically described, the system involves translation of Renin messenger RNA (mRNA), derived in humans from a single gene, to produce Preprorenin in the juxtaglomerular cells of the renal afferent arterioles. Further processing includes glycosilation and removal of a signal peptide in the rough endoplasmic reticulum, yielding to Prorenin. In turn, Prorrenin is packed in immature granules in the Golgi apparatus, where further cleavage leads to Renin in a process probably involving trypsin-like enzymatic activity (Griendling, 1993). Renin, in its mature form, is an approximately 44 KDa glycosilated carboxypeptidase. The catalytic region of Renin contains critical aspartic acid residues, and this protease exhibits high specificity for Angiotensinogen, its natural substrate (Blundell *et al* 1983). Classically, no direct biologic actions other functions besides its catalytic activity have been attributed to Renin, but recently a renin receptor has been cloned in mesangial cells by Nguyen and coworkers, suggesting additional specific cellular functions for this peptide (Nguyen *et al* 2002).

Angiotensinogen, a 55-65 KDa globular glycoprotein belonging to the family of serine protease inhibitors (Serpins), is abundantly produced in the liver, but also has been identified in multiple tissues, including adipose tissue, heart, vasculature, brain and kidney. Angiotensinogen appears also to derive from a single gene in humans. Angiotensinogen undergoes processing before becoming substrate for Renin, which involves co translational removal of a signal peptide (Dickson and Sigmund, 2006). No additional biological functions have been attributed to Angiotensinogen so far, apart from its function as a substrate for Renin in the RAS. Activity of this enzyme leads to formation of the decapeptide Angiotensin I (Ang I).

In turn, Angiotensin Converting Enzyme (ACE) is an approximately 180 kDa glycoprotein with two active carboxy-terminal sites that converts biologically inactive Ang I, through cleavage of its C-terminal dipeptide, into active Angiotensin II (Ang II). This dipeptidyl carboxypeptidase contains a molar equivalent of zinc-hence being included in the family of zinc metallopeptidases-which is active in the hydrolytic step of the catalytic action on Ang I (Bunning *et al* 1983).

ACE consists of a hydrophobic single proteic chain. The majority of the enzyme is membrane-bound, but there is also a significant proportion of soluble ACE. Vascular endothelial cells, brush border of epithelial cells, neuroepithelial cells and endothelial cells express mainly membrane-bound ACE. In addition, the enzyme appears to be derived from a single gene (Griendling *et al* 1993).

As already known, ACE does not only catalyzes the activation of Ang II, but also inactivates Kallidin and the potent vasodilator Bradykinin (1-9), transforming it into the inactive Bradykinin (1-7). The net result of ACEI actions is thus severe vasoconstriction, as Bradykinin's vasoactive effect is mediated via production of NO and vasodilating prostaglandins, such as diverse prostanoids and prostacycline. Ang II is inactivated by specific angiotensinases, which rapidly catalyze the proteolytic degradation of Ang II to Ang (1-7) Ang (2-8) (Ang III), and Ang (3-8) (Ang IV), abrogating its vasoconstricting effect.

3.1. Angiotensin Converting Enzyme 2

The characterization of ACE 2 as an enzyme structurally similar to ACE in the year 2000 indisputably opened new perspectives in our contemporary under-standing of the RAS (Carey *et al* 2003). Tipnis and coworkers (Tipnis *et al* 2000) described human ACE 2 (initially named ACEH for Angiotensin Converting

Enzyme Homolog and also known as ACE-related Carboxypeptidase) as a zinc metalloproteinase with significant homology to ACE, but with predominantly carboxypeptidase instead of dipeptidyl carboxypeptidase. This feature confers ACE 2 a different biologic activity. Indeed, ACE 2 does not contribute to the generation of Ang II. Instead, the result of the activity of ACE 2 on Ang I is Ang (1-9), whereas the product of Ang II cleavage is Ang (1-7), thus providing a degradation pathway for Ang II and counterbalancing the actions of ACE. ACE 2 is encoded by a single gene mapped to Chromosome X (Crackower, 2002), and is widely distributed in diverse tissues, particularly in the kidneys, heart and gonads.

Actions of Ang (1-7) oppose those of Ang II, as it stimulates vasodilatation, inhibition of VSMC growth, through NO production, Ang II inhibition, production of vasodilatory prostaglandins, and enhancement of bradykinin activity (Paula *et al* 1995). Even if specific receptors for Ang (1-7) have not been yet fully characterized, its biologic activity appears to be mediated through binding to endogenous ligands coupled to G Proteins and interactions with Angiotensin II Receptor 1 (AT_1R) (Carey *et al* 2003).

3.2.   Angiotensin II Receptors

Ang II was originally identified as a hormone involved in the regulation of blood pressure, vascular tone, waster as well as electrolyte balance. However, the spectrum of this octapeptide has considerably expanded during the last decades, and now includes modulation of the structure of different tissues, remodeling and fibrosis in diverse tissues, in particular cardiovascular and renal. The actions of Ang II are mediated by interaction with specific receptors. Angiotensin II receptors AT_1R and AT_2R have been identified as G Protein-coupled receptors which however do not share the same intracellular signaling pathways and spectrum of biologic activity. These are not the only receptors characterized, as exemplified by the description of AT4 receptors, but classically most of known activities of Ang II are mediated through interaction with AT_1R, which has two main subtypes identified both in rodent models and in humans: AT_{1a} and AT_{1b} (Konishi *et al* 1994). While AT_{1b} receptors predominate in the pituitary and adrenals and have been more implicated in dipsogenic responses to Ang II, AT_{1a} receptors are more widely distributed and are involved in the regulation of the vascular tone and sodium homeostasis, regulation of endothelial cell function and vascular proliferation.

AT_1R gene has been mapped to chromosome 3, and is highly expressed in smooth muscle cells, fibroblasts, as well as in atrial and ventricular myocytes (Allen *et al* 1999). The amino terminal portion and the first and third loops of the transmembrane domain of this glycoproteic receptor are responsible for the interaction with Ang II (Hjorth *et al* 1994). Upon binding and subsequent activation, AT_1R–mediated responses involve not only direct intracellular signaling, but also cross-talk with other signaling pathways, including AT_2R, other vasoactive substances, cytokines and growth factors (Berry *et al* 2001).

Ang II-AT$_1$R coupling induces the activation of heterotrimetric G proteins in a process that involves exchange of GTP for GDP, which in turn leads to release of activating Gα- GTP and βγ complex. The specific intracellular resultant pathway depends upon the specific subunit activated. For instance, the activation of Gα$_q$ leads to activation of Phospholipase C (PLC) pathway, Gα$_i$ and G$_{aolf}$ induce adenylate cyclase and the cyclic Adenosine Monophospate (cAMP), while Gα$_i$ activation induces cyclic GMP and G$_i$ inhibits cAMP formation.

AT$_1$R activation triggers a series of downstream phosphorylations that elicit multiple vascular responses. In VSMC, proliferation and growth is mediated by intracellular phosphorylation of tyrosine kinase-active molecules, including PLC, Src kinases, Janus Kinases (Jak, Tyk), Focal Adhesion Kinase (FAK), Calcium-dependent tyrosine kinases (PYK2) and Phosphatidyl Inositol 3 Kinase (PI3K). In addition, tyrosine kinase-type growth factors receptors such as Epidermal Growth Factor Receptor (EGFR) and Platelet Derived Growth Factor Receptor (PDGFR) and Insulin Like Growth Factor 1 (IGF-1) are also activated by AT$_1$R.

Interestingly, Ang II/AT$_1$R activates the Jak-STAT pathway, which is also part of the signaling pathway of cytokine receptors, leading to activation of growth response genes which could contribute to cardiac tissue remodeling (Berk, 1999). Cell migration, hypertrophy and adhesion are also stimulated through FAK induction of autophosphorylation and association with surface integrins (Govindarajan *et al* 2000).

PI3K pathway is also activated through AT$_1$R, leading to phosphorylation of inositol lipids to produce 3-phosphoinositides, which affect cellular metabolism, survival, growth and cytoskeletal structure in VSMC (Saward *et al* 1997). Other important mediators of vascular modulation, including Mitogenic Activated Protein Kinase (MAPK), and small GTP-binding molecules such as Ras, Rho, and Cdc42, have been demonstrated to be up-regulated by Ang II/AT$_1$R (Berry *et al* 2001).

3.3.   The Angiotensin II Receptor 2

The Angiotensin II Receptor 2 (AT$_2$R) is also a G protein–coupled protein. Upon stimulation, AT$_2$R-mediated responses appear to counterbalance those mediated through AT$_1$R, and in rodents include increased generation of bradykinin, NO, and cGMP, which share vasodilating properties. AT$_2$R appears to mediate water and sodium homeostasis in the kidney, as well as pressure natriuresis (Ozono *et al* 1997). In addition to the aforementioned actions, hemodynamic responses mediated by AT$_2$R appear to involve in experimental conditions increased production of vasodilating prostaglandins PGE2 PGF2α and PGI$_2$, mediated by activation of Hydroxyeicosatetrenoic acid (HETE), an arachydonic acid-derived metabolite. Also in animal models, active AT$_2$R promotes apoptosis through inhibition of AT$_1$R-mediated dephosphorylation of MAPK, in particular ERK1 and ERK 2 (Huang *et al* 1996), as well as inhibition of the activity of Bcl-2 through its dephosphorylation (Horiuchi *et al* 1997).

Importantly, opposing actions of AT_1R and AT_2R appear to be the result of a balance in their relative tissue expression. Indeed, there is a negative cross-talk between the two receptors subtypes, and the resulting balance contribute to the regulation of cellular growth, as overexpression of AT_2R in animal models results in inhibition of AT_1R intracellular activity (Hirochi *et al* 1999). In rat cardiomyocytes AT_1R-mediated hypertrophy is up-regulated by AT_2R inhibition, while in renal tissue sodium retention mediated by AT_1R is counterbalanced by AT_2R (Booz *et al* 1996, Madrid *et al* 1997).

In humans however, while AT_1R has wide distribution and expression in adult tissues, AT_2R has high expression only in fetal tissues (Aguilera *et al* 1994). Also in human adults, detectable levels of AT_2R are found in the coronaries and aortic vascular tissue, and they can be up-regulated by use of Angiotensin II receptor blockers and in some pathologic conditions, including heart failure and myocardial infarction (Watanabe *et al* 2005). Actually, it has been suggested that AT_2R could exert a bradykinin/NO- mediated vasodilating protective effect against ischemia in vascular tissues, as shown by Tsutsumi et al (Tsutsumi *et al* 1999).

4.   RAS, INFLAMMATION AND OXIDATIVE STRESS

Excessive RAS activity has multiple deleterious effects, including stimulation of oxidative stress through production of Reactive Oxygen Species (ROS), as well as induction of inflammatory, prothrombotic and fibrotic states which ultimately lead to atherosclerosis (Fig. 2).

Inflammatory actions of Ang II appear to be mediated at least partially via AT_1R, as well as through activation of the NF-κB pathway, as been demonstrated in rodent models of abnormally increased RAS activity (Sadoshima, 2000). When inactive, NF-κB is a cytoplasmatic heterotrimeric cytoplasmic protein bound to the inhibitory IκB protein, which is released during activation of this inflammatory pathway. Active NF-κB is then translocated to the nucleus, where it binds to promoter regions of genes involved in inflammation, including intercellular adhesion and vascular cell adhesion molecules. Activation of RAS, through AngII/AT_1R appears to activate NF-κB in VSMC in rodent models, by stimulation of the degradation of IkB, while promoting translocation of NF-κB to the nucleus (Ruiz-Ortega *et al* 2000). On the other hand, these abnormalities are abrogated by AT_1R blockade or by antioxidant therapy.

The link between RAS activation and oxidative stress has been intensively studied over the past several years. Ang II promotes the production of ROS in adipose tissue, skeletal muscle, and cardiovascular tissue (Sowers, 2002). In turn, ROS induce a shift toward proinflammatory and proatherogenic patterns, and mitogenic actions in VSMC (Nickenig and Harrison, 2002).

In mammalian cells, NADPH oxidase, nitric oxide synthase, cytochrome p450 enzymatic complex, the mitochondrial electron transport system, and Xanthine Oxidase systems are all capable of ROS production. However, the NADPH oxidase is probably the most important system implicated in excessive oxidative stress

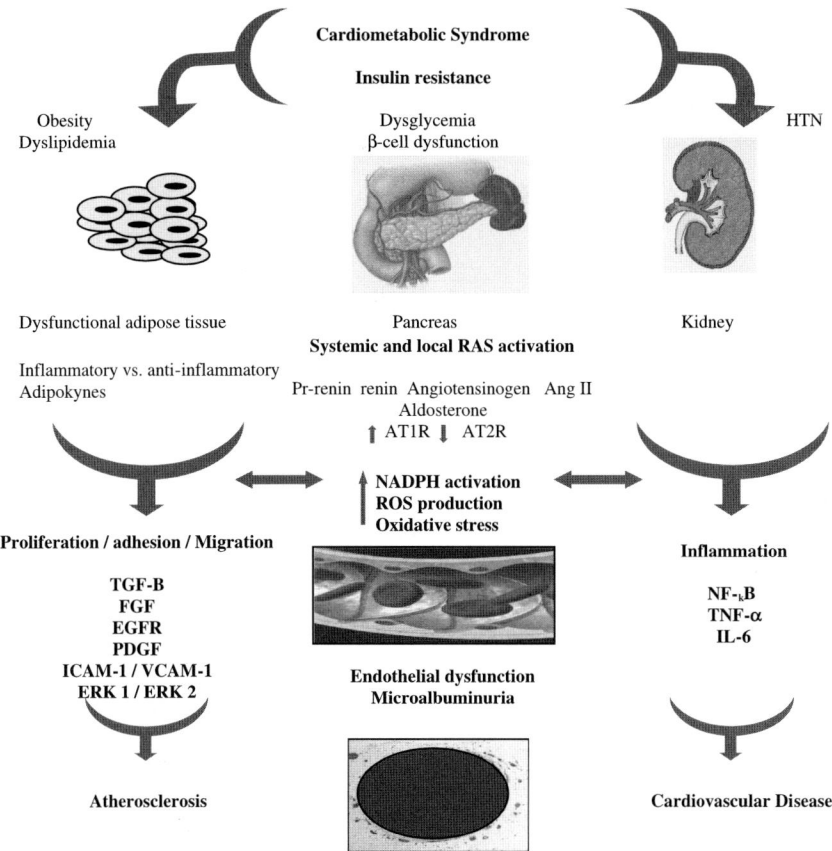

Figure 2. Involvement of RAS activation in atherosclerosis

leading to vascular dysfunction in cardiovascular tissue (Ushio-Fukai *et al* 2002). The NADPH oxidase enzymatic complex is a multisubunit enzyme composed by cytosolic proteins (small GTPase Rac1, p47^{phox}, p67^{phox}), and membrane catalytic proteins Nox 2 (gp 91) and p22^{phox}. (Ushio-Fukai *et al* 2004). Recent studies also show that Nox 2 and the P22^{phox} are abundantly expressed in perinuclear areas of renal cells (Habibi, *et al* unpublished data, 2006) (Fig. 3).

Activation of the NADPH oxidase produces assembly of cytosolic and plasma membrane subunits to generate superoxide ($O_2\cdot^-$) by means of electron transfer from subunit gp 91 of NADPH to O2 molecules.

Ang II, via AT$_1$R, stimulates intracellular pathways that result in translocation of all subunits to the plasma membrane, a key step in NADPH oxidase activation. Zuo *et al* recently demonstrated that Ang II cell stimulation promotes Rac1 association with caveolin 1, as well as its migration into caveolin-enriched lipid rafts (Zuo L *et al* 2004). It is highly likely that in those lipid rafts, Rac1 is activated via exchange

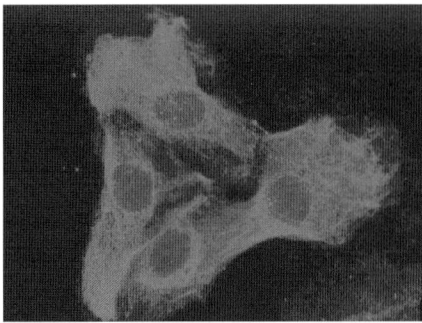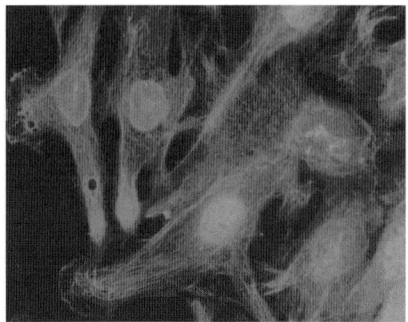

Figure 3. Perinuclear and cytoskeletal distribution of NADPH subunits in proximal tubule OK renal cells. Images courtesy of Dr Javad Habibi, PhD. Research Assistant Professor. University of Missouri at Columbia, U.S.A

of GDP for GTP, and that this activation involves the trafficking of activated AT_1R into the caveolin-enriched lipid rafts (Zuo *et al* 2005). Oxidative stress a key player in the development of atherosclerosis and CVD in the setting of the CMS. RAS, through AT_1R interaction and PKC activation, leads to phosphorylation of phox subunits ($p22^{phox}$) of membrane-bound NADPH oxidase, which is thus activated, leading to generation of superoxide (O^-_2). Experimental studies suggest that Ang II–mediated NADPH activation and production of ROS involve transcriptional as well as non-transcriptional mechanisms (Pagano *et al* 1998). The experimental demonstration of the abrogation of NADPH-induced oxidative stress through AT_1R antagonist therapy in rabbit models supports the role of RAS as an important player in ROS formation (Wang *et al* 1999).

ROS activity has been linked to multiple intracellular signaling pathways regulating vascular cell growth and differentiation. AT_1R–mediated activation of ROS production can induce the inflammatory NF-kB pathway, and can lead to increased expression of Vascular Adhesion molecule 1 (VCAM-1), as demonstrated by Pueyo and coworkers in rat endothelial cells (Pueyo *et al* 2000). In addition, Ang II can activate through a ROS-dependent mechanism different intracellular tyrosine kinase pathways such as extracellular signal-regulated kinase 1 and 2 (ERK1 and ERK2), thus influencing vascular cells growth and proliferation. Furthermore, ROS can also act as second messengers in the transactivation of other growth factors receptors such as EGFR, and in the triggering of the Jak-STAT pathway, which leads to increased production of IL-6, thus favoring additional inflammation (Berry *et al* 2001).

5.   IMPORTANCE OF LOCAL ADIPOSE, PANCREATIC AND RENAL RAS IN THE CMS

The inappropriate activation of RAS in HTN has been classically described and undoubtedly provides much of the rationale for therapy of hypertensive patients. In addition, other components of the CMS have also been shown to be associated with

RAS over activity. Even if obesity is considered as a state of sodium retention and volume expansion, a relationship between body weight and increased levels of Ang II, plasma Renin Activity, ACE and aldosterone in humans has been demonstrated (Licata *et al* 1994). Conversely, weight loss appears to reduce RAS activity as well as blood pressure in obese individuals (Tuck *et al* 1981).

Hyperglycemia can also induce RAS and production of Ang II in mesangial cells in experimental conditions, in this case through up-regulation of renin activity (Vidotti *et al* 2004). Furthermore, an increase in aldosterone production has been detected in diabetic humans, along with increased Ang II, AT_1R and simultaneous down-regulation of AT_2R, leading to increase oxidative stress and vascular remodeling (Giacchetti *et al* 2005).

Dyslipidemia and FA levels elevation, as previously discussed, have also been linked to RAS activation. Blockade of RAS in Zucker Fatty rats through use of Angiotensin Receptor Blockers (ARBs) reduces not only blood pressure, but also diminishes FA concentrations (without affecting circulating triglycerides), improves fatty changes in the liver, while at the same time increasing insulin sensitivity (Ran J *et al* 2004).

The reasons underlying these associations include not exclusively systemic RAS activation, but also involve local RAS systems existing in tissues such as fat, kidneys and pancreas (Fig. 4).

Certainly, the role of adipose tissue RAS in the pathophysiology of CMS is increasingly being recognized, as adipocytes posses the ability to synthesize all components of the RAS, including angiotensinogen, ACE and Ang II receptors. These are found both in white and brown adipose tissues. In humans angiotensinogen, renin, as well as Non-dependent RAS enzymes required for production of Ang I and Ang II,

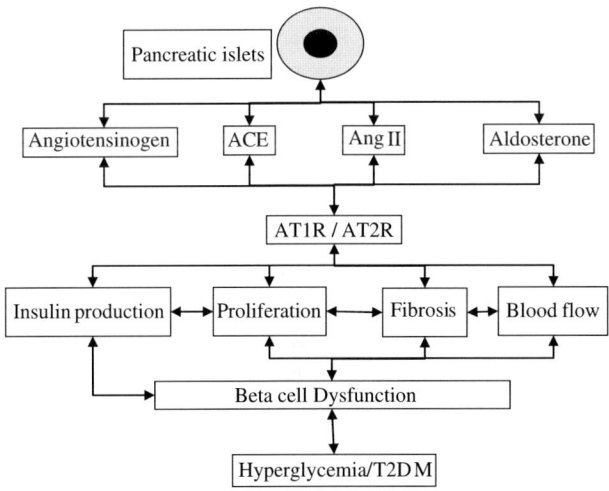

Figure 4. Local adipose and pancreatic role in CMS

including cathepsin D, cathepsin G, tonin and chymase, are expressed (Karlsson *et al* 1998). Moreover, current research indicates that Angiotensinogen messenger RNA expression is higher in abdominal fat compared to subcutaneous fat, a finding that correlates with the differences observed in insulin resistance between the two tissues (Aneja *et al* 2004). Both in rodents and in humans, the most abundant subtype Ang II receptor is AT_1R, in particular $AT_{1A}R$ (Burson *et al* 1994, Crandall *et al* 1994).

From a functional standpoint, in brown rodent adipose tissue Ang II is acutely involved in sympathetic-mediated thermogenic responses during cold acclimation, without activation of the other components of the RAS (Cassis, 1993). In humans, body weight is positively correlated with adipose angiotensinogen mRNA levels (Van *et al* 2000).

As stated above, Ang II is a known growth factor. In human adipose tissue, Ang II stimulation induces cell cycle phase G_1, thus contributing to cellular differentiation of preadipocytes into adipocytes (Crandall *et al* 1999). In addition, Ang II stimulates production of prostacyclin, an arachidonic acid derivative and a potent autocrine trigger for terminal differentiation of adipocytes, while FA activate angiotensinogen gene expression in preadipocytes in a dose-dependent manner (Safonova *et al* 1997). Conversely, in experimental conditions Ang II increases triglycerides in human adipocytes as well as 3T3-L1 cells, through induction of key enzymes of lipogenesis, including Fatty Acid Synthase and Glycerol-3-Phosphate Dehydrogenase (Jones *et al* 1997).

In experimental conditions, targeted expression of angiotensinogen, through generation of rodent models overexpressing adipose angiotensinogen or restricting angiotensinogen expression to adipose tissue, increases fat mass. Overexpression of adipose tissue-derived angiotensinogen can lead to hypertensive animals, postulating an influence of this local RAS both on weight and systemic blood pressure (Massiera *et al* 2001). Interestingly, adipose-derived Ang II increases plasma leptin levels in rats, while sympathetic activation triggered by systemic RAS modulates leptin release (Cassis *et al* 2004). In support of this, studies in rats and humans have shown weight reduction with use of ACE inhibitors (Engeli *et al* 2000). In contrast, Ang II infusions in Sprague-Dawley (SD) rats can induce between 18% and 26% weight loss, in a pressor-independent regulatory mechanism (Brink *et al* 1996). These effects of Ang II in SD rats appear to be dose-dependent and involve an anorexigenic effect of Ang II, as well as alterations in plasma leptin, increased energy expenditure and mobilization of fat (Cassis *et al* 1998). On the other hand, according to work by Frederich *et al* adipose tissue angiotensinogen expression is up-regulated and down-regulated by feeding or fasting, respectively, in SD rats, in a tissue-specific manner. These variations are paralleled by systolic blood pressure changes, which follow a similar trend (Frederich *et al* 1992). The authors suggest that probably adipose tissue RAS could regulate fat blood flow and hence its FA release, thus affecting insulin sensitivity.

Taken together, all mentioned features suggest an active participation of adipose RAS in the regulation of fat mass, body weight and systemic blood pressure, that will contribute to clarifying the relationship between RAS activation and CMS components such as obesity, dyslipidemia, HTN and dysglycemia.

On the other hand, the participation of pancreatic RAS is also gaining mounting interest in the pathophysiology of the CMS and T2DM. The endocrine pancreas is exposed not only to circulating components of the RAS but also to locally produced components; and in conditions such as the CMS, obesity and T2DM, RAS activation is up-regulated. A better understanding of the local pancreatic Renin Angiotensin and Aldosterone System in this regard is of paramount importance, as a role of this system in pathogenesis of T2DM-associated beta cell failure has been proposed by numerous researchers (Tikellis *et al* 2006).

Evidence from animal models and human pancreas is now available. Leung *et al.* recently described the existence of angiotensinogen, ACE, AT_1R and AT_2R in mouse pancreatic islets. In addition, the presence of AT_1R in the membrane of the beta cell has been described, a finding that is different compared to other animal models like the rat (Lau *et al* 2004, Leung *et al* 2001, Leung and Chappell, 2003).

In the human pancreas, AT_1R has been localized in the beta cells, as well as in endothelial cells of the pancreatic vasculature (Tahmasebi *et al* 1999). More recently, Leung *et al* showed, using immunohistochemistry, that in human pancreas angiotensinogen was predominantly localized in the pancreatic islets, while AT_1R protein was localized predominantly in the pancreatic ducts (Lam and Leung, 2002).

Even though not completely clear yet, the physiological role of the pancreatic RAS in mice models seems to involve islet blood flow regulation, effect that ultimately would affect glucose-stimulated insulin secretion and carbohydrates/lipids homeostasis. In mouse pancreatic islets, increasing concentrations of Ang II inhibit in a dose-dependent manner the glucose-stimulated secretion of insulin, mainly through a decrease in insulin synthesis, as is demonstrated by falling Proinsulin production. AT_1R blockade with Losartan seems to reverse these actions (Carlsson *et al* 1998, Lau T *et al* 2004).

According to research by Lupi and coworkers, in isolated human islets hyperglycemia has been shown to increase the expression of mRNA for angiotensinogen, ACE and AT_1R. In addition, there is a significant increase in oxidative stress, while insulin secretion is decreased. In experimental conditions the later effects were blocked by the use of ACE inhibitors (Lupi *et al* 2006).

In addition, recent reports from Chu and coworkers have demonstrated a beneficial effect of RAS blockade with ARBs on pancreatic production and secretion of insulin (Chu *et al* 2006). Indeed, obesity-induced T2DM in *db/db* mice has been shown to impair insulin production, likely through activation of pancreatic RAS and upregulation of AT_1R, which is expressed β-cells. The underlying mechanism appears to involve disturbances in pancreatic regional blood flow and proinsulin synthesis, as demonstrated also in rodents (Carlsson *et al* 1998). The use of ARBs in *db/db* mice significantly increased proinsulin production, as well as insulin secretion. Furthermore, obesity-induced hyperglycemia, glucose intolerance, and onset of T2DM were also delayed in this model, without affecting insulin sensitivity (Chu *et al* 2006). These data suggest a role for pancreatic RAS in the development of β-cell dysfunction in T2DM, and provide important insights into the mechanisms involved in the beneficial effects of RAS blockade on glucose homeostasis. The importance of these observations in human T2DM, and in CMS, will require further specific testing.

On the other hand, hyperglycemia-induced RAS activation has also been involved in the pancreatic fibrosis mediated by pancreatic stellate cells. Even though the role of this effect in diabetes pathogenesis in not clear yet, it is an attractive possibility if one considers that fibrosis secondary to RAS activation has been clearly identified as a pathologic event in tissues such as the heart and kidney (Ko *et al* 2006).

Finally, renal involvement in obesity, CMS and T2DM is well known. Multiples factors converged as causatives agents, and definitively intra-renal RAS activation has demonstrated to play a central role (Lastra *et al* 2006). AT_1R are present in multiple areas of the kidney, including blood vessels, podocytes, proximal tubule and interstitial cells, thick ascending limb epithelia, distal tubules, collecting tubules and *macula densa* (Navar LG, 2004). Meanwhile, AT_2R has been identified in proximal and collecting tubules (Navar, 2004).

Classic actions of the renal RAS include tubular sodium reabsorption, renal vasoconstriction, tubuloglomerular feedback modulation, and pressure-natriuresis (Carey and Siragy, 2003).

Upon interaction with AT_1R, Ang II promotes the production of ROS by up-regulating the activity of the NADPH oxidase enzymatic complex, as well as intrarenal fibrosis through production of profibrotic growing factors like Transforming Growth Factor β1 (TGF-β1) and Connective Tissue Growth Factor (CTGF) (Rodriguez-Vita *et al* 2005). Profibrotic growth factors are implicated in mesangial cell hypertrophy, matrix expansion and fibroblast proliferation. Also, through AT_1R/AT_2R-mediated activation of NF-κB, inflammatory cells and cytokines are recruited into the kidney (Ruiz-Ortega *et al* 2001, Lorenzo *et al* 2002).

Konoshita T *et al*. recently examined the tisular gene expression of RAS components in renal biopsies from diabetic and non diabetic individuals. They reported a significant up-regulation in the ACE gene expression in renal tissue from diabetic patients, without significant changes on the other components of the RAS examined (Konoshita *et al* 2006).

Collectively both systemic and local RAS are abnormally activated in the CMS and have demonstrated to play key roles in the development of obesity, CMS, T2DM – related atherosclerosis that ultimately lead to CVD. Newer research about the exact pathophysiology as well as the impact of local and/or systemic RAS inhibition will undoubtedly provide more effective alternatives for the prevention of CMS-related cardiovascular and renal complications.

6.   THERAPEUTIC IMPLICATIONS FOR THE MANAGEMENT OF THE CMS: THE ROLE OF RAS BLOCKADE IN THE CLINICAL SETTING

As has been extensively discussed, the CMS not only predisposes to T2DM, but also to the development and progression of CVD. From a clinical standpoint, the implication for the management of CMS is that strategies to prevent CVD should go beyond a glucocentric strategy centered on the management of glucose homeostasis disturbance, and a more comprehensive and integral vascular protective strategy should be advocated for. The possibility of pharmacologically modulate the RAS can provide such an opportunity.

At least three different alternatives for RAS blockade are currently available and under intensive widespread use. The Angiotensin Converting Enzyme Inhibitors (ACEI), Angiotensin Receptor Blockers (ARB), and the antagonists of aldosterone, such as spironolactone and eplerenone. Initial evidence provided by studies designed to evaluate cardiovascular outcomes were enlightening regarding the role of RAS blockade in the prevention of diabetes in population with CVD or at high cardiovascular risk (Table 2).

The Captopril Prevention Project (CAPP trial) was a randomized, blinded, prospective, open trial comparing captopril against conventional therapy (diuretics, beta blockers). 10,985 patients were studied and data was analyzed in an intention to treat mode. The primary endpoint was a composite of fatal and non-fatal myocardial infarction, stroke, and CVD-related death. Although no differences were noted on the primary end point favoring ACEI, a significant difference in the prevention of diabetes was seen favoring the group treated with captopril, showing a significant 14% lower incidence of T2DM (Hansson *et al* 1999).

Later, in 2000, results from the HOPE trial became available. 9,297 high risk patients with decreased left ventricle ejection fraction or overt heart failure were randomized to ramipril treatment (10 mg) or to matching placebo. The patients were followed-up for 5 years and the primary end-point was a composite of myocardial infarction, stroke, or death from cardiovascular causes. This study not only showed positive results regarding cardiovascular outcomes, but also revealed a significantly decreased incidence of newly diagnosed T2DM (Relative Risk 0.66, 0.51–085, $p < 0.001$) (Heart Outcomes Prevention Evaluation Study Investigators, 2000).

On the other hand, similar evidence in terms of T2DM prevention is also available with angiotensin receptor blockers (Table 2). The VALUE trial, whose results were published in 2004, analyzed cardiac morbidity and mortality in a group on 15,245 hypertensive individuals with cardiovascular risk factors. Participants were randomized to antihypertensive regimens with valsartan or amlopidine. Despite the negative outcome for the angiotensin receptor blocker, probably related to a smaller reduction in blood pressure, again a positive metabolic effect was seen: 23% reduction in the incidence of diabetes in the group assigned to therapy with valsartan. Even thought this is encouraging, question remains regarding the significance of

Table 2. Relevant clinical trial showing an influence of RAS blockade on the development of Type 2 Diabetes Mellitus

Trial	Number of participants	Population cardiovascular status	Mean follow up time (years)	RAS blockade strategy	Primary outcome	Relative Risk
CAPPP (1999)	10985	Hypertensives	6.1	Captopril	Composite of myocardial infarction, stroke, and other cardiovascular deaths.	0.79 (0.67–0.94)
HOPE (2000)	9297	Vascular disease or diabetes + one other cardiovascular risk factor + low ejection fraction or heart failure	5	Ramipril	Composite of myocardial infarction, stroke, and other cardiovascular deaths.	0.66 (0.51–0.85)
ALLHAT (2003)	33357	Hypertension and atleast 1 other CHD risk factor	4.9	Lisinopril	Combined fatal CHD or nonfatal myocardial infarction	0.70 (0.56–0.86)
CHARM (2003)	7601	Heart failure	3.2	Candesartan	All-cause mortality	0.78 (0.64–0.96)
VALUE (2004)	15245	Hypertensive patients at high cardiovascular risk	4.2	Valsartan	Composite of cardiac mortality and morbidity	0.77 (0.69–0.86)
DREAM (2006)	5269	No cardiovascular disease	3	Ramipril	Development of diabetes or death	0.91 (0.81–1.03) Non significant

preventing elevation in blood glucose readings versus preventing cardiovascular outcomes (Julius *et al* 2004).

As part of the CHARM trial (Candesartan in Heart Failure-Assessment of Reduction in Mortality and Morbidity Program), the incidence of newly diagnosed diabetes was analyzed as a predefined secondary outcome. This trial was a randomized, controlled, double-blind study with 5436 of the 7601 patients with heart failure who did not have a diagnosis of T2DM on admission to the study. Candesartan treatment (dose titrated up to 32 mg daily) or matching placebo was examined. Six percent of the patient in the candesartan group developed diabetes as compared with 7.4% in the placebo group (P = 0.020). The authors reported that this benefit was less marked in patients that were already taking ACEI (Yusuf *et al* 2005).

Looking for an answer for the questions surrounding how RAS blockade affects T2DM incidence, as it is usual when no clear cut evidence is found in the randomized trials, a meta-analysis was done by Abuissa *et al*. Twelve randomized controlled clinical trials were examined, 7 used ACEIs and 5 used ARBs. This meta-analysis compiled data regarding 72.333 non-diabetic patients, and showed that ACE inhibitors or ARBs produced a significant 25% over-all reduction in the incidence of new-onset diabetes (27% for ACEI, and 23% for the ARB) (Abuissa *et al* 2005).

However many questions remain unanswered. One of the most intensively debated points on the above mentioned trials is probably that none of them were specifically designed with a primary end point of T2DM prevention. In an attempt to shed light on this, the DREAM trial (Diabetes Reduction Assessment with Ramipril and Rosiglitazone Medication) results were published earlier in 2006.

The DREAM trial was a prospective randomized trial which enrolled 5.269 people with impaired fasting plasma glucose levels ($\geq$110 mg/dL and <126mg/dL) or impaired glucose tolerance (plasma glucose level $\geq$140 mg/dL but <200mg/dL 2 hours after an oral 75 grams glucose load) but who did not have a history of diabetes, intolerance, CVD, or history of prior therapy with either ACEI or thiazolidinediones. This study had a 2 by 2 factorial design, and patient were randomized to ramipril (target dose 15 mg) or matching placebo. A second arm of the study randomized patients to rosiglitazone or placebo. Primary outcome was newly diagnosed T2DM or death. Secondary outcomes were a composite of cardiovascular and renal events, data which is not yet available. The patients were followed-up for a median of 3 years. By the end of this period primary outcome was reached in 18.1% of patients in the ramipril group and in 19.5% in the placebo group (hazard ratio, 0.91; 95% confidence interval [CI], 0.81 to 1.03; P = 0.15), showing a trend but not significant protection against development of T2DM. Results were similar for participants with Impaired Fasting Glucose and/or with Impaired Glucose Tolerance. The authors reported a positive effect of ramipril on glucose homeostasis, in terms of return to normoglycemia. Accordingly, 42.5% of participants in the treatment group compared to 38.2% in the placebo group had normal fasting plasma glucose levels and normal 2-hour plasma glucose levels (Hazard Ratio, 1.16; 95% CI, 1.07 to 1.27; P = 0.001) (The DREAM Trial Investigators, 2006).

How to reconcile the results of this study with the beneficial metabolic effects of the RAAS blockade seen in previous reports? The authors of the DREAM trial propose several possible explanations, including that probably the studied population was younger, without overt CVD in contrast to previously mentioned studies, the use of stringent glycemic criteria was on admission to the study, and of course the fact that the trial was primarily designed to detect diabetes prevention. Newer studies, more specifically targeted, as well as further analysis of the data provided by the Dream trial investigators will surely help to clarify the impact of RAS blockade on insulin resistance, glucose homeostasis and probably the CMS.

7.   CONCLUSIONS AND PERSPECTIVES

The epidemic of obesity and CMS that affects the modern world requires intensive and dynamic research directed towards uncovering the key players that ultimately will lead to CVD. Proteases of the System tightly regulate processes that lead to production of generation of active mediators involved in multiple cellular processes. Indeed, the growing knowledge about RAS components and physiology expands the concept of RAS beyond their role as mere modulators of blood pressure, to encompass regulation of cell differentiation, growth, and vascular homeostasis. Importantly mechanisms of RAS cross talk with diverse intracellular signaling systems allow better understanding the development of CMS-mediated insulin resistance, oxidative stress atherogenesis and CVD. In addition, research has uncovered new elements of RAS, including Ang (1-7) ACE 2, and AT_2R, which maintain a balance between vascular constriction, cellular proliferation, migration and vasodilatation, tissue repair, growth inhibition and apoptosis. Also, the current concept of RAS acknowledges the existence of several local systems located in tissues such as adipose tissue and pancreas, which possess complex regulatory mechanisms that contribute to modulate glucose and lipids homeostasis, body weight, energy expenditure and vascular function.

Available research actively provides the foundations for current therapy of CMS and prevention of associated CVD. Importantly, non-pharmacologic therapies, which involve regular physical activity and healthy dietary habits, provide the foundations for controlling weight gain, HTN, dysglycemia and atherogenic dyslipidemia. From a pharmacologic standpoint, the blockade of RAS through use of ACEI and ARBs has proven to improve individual components of the CMS beyond the effect that could be attributable to HTN control, as well as overall CVD morbidity and mortality on the long term (Nickenig et al 2006). Of particular interest are the results of previously mentioned trials including CAPP, HOPE, CHARM, and LIFE, in which prevention of T2DM was achieved. As previously discussed, the DREAM trial did not replicate these findings in terms of T2DM prevention, but did show a positive effect of ACEI in glucose homeostasis and return to normoglycemia.

Exciting research will shed more light on the importance of RAAS blockade in the management and prevention of CMS and CMS-related CVD. New trials are currently ongoing, including the Nateglinide and Valsartan in Impaired Glucose Tolerance Outcomes research (NAVIGATOR) trial, which specifically is addressing the role of these two medications in the prevention of both T2DM and CVD in patients with impaired glucose tolerance. In addition, the ONTARGET trial (ONgoing Telmisartan Alone and in Combination with Ramipril Global Endpoint Trial) explores ACEI and ARBs as monotherapy or combined in participants at high CVD risk. Numerous other studies are in progress, and different strategies to inhibit the RAS are studied, such as direct renin inhibition with aliskiren. All these and others will allow in the future a more comprehensive and effective approach to modulation of RAS and management of the CMS, with the aim of controlling CVD and the burden it imposes on public health.

REFERENCES

Abuissa H, Jones PG, Marso SP, O'Keefe JH Jr, 2005, Angiotensin-converting-enzyme inhibitors or angiotensin receptor blockers for prevention of type 2 diabetes: a meta-analysis of randomized clinical trials. *J Am Coll Cardiol.* **46**: 821–826

Aguilera G, Kapur S, Feuillan P, Sunar-Akbasak B, Bathia AJ, 1994, Developmental changes in angiotensin II receptor subtypes and AT1 receptor mRNA in rat kidney. *Kidney Intl.* **46**: 973–979

Albu JB, Kovera AJ, Johnson JA, 2000. Fat distribution in health and obesity. *Ann N.Y. Acad Sci.* **904**: 491–501

Alexander CM, Landsman PB, Teutsch SM, Haffner SM, 2003, NCEP-Defined Metabolic Syndrome, Diabetes, and Prevalence of coronary artery disease among NHANES III participants age 50 years and older. *Diabetes.* **52**: 1210–1214

Allen AM, Zhuo JL, 1999, Mendelsohn FAO. Localization of angiotensin II AT1 and AT2 receptors. *J Am Soc Nephrol.* **10**: S23–S29

Aneja A, El-Atat F, McFarlane SI, Sowers JR, 2004, Hypertension and obesity. *Recent Prog Horm Res.* **59**: 169–205

Avogaro P, Crepaldi G, Enzi G, Tiengo A, 1967, Associazione di hiperlipidemia diabete mellito e obesita di medio grado. *Acta Diabetol Lat.* **4**: 36–41

Bays H, Mandarino L, De Fronzo R, 2004, Role of the adipocyte, free fatty acids and ectopic fat in the pathogenesis of type 2 diabetes mellitus: Peroxisomal proliferators-activated receptor agonists provide a rationale therapeutic approach. *J Clin Endocrinol Metab.* **89**: 463–478

Bergman RN, Van Citters GW, Mittelman SD, *et al* 2001, Central role of the adipocyte in the Metabolic Syndrome. *J Investig Med.* **49**: 119–126

Berk BC, Corson MA, 1999, Angiotensin II signal transduction in vascular smooth muscle: role of tyrosine kinases. *Circ Res.* **80**: 607–616

Berry C, Touyz R, Dominiczak AF, Webb RC, Johns DG, 2001, Angiotensin receptors: signaling, vascular pathophysiology, and interactions with ceramide. *Am J Physiol Heart Circ Physiol.* **281**: H2337–H2365

Blundell T, Sibanda BLK, Pearl L, 1983, Three dimensional structure, specificity and catalytic mechanism of renin. *Nature.* **304**: 273–275

Booz GW, Baker KM, 1996, Role of type 1 and type 2 angiotensin receptors in angiotensin II – induced cardiomyocyte hypertrophy. *Hypertension.* **28**: 635–640

Brink M, Welen J, Delafontaine P, 1996, Angiotensin II causes weight loss and decreases Insulin-Like Growth Factor in rats through a pressor-independent mechanism. *J Clin Invest.* **97**: 2509–2516

Bunning P, Holmquist B, Riordan JF, 1983, Substrate, specificity and kinetic characteristics of angiotensin converting enzyme. *Biochemistry.* **22**: 103–110

Burson JM, Aguilera G, Gross KW, Sigmund CD, 1994, Differential expression of angiotensin receptor 1A and 1B in mouse. *Am J Physiol Endocrinol Metab.* **267**: E260–E267

Carey RM, Siragy HM, 2003, Newly recognized components of the Renin-Angiotensin System: Potential Roles in cardiovascular and renal regulation. *Endocrine Reviews.* **24**: 261–271

Carlsson PO, Berne C, Jansson L, 1998, Angiotensin II and the endocrine pancreas: effects on islet blood flow and insulin secretion in rats. *Diabetologia.* **41**: 127–133

Cassis LA, 1993, Role of angiotensin II in brown adipose thermogenesis during cold acclimation. *Am J Physiol Endocrinol Metab.* **265**: E680–E685

Cassis LA, English VL, Bharadwaj K, Boustany CM, 2004, Differential effects of local *versus* systemic angiotensin II in the regulation of leptin release from adipocytes. *Endocrinology.* **145**: 169–174

Cassis LA, Marshall DE, Fettinger MJ, Rosenbluth B, Lodder RA, 1998, Mechanisms contributing to angiotensin II regulation of body weight. *Am J Physiol Endocrinol Metab.* **274**: 867–876

Chu KY, Lau T, Carlsson P, Leung PS, 2006, Angiotensin II type 1 receptor blockade improves β-cell function and glucose tolerance in a mouse model of type 2 diabetes. *Diabetes.* **55**: 367–374

Crackower MA, Sarao R, Oudit GY, *et al* 2002, Angiotensin-converting enzyme 2 is an essential regulator of heart function. *Nature.* **417**: 822–828

Crandall DL, Armellino DC, Busler DE, Mc Hendry-Rinde B, Kral JG, 1999, Angiotensin II receptor in human preadipocytes: role in cell cycle regulation. *Endocrinology.* **140**: 154–158

Crandall DL, Herzlinger HE, Saunders BD, Armellino DC, Kral JG, 1994, Distribution of angiotensin receptors in rat and human adipocytes. *J Lipid Res.* **35**: 1378–1385

Dickson ME, Sigmund CD, 2006, Genetic basis of hypertension: revisiting Angiotensinogen. *Hypertension.* **48**: 14–20

Duncan GE, Sierra ML, Zhou XH, 2004, Prevalence and trends of a Metabolic Syndrome phenotype among U.S. adolescents, 1999–2000. *Diabetes Care.* **27**: 2438–2443

Engeli S, Negrel R, Sharma AM, 2000, Physiology of the adipose tissue renin-angiotensin system. *Hypertension.* **35**: 1270–1277

Fernández-Real JM, Ricart W, 2003, Insulin resistance and chronic cardiovascular inflammatory syndrome. *Endocrine Reviews.* **24**: 278–301

Flegal KM, Carroll MD, Ogden CL, *et al* 2002, Prevalence and trends in obesity among US adults, 1999–2000. *JAMA.* **288**: 1723–1727

Ford ES, 2005, Prevalence of the Metabolic Syndrome defined by the International Diabetes Federation among adults in the US. *Diabetes Care.* **28**: 2745–2749

Frederich RC, Kahn BB, Peach MJ, Flier JS, 1992, Tissue-specific nutritional regulation of angiotensinogen in adipose tissue. *Hypertension.* **19**: 339–344

Giacchetti G, Sechi LA, Rilli S, Carey RM, 2005, The renin angiotensin-aldosterone system, glucose metabolism and diabetes. *Trends Endocrinol Metab.* **16** (3): 120–126

Goldstein BJ, Scalia R, 2004, Adiponectin: A novel Adipokyne linking adipocytes and vascular function. *Journal of Clinical Endocrinology and Metabolism.* **89**: 2563–2568

Goodpaster BH, Krishnaswami S, Harris TB, *et al* 2005, Obesity, regional body fat distribution, and the Metabolic Syndrome in older men and women. *Arch Intern Med.* **165**: 777–783

Goodpaster BH, Thaete FL, Kelley DE, 2000, Thigh adipose tissue distribution is associated with insulin resistance in obesity and in type 2 diabetes mellitus. *Am J Clin Nutr.* **71**: 885–892

Govindarajan G, Eble DM, Lucchesi PA, Samarel AM, 2000, Focal adhesion kinase is involved in angiotensin II-mediated protein synthesis in cultured smooth vascular cells. *Circ Res.* **87**: 710–716

Griendling KK, Murphy TJ, Alexander RW, 1993, Molecular Biology of the rennin-angiotensin system. *Circulation.* **87**: 1816–1828

Hansson L, Lindholm LH, Niskanen L, *et al* 1999, Effect of angiotensin-converting-enzyme inhibition compared with conventional therapy on cardiovascular morbidity and mortality in hypertension: the Captopril Prevention Project (CAPP) randomized trial. *Lancet.* **353**: 611–6

Hardie DG, 2004, The AMP-activated protein kinase pathway - New players upstream and downstream. *J Cell Sci.* **117**: 5479–5487

Heart Outcomes Prevention Evaluation Study Investigators, 2000, Effects of an angiotensin-converting-enzyme inhibitor, ramipril, on cardiovascular events in high-risk patients. *N Engl J Med.* **342**: 145–153

Hirochi M, Hayashida W, Akishita M, *et al* 1999, Stimulation of different subtypes of angiotensin II receptors, AT1 and AT2 receptors, regulates STAT activation by negative cross talk. *Circ Res.* **84**: 876–882

Hjorth SA, Schambye HT, Greenlee WJ, Schwartz TW, 1994, Identification of peptide binding residues in the extracellular domains of the AT1 receptor. *J Biol Chem.* **269**: 30953–30959

Horiuchi M, Hayashida W, Kambe T, Yamada T, Dzau VJ, 1997, Angiotensin type 2 receptor dephosphorylates Bcl-2 by activating mitogen-activating protein kinase phosphatase-1 and induces apoptosis. *J Biol Chem.* **272**: 19022–19026

Hotamisligil GS, Spiegelman BM, 1994, Tumor necrosis factor a: a key component of the obesity-diabetes link. *Diabetes.* **43**: 1271–1278

Huang XC, Richards EM, Sumners C, 1996, Mitogen-activated protein kinases in rat brain neuronal cultures are activated by angiotensin II type 1 receptors and inhibited by angiotensin II type 2 receptors. *J Biol Chem.* **271**: 15635–15641

James PT, Leach R, Kalamara E, Shayeghi M, 2001, The Worldwide obesity epidemic. *Obes Res.* **9**: 228S–233S

Jones BH, Stanridge MK, Moustaid N, 1997, Angiotensin II increased lipogenesis in 3T3-L1 and human adipose cells. *Endocrinology.* **138**: 1512–1519

Julius S, Kjeldsen SE Webel, M, *et al* 2004, Outcomes in hypertensives patients at high risk of cardiovascular risk treated with regimens based on valsartan and amlodipine: the VALUE randomized trial. *Lancet.* **363**: 2022–2231

Kadowaki T, Yamauchi T, Kubota N, Hara K, Ueki K, Tobe K, 2006 Adiponectin and adiponectin receptors in insulin resistance, diabetes, and the metabolic syndrome. *J Clin Invest.* **116**: 1784–1792

Karlsson C, Lindell K, Ottosson M, Sjostrom L, Carlsson B, Carlsson MS, 1998, Human adipose tissue expresses angiotensinogen and enzymes required for its conversion to Angiotensin II. *J Clin Endocrinol Metab.* **83**: 3925–3929

Ko SH, Hong OK, Kim JW, Ahn YB, Song KH, Cha BY, Son HY, Kim MJ, Jeong IK, Yoon KH, 2006, High glucose increases extracellular matrix production in pancreatic stellate cells by activating the renin-angiotensin system. *J Cell Biochem.* **98**: 343–55

Konishi H, Kuroda S, Inada Y, Fujisawa Y, 1994, Novel subtype of human angiotensin II type 1 receptor: cDNA cloning and expression. *Biochem Biophys Res Commun.* **199**: 467–474

Konoshita T, *et al* 2006, Tissue gene expression of renin-angiotensin system in human type 2 diabetic nephropathy. *Diabetes Care.* **29**: 848–52

Kristiansen OP, Mandrup-Poulse T, 2005, Interleukin-6 and Diabetes: The good, the bad, or the indifferent? *Diabetes.* **54** (Suppl 2): S114–S124

Krssak M, Falk Petersen K, Dresner A, *et al* 1999, Intramyocellular lipid concentrations are correlated with insulin sensitivity in humans: a 1H NMR spectroscopy study. *Diabetologia.* **42**: 113–116

Lam KY, Leung PS, 2002, Regulation and expression of a rennin-angiotensin system in human pancreas and pancreatic endocrine tumors. *Eur J Endocrinol,* **146**: 567–572

Lau T, Carlsson PO, Leung PS, 2004, Evidence for a local angiotensin system and dose-dependent inhibition of glucose-stimulated insulin release by angiotensin II in isolated pancreatic islets. *Diabetologia.* **47**: 240–248

Lastra G, Manrique C, Sowers, JR, 2006, Obesity and chronic kidney disease: The weight of the evidence. *Adv Chronic Kidney Dis.* **13**: 365–373

Leung PS, Carlsson PO, 2001, Tissue renin-angiotensin system: its expression, localization, regulation and potential role in the pancreas. *J Mol Endocrinol.* **26**: 155–164

Leung PS, Chappell MC, 2003, A local pancreatic renin-angiotensin system: endocrine and exocrine roles. *Int J Biochem Cell Biol.* **35**: 838–846

Licata G, Scaglione R, Ganguzza A, *et al* 1994, Central obesity and hypertension. Relationship between fasting serum insulin, plasma renin activity, and diastolic blood pressure in young obese subjects. *Am J Hypertens.* **7**: 314–320

Lorenzo O, Ruiz-Ortega M, Suzuki Y, *et al* 2002, Angiotensin III Activates Nuclear Transcription Factor-kB in Cultured Mesangial Cells Mainly via AT_2 Receptors: Studies with AT_1 Receptor-Knockout Mice. *J. Am. Soc. Nephrol.* **13**: 1162

Lorenzo, C, Serrano-Rios M, Martinez-Larrad MT, *et al* 2006, Geographic variations of the International Diabetes Federation anf the National Cholesterol Education Program – Adult Treatment Panel III Definitions of the metabolic syndrome in nondiabetic subjects. *Diabetes Care.* **29**: 685–691

Lupi *et al* 2006, The direct effects of the angiotensin converting enzyme inhibitors, zofenoprilat and enalaprilat, on isolated human pancreatic islets. *Eur J of Endocrinol.* **154**: 355–361

Madrid MI, Garcia-Duran M, Tornel J, De Gasparo M, Fenoy FJ, 1997, Effect of interactions between nitric oxide and angiotensin II on pressure natriuresis. *Am J Physiol Regulatory Integrative Comp Physiol.* **273**: R1676–R1682

Manrique C, Lastra G. Sowers JR, 2005, Hypertension and the Cardiometabolic Syndrome. *Journal of Clinical Hypertension.* **7**: 471–476

Massiera F, Bloch-Faure M, Ceiler D, *et al* 2001, Adipose angiotensinogen is involved in adipose tissue growth and blood pressure regulation. *FASEB J.* **15**: 2727–2729

Navar LG, 2004, The intrarenal renin-angiotensin system in hypertension. *Kidney Intl.* **65**: 1522–1532

Nguyen G, Bouzhir L, Delarue F, Rondeau E, Giller T, Sraer JD, 2002, Pivotal role of the renin/Prorenin receptor in Angiotensin II production and cellular responses to Renin. *J Clin Invest.* **109**: 1417–1427

Nickenig G, Harrison DG, 2002, The AT1-type angiotensin receptor in oxidative stress and atherogenesis. Part I: Oxidative stress and atherogenesis. *Circulation.* 105: 393–396

Nickenig G, Ostergren J, Struijke-Boudier H, 2006, Clinical evidence for the cardiovascular benefits of angiotensin receptor blockers. *JRAAS.* **7**: S1–S7

Ouchi N, Ohishi M, Kihara S, *et al* 2003, Association of hypoadiponectinemia with impaired vasoreactivity. *Journal of Hypertension.* **42**: 231–234

Ozono R, Wang ZQ, Moore AF, Inagami T, Siragy HM, Carey RM, 1997, Expression of the subtype 2 angiotensin (AT2) receptor protein in rat kidney. *Hypertension.* **30**: 1238–1246

Pagano PJ, Chanock SJ, Siwik DA, Colucci WS, Clark JK, 1998, Angiotensin II induces p67phox mRNA expression and NADPH oxidase superoxide generation in rabbit aortic adventitial fibroblasts. *Hypertension.* **32**: 331–337

Park YW, Zhu S, Palaniappan L, Heshka S, Carnethon MR, Heymsfield SB, 2003, The metabolic syndrome: Prevalence and risk factor findings in the US population from the third national health and nutrition examination survey, 1988 1994. *Arch Int Med.* **163**: 427–436

Paula RD, Lima CV, Khosla MC, 1995, Angiotensin (1–7) potentiates hypotensive effect of bradykinin in conscious rats. *Hypertension.* **26**: 1154–1159

Peach MJ, 1977, Renin-angiotensin system: Biochemistry and mechanisms of action. *Physiol Rev.* **57**: 313–370

Pickup JC, 2004, Inflammation and activated innate immunity in the pathogenesis of type 2 diabetes. *Diabetes Care.* **27**: 813–823

Pittas AG, Joseph NA, Greenberg AS, 2004, Adipocytokines and insulin resistance. *J Clin Endocrinol Metab.* **89**: 447–452

Pueyo ME, Gonzalez W, Nicoletti A, Savoie F, Arnal J, Michel J, 2000, Angiotensin II stimulates endothelial vascular cell adhesion molecule – 1 via nuclear factor κB activation induced by intracellular oxidative stress. *Arterioscler thromb Vasc Biol.* **20**: 645–654

Ran J, Hirano T, Adachi M, 2004, Angiotensin II type 1 receptor b locker ameliorates overproduction and accumulation of triglyceride in the liver of Zucker fatty rats. *Am J Physiol Endocrinol Metab.* **287**: E227–E232

Ravussin E, Smith SR, 2002, Increased fat intake, impaired fat oxidation, and failure of fat cell proliferation result in ectopic fat storage, insulin resistance and type 2 diabetes mellitus. *Ann N.Y. Acad Sci.* **967**: 363–378

Rodriguez-Vita J, Sanchez-Lopez E, Esteban V, Ruperez M, Egido J, Ruiz-Ortega M, 2005, Angiotensin II activates the Smad pathway in vascular smooth muscle cells by a transforming growth factor-beta-independent mechanism. *Circulation.* **111**: 2509–2517

Ruiz-Ortega M, Lorenzo O, Ruperez M, *et al* 2001, Systemic infusion of angiotensin II into normal rats activates nuclear factor κ-B and AP-1 in the kidney. Role of AT1 and AT2 receptors. *Am J Pathol.* **158**: 1743–175

Ruiz-Ortega M, Lorenzo O, Ruperez M, Kong S, Wittig B, Egido J, 2000, Angiotensin II activates nuclear transcription factor kB through AT1 and At2 in vascular smooth cells: molecular mechanisms. *Circ Res.* **86**: 1266–1272

Sadoshima J, 2000, Cytokine actions of angiotensin II. *Circ Res.* **86**: 1187–1189

Safonova I, Aubert J, Negrel R, Ailhaud G, 1997, Regulation by fatty acids of angiotensinogen gene expression in preadipose cells. *Biochem J.* **322** (Pt 1): 235–239

Saward L, Zahradka P, 1997, Angiotensin II activates phosphatidylinositol 3-kinase in vascular smooth cells. *Circ Res.* **81**: 249–25

Schneider BS, Faust IM, Hemmes R, Hirsch J, 1981, Effects of altered adipose tissue morphology on plasma insulin levels in the rat. *Am J Physiol.* **240**: E358–E362

Senn JJ, Klover PJ, Nowak IA, *et al* 2003, Suppressor of Cytokine Signaling – 3 (SOCS-3), a potential mediator of Interleukin-6-dependent insulin resistance in hepatocytes. *J Biol Chem.* **278**: 13740–13746

Sowers JR, 2002, Hypertension, angiotensin II and oxidative stress. *N Engl J Med.* **346**: 1999–2001

Stein CJ, Colditz GA, 2004, The epidemic of obesity. *J Clin Endocrinol Metab.* **89**: 2522–2525

Tahmasebi M, Puddefoot JR, Inwang ER, *et al* 1999, The tissue renin-angiotensin system in human pancreas. *J Endocrinol.* **161**: 317–322

The DREAM Trial Investigators, 2006, Effect of ramipril on the incidence of diabetes. N *Engl J Med.* **355**: 1551–62

Tikellis C, Cooper ME, Thomas MC, 2006, Role of the renin-angiotensin system in the endocrine pancreas: implications for the development of diabetes. *Int J Biochem Cell Biol.* **38**: 737–51

Tipnis SR, Hooper NM, Hyde R, Karran E, Christie G, Turner AJ, 2000, A human homolog of angiotensin-converting enzyme. Cloning and functional expression as a captopril-insensitive carboxypeptidase. *J Biol. Chem.* **275**: 33238–33243

Tsutsumi Y, Matsubara H, Masaki H, *et al* 1999, Angiotensin II type 2 receptor overexpression activates the vascular kynin system and causes vasodilatation. *J Clin Invest.* **104**: 925–935

Tuck ML, Sowers J, Dornfield L, Kledzik G, Maxwell M, 1981, The effect of weight reduction on blood pressure plasma renin activity and aldosterone levels in obese patients. *N Eng J Med.* **304**: 930–933

Ushio-Fukai M, Alexander W, 2004, Reactive oxygen species as mediators of angiogenesis signaling: Role of NADPH oxidase. *Mol Cell Biochem* **264**: 85–97

Ushio-Fukai M, Tabg Y, Fukai T, *et al* 2002, Novel role of gp91phox containing NADPH oxidase in vascular endothelial growth factor induced signaling and angiogenesis. *Circ Res.* **91**: 1160–1167

Van HV, Ariapart P, Hoffstedt J, Lundkvist I, Bringman S, Arner P, 2000, Increased adipose angiotensinogen gene expression in human obesity. *Obes Res.* **8**: 337–341

Vidotti, DB, Casarinin DE, Cristovam PC, Leite CA, Boim MA, 2004, High glucose concentration stimulates renin activity and angiotensin II generation in mesangial cells. *Am J Physiol Renal Physiol.* **286**: F1039–F1045

Wang HD, Hope SK, Du Y, Quinn MT, Cayatte AJ, Cohen RA, 1999, Paracrine role of adventitial superoxide anion in spontaneous tone in the isolated rat aorta in angiotensin II – induced hypertension. *Hypertension.* **33**: 1225–1232

Watanabe, T, Thomas A, Barker CB, 2005, Angiotensin II and the endothelium: Diverse signals and effects. *Hypertension.* **45**: 163–169

Yusuf S, Ostergren JB Gerstein HC, *et al* 2005, Candesartan in Heart Failure-Assessment of Reduction in Mortality and Morbidity Program Investigators. Effects of candesartan on the development of a new diagnosis of diabetes mellitus in patients with heart failure. *Circulation.* **112**: 48–53

Zuo L Ushio-Fukai M, Hilenski LL, Alexander RW, 2004, Microtubules regulate angiotensin II type 1 receptor and Rac1 localization in caveolae/lipid rafts: role in redox signaling. *Arterioscler Thromb Vasc Biol.* **24**: 1223–1228

Zuo L, Ushio-Fukai M, Ikeda S, Hilenski L, Patrushev N, Alexander RW, 2005, Caveolin 1 is Essential for Activation of Rac-1 and NADPH oxidase After Angiotensin II Type 1 receptor stimulation in Vascular Smooth Muscle Cells: Role in Redox Signaling and Vascular Hyperthophy. *Arterioscler Thromb Vasc Biol.* **25**: 1824–1830

CHAPTER 6

THE ROLE OF THE RENIN-ANGIOTENSIN SYSTEM IN HEPATIC FIBROSIS

J.S. LUBEL[1], F.J. WARNER[2], AND P.W. ANGUS[1]

[1]*Department of Gastroenterology, Austin Health, Studley Road, Heidelberg, Melbourne, Victoria, Australia*
[2]*A.W. Morrow Gastroenterology and Liver Centre, Centenary Institute of Cancer Medicine and Cell Biology, University of Sydney, Sydney, Australia*

1. INTRODUCTION

The liver is the second largest organ of the body and has a multitude of functions including carbohydrate and fatty acid metabolism, lipid transport, protein synthesis, storage of fat-soluble vitamins as well as detoxification and modification of compounds absorbed from the small intestine. It has a dual blood supply, with approximately 75% coming from the portal vein and 25% from the hepatic artery. The primary functional unit of the liver, the hepatic lobule, consists of a hexagonal zone of hepatic parenchyma surrounding a central hepatic vein with a number of portal tracts at the periphery which contain a terminal portal vein, bile ductule and hepatic arteriole. In the normal liver, blood flows from portal venous branches through specialised vascular channels called hepatic sinusoids, into the centrilobular hepatic vein. Hepatic sinusoids lack a distinct basement membrane and their endothelial cells have fenestrations which permit bidirectional free passage of solutes between the sinusoid and a sub-sinusoidal space known as the space of Disse. Hepatocytes, account for 70% of liver mass. These cells, which have microvilli on their basolateral surface to facilitate the interchange of nutrients with the sinusoid, are responsible for most of the metabolic and synthetic functions of the liver.

Chronic liver diseases disturb the normal structure and function of the liver by initiating hepatic fibrosis, a process that can eventually lead to progressive destruction of the normal hepatic architecture, loss of functioning hepatocytes and the development of liver cirrhosis. Angiotensin II, the main effector peptide of the renin-angiotensin system (RAS), is known to play an important role in chronic tissue injury and fibrosis in cardiovascular disease, chronic renal disease and diabetes. Its

113

Po Sing Leung (ed.), Frontiers in Research of the Renin-Angiotensin System on Human Disease, 113–134.
© 2007 *Springer.*

role in liver disease is less well established, however, recent studies indicate that, as in other organs, there is a renin-angiotensin-system within the liver and that locally generated angiotensin II plays an important role in the pathogenesis of liver injury and hepatic fibrosis. There is also evidence that in the fibrotic liver angiotensin II contributes to portal hypertension by stimulating contraction of perisinusoidal myofibroblasts and increasing sinusoidal resistance to portal flow. In addition to these local effects in the liver, the systemic RAS is activated in patients with advanced liver disease in response to mesenteric and systemic vasodilatation and has an important homeostatic role in maintaining adequate perfusion pressure to the kidney and other vital organs. It also contributes to renal sodium and water retention by releasing aldosterone and by stimulating secretion of antidiuretic hormone (ADH) from the posterior pituitary. These multiple roles of the RAS in liver disease have lead to major interest in the potential role of RAS antagonists in the prevention of liver fibrosis and the treatment of chronic liver disease and its complications.

2.   PATHOGENESIS AND SIGNIFICANCE OF HEPATIC FIBROSIS

There are a large number of chronic liver diseases which cause hepatic fibrosis, including chronic viral hepatitis, alcoholic liver disease, non-alcoholic fatty liver disease, iron overload, diseases of the biliary tract and immune and metabolic liver diseases. Cirrhosis, the end stage of hepatic fibrosis, is characterised by the presence of extensive fibrotic septa separating and surrounding parenchymal nodules of regenerating hepatocytes. This disturbance of the normal hepatic architecture, in conjunction with vasoconstriction within the liver, impedes portal blood flow causing portal hypertension; this is the cause of many of the serious complications of cirrhosis including variceal bleeding, hepatic encephalopathy and ascites. Hepatitis B infection is the most common cause of cirrhosis worldwide. It is also the single most important cause of hepatocellular carcinoma, a disease responsible for nearly one third of the world's cancer-related deaths (Lodato et al 2006).

Currently the only proven treatment for hepatic fibrosis is to remove the responsible injurious agent. Recent studies have shown that if this can be achieved, for example by eliminating viral replication in patients with chronic hepatitis B or C, hepatic fibrosis and even early stage cirrhosis can resolve. In patients with end-stage cirrhosis and liver failure, therapy is limited to symptom control and the prevention of life threatening complications such as variceal bleeding whilst cure can only be achieved with liver transplantation. Unfortunately despite major advances in antiviral therapy in recent years, many patients with chronic hepatitis do not respond to therapy. There are also a number of chronic liver diseases for which we currently do not have effective treatment. There is therefore an ongoing need to develop anti-fibrotic therapies that can be used to prevent fibrosis progression and the development of cirrhosis.

In the healthy liver, extracellular matrix (ECM) consists of collagens (predominantly type IV), glycoproteins, proteoglycans and glycosaminoglycans which provide a structural and functional framework for cellular migration, adhesion, differentiation, proliferation and fibrogenic activation (Schuppan *et al* 2001). The space of Disse contains a delicate ECM with basement membrane-like composition, which permits solute diffusion from blood within the sinusoids to the surrounding cells. Hepatic fibrosis results in major changes to both the volume and composition of ECM. There are increases in the interstitial fibrillar collagens types I and III as well as non-fibrillar collagens (types IV and VI). Proteoglycan and glycosamino-glycan content also increases with the overall composition of the ECM changing from a low-density form to a denser more complex interstitial type. The collagenous and non-collagenous ECM content of the liver is increased by at least 3-5 fold in the cirrhotic liver. There is an associated loss of hepatocyte microvilli and struc-tural changes to the sinusoidal endothelium which include loss of fenestrations, and deposition of fibrillar collagen in the space of Disse. These changes impair the transfer of sinusoidal nutrients to hepatocytes facilitating further hepatocyte injury and liver dysfunction.

The pattern of liver fibrosis ultimately depends on the site and intensity of injury. Hence, biliary obstruction results in bile ductular and periductular myofi-broblast proliferation and initially produces periportal and then linking portal-portal fibrosis, viral hepatitis infection leads to portal and then portal-central fibrosis whilst disruption to hepatic venous outflow (as occurs in right ventricular failure or Budd Chiari syndrome) causes centrolobular hepatocyte necrosis and leads to centrolobular fibrosis (central to central septa) (Cassiman and Roskams 2002).

The cell type involved in hepatic fibrosis which has been most studied is the hepatic stellate cell (HSC). In part, this is due to the relative ease with which this cell can be isolated, purified and subcultured from both human and animal liver tissue. However, it has become clear from characterisation of cellular markers and electron microscopic studies that there is a diverse population of myofibroblasts within the liver that may also contribute to hepatic fibrosis. These include portal and septal myofibroblasts, cells residing in vessel walls, centrilobular myofibroblasts, and even marrow-derived HSC and myofibroblasts (Cassiman 2002, Kallis, Alison and Forbes 2006, Russo *et al* 2006). It is likely that the expression and importance of these myofibroblast subtypes vary in different human diseases and animal models.

The HSC normally resides in the space of Disse and is responsible for the storage of vitamin A. It is maintained in a quiescent, non-fibrogenic phenotype, in part, by the surrounding ECM composed predominantly of collagen IV (the collagen type present within the lamina densa of the basal lamina) and other non-collagenous components such as laminins. Following repetitive injury, changes in composition of the ECM in conjunction with the release of proinflammatory and profibrotic cytokines released from damaged hepatocytes, Kuppfer cells and inflammatory cells, leads to a cascade of events culminating in the transformation of HSCs into activated myofibroblasts. These activated cells deposit extracellular matrix (ECM) but in addition express contractile proteins which enable them to modulate sinusoidal blood flow. HSCs are capable of producing a broad array of profibrotic and proin-flammatory cytokines and chemokines including tansforming growth factor beta-1 (TGFβ1), platelet derived growth factor (PDGF) and angiotensin II, all of which can act in both a paracrine and autocrine manner to further perpetuate fibrosis (Friedman, Maher and Bissell 2000). As will be discussed below, recent data have shown that angiotensin II is involved in both the recruitment of inflammatory cells in response to liver injury (Sewnath *et al* 2004) and transformation of hepatic stellate cells to their activated phenotype (Bataller *et al* 2003).

Hepatic fibrosis is a dynamic process and the end result reflects a balance between pathways which lead to matrix accumulation and those which result in matrix degradation and fibrosis resolution. Matrix metalloproteinases (MMPs) capable of enzymatically degrading ECM are secreted from many liver cells including HSCs, Kuppfer cells, hepatocytes and macrophages (Knittel *et al* 1999). Certain MMPs (MMP-2, MMP-9 and MMP-3) may contribute to the pathogenesis of fibrosis by facilitating liver remodelling, altering both the quantity and the composition of the ECM. Other MMP subtypes (MMP-1, MMP-8) degrade fibrillar collagens in the fibrotic liver and therefore drive fibrosis resolution. Counterbalancing the effects of MMPs is a group of tissue inhibitors of metalloproteinases (TIMPs), which promote collagen and matrix deposition by preventing ECM degradation by matrix proteinases (Arthur 2000).

3.   THE RENIN-ANGIOTENSIN SYSTEM

3.1.   The Circulating Renin-Angiotensin System

Since the discovery of renin from kidney extracts by Tigerstedt and Bergman in 1898 our understanding of the intricacies of the organisation and function of the renin-angiotensin system (RAS) has expanded considerably (Tigerstedt R 1898, Basso and Terragno 2001). The circulating RAS is best known for its role as a regulator of blood pressure, and fluid and electrolyte homeostasis. Angiotensin II, the principal effector of the RAS, causes vasoconstriction directly by stimulating angiotensin type 1 (AT_1) receptors present on the surface of vascular smooth muscle cells and indirectly by potentiating the release of norepinephrine from postganglionic sympathetic fibres and stimulating antidiuretic hormone (ADH) release from the posterior pituitary. Long-term, angiotensin II regulates blood pressure by modulating sodium and water reabsorption through stimulation of AT_1 receptors in the kidney, and by stimulating the production and release of aldosterone from the adrenal glands. In addition, angiotensin II increases thirst sensation through stimulation of the subfornical organ within the diencephalon (Timmermans *et al* 1992). Other effects that may be important in chronic organ damage include promotion of thrombosis, cardiac hypertrophy and angiogenesis.

The classical enzymatic pathway generating angiotensin II begins with the cleavage of the peptide bond between the leucine and valine residues on angiotensinogen producing the biologically inactive decapeptide, angiotensin I. This process is mediated by renin, an aspartic protease released from juxtaglomerular cells of the kidney into the circulation. The cascade continues with Angiotensin Converting Enzyme (ACE) found predominantly in the capillaries of the lung cleaving a dipeptide from the C-terminus of angiotensin I to form angiotensin II. The actions of angiotensin II are mediated via specific seven transmembrane G protein-coupled receptors. In humans, two angiotensin receptors (AT_1 and AT_2) with differing affinities for angiotensin II have been described (Timmermans *et al* 1992). Angiotensin II can further be cleaved at either its carboxy- or amino-terminus to produce biologically active angiotensin fragments. Thus, from the amino-terminus, Angiotensin III (2-8) can be formed following cleavage of the aspartate-arginine bond of angiotensin II by aminopeptidase A and angiotensin IV (3-8) can be formed following further cleavage of angiotensin III by aminopeptidase B and N (Ardaillou 1997). Angiotensin III shares many of the properties of angiotensin II with 40% of the pressor activity and 100% of the aldosterone stimulating activity of angiotensin II. Angiotensin IV has its own distinct receptor (AT_4) and has central nervous system effects together with some opposing actions to angiotensin II (von Bohlen und Halbach 2003). Enzymatic cleavage of the carboxy-terminus of angiotensin II or angiotensin I can produce the biologically active fragment angiotensin (1-7).

There has been renewed interest in the circulating RAS following the simultaneous discovery by two independent research groups in 2000 of an ACE homologue called ACE2. These two enzymes share 61% protein sequence similarity but have distinct enzymatic actions and tissue distributions (Donoghue *et al* 2000, Tipnis *et al* 2000). Like ACE, ACE2 is a zinc metalloprotease and a type 1 integral membrane protein expressed predominantly on the cell surface and as such acts as an ectoenzyme (Warner *et al* 2005). In its membrane bound form it comprises an extracellular N-terminal domain containing the active site and a short intracellular C-terminal anchor. The highest levels of ACE2 are seen in the kidney, heart, testis and gastrointestinal tract (particularly ileum, duodenum, jejunum, caecum and colon) with lower levels expressed in liver and lung (Harmer *et al* 2002, Hamming *et al* 2004, Donoghue 2000, Tipnis 2000). ACE2 can be released from the cell surface by the action of a secretase-like enzyme and the soluble ACE2 formed can be detected in plasma and urine (Lambert *et al* 2005, Lew *et al* 2006, Ocaranza *et al* 2006, Rice *et al* 2006). In contrast to ACE, ACE2 contains only a single catalytic domain compared with the two active sites (N- and C-domains) of somatic ACE. Furthermore, ACE2 is a carboxypeptidase rather than a peptidyl dipeptidase. As a consequence of its mechanism of action, ACE2 has different substrate specificity to that of ACE (Warner *et al* 2004) and also is not inhibited in-vitro by ACE inhibitors such as captopril, lisinopril or enalaprilat (Tipnis 2000).

ACE2 has activity on a number of biologically active peptides including angiotensin I and angiotensin II, des Arg[9] bradykinin, apellin 13 and dynorphin A (1-13) (Vickers *et al* 2002). The enzyme has a preference for hydrophobic or basic residues at the carboxy-terminus as well as for propyl residues at the penultimate position (Table 1) (Turner 2003).

The many diverse functions and interactions of ACE2 are only now being realised (Burrell *et al* 2004, Thomas and Tikellis 2005). This enzyme is not only crucial in cardiovascular and renal injury, but also has been identified as the receptor for the SARS coronavirus (W. Li *et al* 2003). Of particular interest over the past 5 years

Table 1. Peptide substrates for ACE2 showing catalytic efficiency in descending order. Note that ACE2 catalytic efficiency for angiotensin II is 400 fold that of angiotensin I (Vickers 2002)

Substrate	Site of cleavage	Catalytic efficiency (k_{cat}/K_m)
Dynorphin A (1-13)	L-K	3.1×10^6 m^{-1}.s^{-1}
Apelin-13	P-F	2.1×10^6 m^{-1}.s^{-1}
Angiotensin II	P-F	$\mathbf{1.9 \times 10^6}$ **m**$^{-1}$.**s**$^{-1}$
Des-Arg^9-bradykinin	P-F	1.3×10^5 m^{-1}.s^{-1}
Angiotensin I	H-L	$\mathbf{4.9 \times 10^3}$ **m**$^{-1}$.**s**$^{-1}$

has been the role of ACE2 in the formation of the biologically active fragment angiotensin (1-7). ACE2 can generate angiotensin (1-7) directly through enzymatic cleavage of angiotensin II or indirectly by cleaving angiotensin I into the inactive peptide fragment angiotensin (1-9), which is then further enzymatically cleaved by ACE to angiotensin (1-7) (Zisman *et al* 2003, Zisman *et al* 2003). Of these two pathways, the conversion of angiotensin II to angiotensin (1-7) by ACE2 is kinetically favoured *in-vitro* (Vickers 2002, Rice *et al* 2004). Furthermore, in-vitro studies show ACE2 to be 10- to 600-fold more potent in hydrolysing Angiotensin II to Angiotensin (1-7) than propyl endopeptidase and propyl carboxypeptidase, peptidases with similar carboxypeptidase actions (Ferrario 2003). These findings suggest that ACE2 is a major angiotensin (1-7) generating enzyme as well as an important enzyme for the degradation of angiotensin II.

The biological effects of angiotensin (1-7) were first described in the rat hypothalamic-hypophysial implant in 1988 in which angiotensin (1-7) stimulated release of vasopressin (Schiavone *et al* 1988). Subsequent animal experiments have shown angiotensin (1-7) to have antihypertensive (Benter *et al* 1995), antiarrhythmic (Ferreira, Santos and Almeida 2001) and cardioprotective properties (Ferreira, Santos and Almeida 2002). The vasodilatory effects of angiotensin (1-7) are mediated through the release of nitric oxide (NO) (Nakamoto *et al* 1995, P. Li *et al* 1997, Brosnihan, Li and Ferrario 1996), prostaglandins (Freeman *et al* 1996, Iyer *et al* 2000) and the release and interaction with bradykinin (P. Li 1997, Gorelik, Carbini and Scicli 1998, Fernandes *et al* 2001, Ueda *et al* 2001). Angiotensin (1-7) has also been shown to have anti-trophic properties in vascular endothelial, smooth muscle cells, cardiac myocytes, and cardiac fibroblasts (Freeman 1996, Strawn, Ferrario and Tallant 1999, Iwata *et al* 2005, Tallant, Ferrario and Gallagher 2005). In addition, anti-inflammatory, anti-fibrotic (Grobe *et al* 2006, Grobe *et al* 2006) and anti-thrombotic properties (Kucharewicz *et al* 2000, Kucharewicz *et al* 2002) have been attributed to angiotensin (1-7).

The putative receptor for angiotensin (1-7) is the G protein-coupled receptor encoded by the *Mas* proto-oncogene (Santos *et al* 2003). This receptor has been shown in-vitro to hetero-oligomerize with the AT$_1$ receptor and act as a physiological antagonist to angiotensin II as well as interact with the AT$_2$ receptor (Castro *et al* 2005, Kostenis *et al* 2005). Evidence is emerging that AT$_2$ receptors and other yet unidentified angiotensin (1-7) receptor subtypes may be important in the biological action of angiotensin (1-7) (Walters, Gaspari and Widdop 2005, Silva *et al* 2006). Some of the actions of angiotensin (1-7) clearly oppose those of angiotensin II and consequently it has been proposed that the RAS can be divided on this basis into two distinct arms that are capable of producing complementary effects (Fig. 1). Thus our conceptual understanding of the RAS has evolved from an endocrine system consisting of a linear sequence of enzymatic reactions yielding the effector peptide angiotensin II to a complex system closely integrated with other systems (such as the kinin-kallikrein system) with the potential of producing effector peptides with counterbalancing effects (angiotensin (1-7) and angiotensin II). Importantly, the RAS is not just a systemic endocrine system but also can function autonomously as a paracrine system within certain organs.

3.2.   The Intra-hepatic RAS

Local or intra-organ renin-angiotensin systems have been described in a number of organs including the heart, kidney, liver and pancreas (Bataller 2003, Leung and Chappell 2003). These local systems have been shown to be responsive to various stimuli of physiological and pathophysiological importance. Moreover, the locally generated angiotensin peptides fragments have a plethora of actions and have been

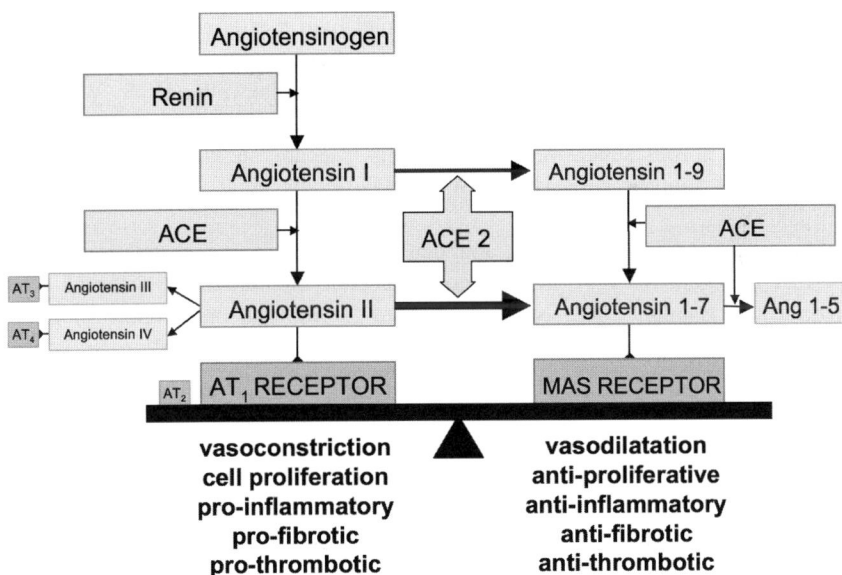

Figure 1. The Renin-Angiotensin System. Peptides are shown in blue boxes, enzymes in yellow boxes and target receptors in pink boxes. The system has four known biologically active peptides, angiotensin II, III, IV and angiotensin 1-7, which act through distinct cellular receptors (AT_{1-4} and Mas). The two principal arms of this system act via the AT_1 and Mas receptors and have opposing actions

implicated in cell growth, anti-proliferation, apoptosis, reactive oxygen species generation, hormonal secretion, pro-inflammatory, and pro-fibrogenic actions.

The role of the hepatic RAS in normal and diseased liver is less well described than that of the heart and kidney. However, it is clear that most of the key components of the enzymatic cascade that lead to the formation of angiotensin II in other organs are present in the liver. One common theme throughout the literature is the observation that liver injury is associated with an up-regulation and/or redistribution of RAS components including angiotensinogen, renin, ACE, angiotensin II and AT_1 receptors (Sakata et al 1991, Paizis et al 2002, Bataller 2003). The main source of the RAS precursor, angiotensinogen, is the hepatocyte (Morris, Iwamoto and Reid 1979, Paizis 2002), but low levels of protein have also been detected in Kupffer cells, and in the bile duct epithelium (Sawa 1990). Studies in humans and rodents show plasma renin concentration and activity and its substrate angiotensinogen are increased in cirrhotic livers compared to controls (Morris 1979, Richoux et al 1983, Kojima et al 1998, Rincon-Sanchez et al 2005, Rivera-Huizar et al 2006). The product of angiotensiogen cleavage by renin, angiotensin I, has not been demonstrated in liver tissue, however, there is evidence to suggest de novo generation of angiotensin I may occur locally in hepatomesenteric vascular beds as well as in circulating plasma (Admiraal et al 1990). In contrast, angiotensin II is present in both plasma and liver tissue from normal animals and increases significantly in rat models of liver disease and in cirrhotic patients (Asbert et al 1992, Wang et al 2003, Herath et al 2006). Other RAS components expressed in the normal liver tissue include ACE and the AT_1 receptor which are both predominantly localised to vascular endothelia, but are also observed in hepatocytes and bile duct epithelial cells (H. S. Wei et al 2000, Ikura et al 2005). In the fibrotic liver, ACE and AT_1 protein expression is also found in fibrous septa, mesenchymal cells (hepatic stellate cells and myofibroblasts) and Kupffer cells (H. S. Wei 2000, Paizis 2002, Leung et al 2003, Ikura 2005).

Although the AT_1 receptor is abundant in the liver, the expression of the AT_2 receptor gene is very low or not detectable in normal or diseased liver (Paizis 2002, Bataller 2003, Nabeshima et al 2006). The only report so far to attribute AT_2 receptor gene expression to a particular liver cell type is that of Bataller and co-workers who detected low levels of the receptor messenger RNA in isolated human hepatocytes and all HSC phenotypes (quiescent, culture activated and in vivo activated) (Bataller 2003). Despite the possible existence of AT_2 receptors in the liver, and a recent study showing that ablation of AT_2 receptors augments liver injury and fibrosis (Nabeshima 2006), the vast majority of reports support the concept that AT_1 receptors mediate most of the inflammatory, proliferative and vascular effects of angiotensin II in the liver (Bataller 2003, Kanno, Tazuma and Chayama 2003, Yoshiji et al 2003, Bataller et al 2005). Moreover, the gene expression of AT_1 on human myofibroblasts has been shown to correlate with the extent of fibrosis and degree of portal hypertension (Ikura 2005).

4.   HEPATIC FIBROSIS AND THE RAS

There is increasing evidence that in the liver, angiotensin II regulates cell growth and fibrosis and is involved in key events of inflammation and wound healing. One cell type that is pivotal in these processes is the activated hepatic stellate cell. Following injury, expression of AT_1 receptors is increased on activated hepatic stellate cells and these cells demonstrate increased responsiveness to angiotensin II compared to quiescent HSC (Bataller *et al* 2000). Incubation of the activated HSCs with angiotensin II results in a dose dependent increase in intracellular calcium concentration, cell contraction and cellular proliferation through a mitogen-activated protein kinase (MAPK) -dependent pathway and these effects are blocked by losartan, an angiotensin II type 1 receptor antagonist (ARB), (Bataller 2000). ARBs block other dose dependent profibrotic and proinflammatory effects of angiotensin II on HSCs including the expression of inflammatory cytokines and growth factors such as TGF-β1, IL-1β, CTGF, and NF-$\kappa\beta$, production of extracellular matrix (ECM) and fibrotic markers, smooth muscle α-actin and collagen (H. S. Wei 2000, Ohishi *et al* 2001, Yoshiji *et al* 2001, Bataller 2003, Kurikawa *et al* 2003, Y. Zhang *et al* 2003, Y. J. Zhang *et al* 2003). Angiotensin II is also a powerful chemo-attractant for activated HSCs concentrating these cells at the site of hepatic injury (Bataller *et al* 2003). These effects may be amplified by upregulation of key components of a local RAS by liver injury (Paizis 2002, Bataller 2003), creating an autocrine loop in which liver injury increases angiotensin II production and this in turn perpetuates liver damage and fibrosis.

A recent study showed that these profibrogenic effects of angiotensin II in human hepatic stellate cells are at least in part mediated via the generation of reactive oxygen species (ROS) by NADPH oxidase. This proposed mechanism is supported by the finding that hepatic fibrosis following bile duct ligation is markedly attenuated in NADPH oxidase-deficient mice (Bataller 2003). NADPH oxidase is expressed in other hepatic cell types including Kupffer cells and sinusoidal endothelial cells and these cells may also contribute to fibrogenesis through the formation of ROS (Whalen *et al* 1999, Kono *et al* 2000).

The importance of the RAS in hepatic fibrosis is supported by studies which have shown that inflammation and fibrosis in response to both CCL4 treatment (Kanno 2003) and bile duct ligation (Yang *et al* 2005) are attenuated in AT_1 knockout mice. Supporting evidence has also come from *in-vivo* studies which have shown that angiotensin II infusion stimulates proliferation of bile duct cells, exacerbates liver fibrosis and increases serum transaminases and endotoxin levels in BDL rat livers (Bataller *et al* 2005). Interestingly, angiotensin II infusion increases the number of vascular thromboses of small hepatic vessels within portal tracts in both BDL and sham operated animals, the putative mechanism being an increase in tissue factor procoagulant activity (Bataller 2005). This prothrombotic effect of angiotensin II may contribute to further liver injury and collagen deposition by causing local hypoxia (Corpechot *et al* 2002).

In addition to its direct profibrotic effects, angiotensin II is an amplifier of the general inflammatory response to chronic liver injury and induces acute phase reactants, oxidative stress, the release of inflammatory and fibrogenic cytokines (IL-6, IL-1, TGFβ1, TNFα) and ECM deposition (Bataller 2003, Miyoshi *et al* 2003, Bataller 2005, Sasaki *et al* 2005). In addition to complex interactions with other cell types, angiotensin II induces the secretion of monocyte chemoattractant protein (MCP-1) and IL-8 from activated HSCs (Marra *et al* 1998, Kanno *et al* 2005). MCP-1 is a low molecular weight secretory protein that potently stimulates leukocyte recruitment and activation. Upregulation of MCP-1 gene expression is though to be mediated via Rho intracellular signalling pathways following angiotensin II binding to the AT_1 receptor (Kanno 2005). Other events that occur as a result of AT_1 receptor activation include the release of a number of transcription factors; activator Protein 1 (AP-1), signal transducer and activator of Transcription (STATs) and NFκB (Jamaluddin *et al* 2000, McAllister-Lucas *et al* 2006), which are crucial for many of the downstream pro-inflammatory effects of angiotensin II such as the production of cytokine, IL-6. Furthermore, activation of the transcription factor NFκB is a fundamental positive feedback mechanism by which angiotensin II acting at AT1 receptors located on hepatocytes stimulates the transcription of angiotensinogen, the precursor of angiotensin (Ron, Brasier and Habener 1990, Brasier, Li and Copland 1994). A number of cell types present within the liver express AT_1 receptors and may contribute to these proinflammatory effects of AngII (Leung 2003, X. Zhang *et al* 2004). For example, Kupffer cells, the resident hepatic macrophage, are activated in alcoholic liver disease and are stimulated by angiotensin II to produce TNF-α and TGF-β1 (Enomoto *et al* 2000). The production of these cytokines by Kuppfer cells is significantly reduced by the angiotensin receptor antagonist (ARB), losartan but not the ACE inhibitor captopril, confirming the role of the AT_1 receptor in this cell type (Y. H. Wei, Jun and Qiang 2004).

The hepatic RAS also appears to affect the balance between ECM deposition and degradation which depends on the relative activity of matrix metalloproteinases (MMPs) and their inhibitors, tissue inhibitors of metalloproteinases (TIMPs). TIMP-1 is a broad specificity inhibitor of MMPs which acts by forming 1:1 complexes with MMPs. Angiotensin II upregulates TIMP-1 mRNA expression in activated HSCs through AT_1 receptor binding and subsequent protein kinase C (PKC) intracellular signalling pathways. This has been verified in two animal models of fibrosis (pig serum and CCL_4) where down-regulation of TIMP-1 gene expression followed administration of ACE inhibitors or ARB (Yoshiji 2003).

Paizis et al, recently demonstrated that ACE2 gene expression and protein levels are markedly elevated in the BDL liver and cirrhotic human liver tissue, opening the possibility that this putative counter-regulatory arm of the RAS is actively involved in chronic liver disease (Paizis *et al* 2005). In addition angiotensin (1-7), ACE2 and Mas, have recently been shown to increase progressively following bile duct ligation in rats (Herath 2006, Lubel *et al* 2006, Pereira *et al* 2006). Furthermore in this same model, pharmacological blockade of the Mas receptor may worsen liver fibrosis (Pereira 2006). The potential benefits of angiotensin (1-7) are of particular clinical relevance because both ACE inhibitors and angiotensin receptor blockers (ARBs) can result in elevations in angiotensin (1-7) raising the possibility that some of the beneficial effects of these drugs are mediated by this peptide (Iyer, Ferrario and Chappell 1998, Collister and Hendel 2003).

4.1.   Effects of RAS Inhibition on Hepatic Fibrosis in vivo

ACE inhibitors have been found to have multiple benefits in both cardiovascular and renal disease (hypertension, prevention of myocardial infarction and stroke, preventing heart failure, arrhythmias, renal failure, proteinuria and diabetic nephropathy). Losartan was the first drug of an alternative class of RAS antagonists which block the angiotensin II type 1 receptor. Subsequently a large number of ACE inhibitors and angiotensin receptor blockers (ARBs) have been developed. These two classes of drug collectively have been shown to reduce chronic end-organ damage in cardiovascular and renal disease and diabetes. The benefits of these drugs appear to be independent of their antihypertensive effects suggesting that they have direct antifibrotic or tissue protective effects in these diseases.

4.2.   Studies in Animal Models

Interventional animal studies using RAS inhibitors have provided compelling evidence that the RAS plays a major role in the pathogenesis of hepatic fibrosis. Most of these studies have been performed in rodents and several established models of hepatic fibrosis have been used (Table 2) (Ramos *et al* 1994, H. Wei *et al* 2000, Jonsson *et al* 2001, Ohishi 2001, Paizis *et al* 2001, Yoshiji *et al* 2001, Croquet *et al* 2002, Ramalho *et al* 2002, Toblli *et al* 2002, Yoshiji *et al* 2002, Kurikawa 2003, X. Li *et al* 2003, Tuncer *et al* 2003, Yoshiji 2003, X. Li *et al* 2004, Y. H. Wei 2004, Yoshiji *et al* 2005). Although methodologies have differed widely, there is a surprising degree of uniformity in the results. In almost all published studies, both ACE inhibitors and AT1 receptor blockers have been shown to have beneficial effects. These include both the attenuation of fibrosis and down-regulation of key inflammatory and profibrotic cytokines known to be involved in the pathogenesis of hepatic fibrosis. A summary of the major findings of these studies is provided in Table 2.

One of the most common and serious complications of cirrhosis is the development of hepatocellular carcinoma. In keeping with the known proliferative and angiogenic effects of angiotensin II, there is increasing evidence that the RAS is involved in the development and growth of this neoplasm. Experiments in mice have shown that the potent angiogenic factor vascular endothelial growth factor (VEGF) is induced by angiotensin II and that the ACE inhibitor, perindopril, significantly attenuates VEGF-mediated tumour development. (Yoshiji, Kuriyama and Fukui 2002, Yoshiji et al 2002)

4.3.   Human Studies

The efficacy, ease of use and excellent safety profile of RAS blockers in the treatment of patients with cardiovascular and renal disease makes them an attractive

Table 2. In-vivo animal evidence of RAS involvement in hepatic fibrosis using either ACE inhibitors (ACEi) or angiotensin receptor blockers (ARBs)

Model	Strain/Species	RAS Blocker	Histological improvement	OH Proline	Fibrosis markers	Collagen expression	Portal pressure/flow	TGFB	MMP	PDGF	α-SMA	Author
Bile Duct Ligation (BDL)	SD Rat	Losartan	✓	✓	×		✓					(Croquet et al. 2002)
	Lewis Rats	Captopril	✓	✓	✓			✓	✓		✓	(Jonsson et al. 2001)
	SD Rat	Olmesartan	✓	✓		✓		✓			✓	(Kurikawa et al. 2003)
	SD Rat	Irbesartan	×	×								(Paizis et al. 2001)
	Wistar Rat	Losartan	✓	✓	✓	✓	✓	✓			✓	(Ramalho et al. 2002)
	SD Rat	Losartan	✓		✓	✓	✓					(Croquet et al. 2002)
	Wistar Rat	Perindopril	✓		✓			✓	✓	✓		(X. Li et al. 2003)
	Wistar Rat	Losartan	✓		✓			✓	✓	✓		(X. Li et al. 2003)
	Wistar Rat	Perindopril	✓		✓			✓	✓	✓		(X. Li et al. 2004)
	SD Rat	Lisinopril	✓		✓	✓						(Ohishi et al. 2001)
Carbon Tetrachloride (CCL₄)	SD Rat	Captopril	×								×	(Tuncer et al. 2003)
	SD Rat	Candesartan	✓								✓	
	SD Rat	Enalapril	✓									(H. S. Wei et al. 2000)
		Losartan	✓									
		Losartan & Enalapril	✓									
	SD Rat	Losartan	✓	✓	✓	✓						(Y. H. Wei et al. 2004)
		Captopril	✓	✓	✓	✓						
		Candesartan	✓									
	Fisher Rats	Perindopril	✓			✓						(Yoshiji et al. 2003)
	BALB/c mice	Perindopril	✓			✓					✓	(Yoshiji et al. 2005)

Portal Vein Ligation (PVL)	SD Rat	Losartan	×						(Croquet et al. 2002)
Adriamycin induced nephrotic syndrome	SD Rat	Enalapril	✓	×	×	×			(Tobli et al. 2002)
Choline deficient L-amino aci12fd (CDAA) diet	Fisher Rat	Perindopril	✓	✓	✓			✓	(Yoshiji et al. 2002)
	Wistar Rat	Captopril	✓	✓					(Ramos et al. 1994)
Pig serum injection	Fisher Rats	Candesartan	✓		✓	✓		✓	(Yoshiji et al. 2001)
		Perindopril	✓		✓	✓		✓	
	Fisher Rats	Candesartan	✓	✓					(Yoshiji et al. 2003)
		Perindopril	✓	✓					

SD, Sprague Dawley; OH Proline, hydroxyproline; ✓ denotes a positive finding; × denotes a negative finding.

potential therapy for the treatment of human liver disease. The effects of AT_1 blockade on portal hypertension have been examined in a number of studies. The rationale for these studies is that angiotensin II increases intra hepatic resistance to portal flow in the cirrhotic liver by mediating contraction of perisinusoidal myofibroblasts and thus contributes to the variable component of portal hypertension (Vlachogiannakos et al 2001). Although some studies have shown that these drugs can lower portal pressure, their use has been associated with unacceptable drops in systemic blood pressure and renal blood flow, particularly in patients with advanced liver disease. This is because the systemic renin angiotensin system is activated in such patients in response to systemic and mesenteric vasodilation (Arroyo et al 1979, Bosch et al 1980, Sakata 1991) and plays a central role in the maintenance of renal perfusion pressure and glomerular filtration.

There have been only a small number of studies examining the effects of RAS inhibition on fibrosis in human liver disease and there are no large randomised trials. This may at first seem surprising considering the wealth of supportive evidence that has come from animal and in-vitro studies. However, studies of antifibrogenic therapies are difficult to perform in man because of the need to perform multiple biopsies. In addition, fibrosis progresses very slowly in most common diseases such as hepatitis C and non-alcoholic fatty liver disease making it difficult to detect possible beneficial effects of antifibrotic therapy unless studies are conducted over a number of years.

One small study (n=7) found that administration of the angiotensin II receptor antagonist losartan 50mg/day for 48 weeks in patients with non-alcoholic steatohepatitis (NASH) reduced serum TGF-β, ferritin and aminotransferases. Five patients showed improvement in the grade of hepatic necro-inflammation. Importantly, this small study had no control group and was not analysed on an intention to treat basis (Yokohama et al 2004). In a subsequent study the pre and post treatment biopsies of seven patients with non-alcoholic steato-hepatitis treated with losartan (50mg/day for 48 weeks) were compared with eight patients with non-alcoholic fatty liver disease who acted as a control group. The treatment group showed a significant improvement in necro-inflammatory grade, stage of fibrosis, significantly fewer activated HSCs and a mild increase in quiescent HSCs (Yokohama et al 2006) at the end of 48-weeks. However, the lack of a proper randomised control group is a particular problem in studies of patients with NASH since the disease can improve in response to changes in life style.

A number of studies have reported possible antifibrotic effects of RAS blockers in patients with hepatitis C. In one study, 30 HCV infected patients with mild fibrosis were treated with losartan 50mg/day and ursodeoxycholic acid 600mg/day whilst controls received ursodeoxycholic acid alone. There were significant differences in serum markers of hepatic fibrosis (TGF-β1 and type IV collagen) in the losartan and ursodeoxycholic acid group, but no significant changes in fibrosis score (METAVIR scoring system) were observed. The full details of this study have not been published (Rimola et al 2004). Another report published in letterform only described outcomes in patients with hepatitis C treated with low-dose interferon

(IFN alpha 3×10^6 IU 3 times a week for 12 months) in combination with the ACE inhibitor, perindopril (4mg/day). Treatment was accompanied by significant improvement in serum markers of fibrosis (hyaluronic acid, type IV collagen 7S and procollagen III-N-peptide), however, histological analysis was not performed. Unfortunately, it is impossible to determine from this study whether any of the observed effects were due to perindopril itself as a perindopril monotherapy group was not included (Yoshiji, Noguchi and Fukui 2005). Finally, a retrospective review which compared liver histology in liver transplant patients with recurrent hepatitis C who were taking RAS blocking drugs (n=27) with those who were not (n=101) showed that the group taking RAS blockers were less likely to develop severe hepatic fibrosis (bridging fibrosis or cirrhosis) at 1 and 10 years post transplantation compared to the control group (15% vs. 35% at 1 year (P<0.05), and 35% vs. 70% at 10 years (P<0.005), respectively) (Rimola 2004).

5.   CONCLUSIONS

Recent studies have provided clear evidence that there is an hepatic RAS that may be of major importance in the pathogenesis of chronic liver disease. This system is upregulated by chronic liver injury and contributes to oxidative stress, recruitment of inflammatory cells and the development of fibrosis. The RAS also plays a role in the pathogenesis of portal hypertension and many of the systemic complications of cirrhosis. There is ample evidence from *in-vitro* studies and work in a number of animal models of liver disease to suggest that blockade of the RAS can ameliorate liver injury, inhibit hepatic fibrosis and lower portal pressure. Whilst ACE inhibitors and ARB have proven to be invaluable pharmacological tools, most studies have employed higher doses of these drugs than are used clinically. It remains to be determined whether RAS inhibition will prove to be an effective therapeutic approach for the treatment and prevention of hepatic fibrosis and its complications in human liver disease.

ACKNOWLEDGEMENTS

J.S. Lubel is the recipient of an Australian Postgraduate National Health and Medical Research Council (NHMRC) Scholarship and F.J. Warner is supported by a Rolf Edgar Lake Fellowship. This work was facilitated by funding from the NHMRC (Australia).

REFERENCES

Admiraal PJ, Derkx FH, Danser AH, Pieterman H and Schalekamp MA 1990 Metabolism and production of angiotensin I in different vascular beds in subjects with hypertension *Hypertension* 15 **1** 44–55
Ardaillou R 1997 Active fragments of angiotensin II: enzymatic pathways of synthesis and biological effects *Curr Opin Nephrol Hypertens* 6 **1** 28–34
Arroyo V, Bosch J, Mauri M, Viver J, Mas A, Rivera F and Rodes J 1979 Renin, aldosterone and renal haemodynamics in cirrhosis with ascites *Eur J Clin Invest* 9 **1** 69–73

Arthur MJ 2000 Fibrogenesis II. Metalloproteinases and their inhibitors in liver fibrosis *Am J Physiol Gastrointest Liver Physiol* 279 **2** G245–9

Asbert M, Jimenez W, Gaya J, Gines P, Arroyo V, Rivera F and Rodes J 1992 Assessment of the renin-angiotensin system in cirrhotic patients. Comparison between plasma renin activity and direct measurement of immunoreactive renin *J Hepatol* 15 **1-2** 179–83

Basso N and Terragno NA 2001 History about the discovery of the renin-angiotensin system *Hypertension* 38 **6** 1246–9

Bataller R, Gabele E, Parsons CJ, Morris T, Yang L, Schoonhoven R, Brenner DA and Rippe RA 2005 Systemic infusion of angiotensin II exacerbates liver fibrosis in bile duct-ligated rats *Hepatology* 41 **5** 1046–55

Bataller R, Gines P, Nicolas JM, Gorbig MN, Garcia-Ramallo E, Gasull X, Bosch J, Arroyo V and Rodes J 2000 Angiotensin II induces contraction and proliferation of human hepatic stellate cells *Gastroenterology* 118 **6** 1149–56

Bataller R, Sancho-Bru P, Gines P and Brenner DA 2005 Liver fibrogenesis: a new role for the renin-angiotensin system *Antioxid Redox Signal* 7 **9-10** 1346–55

Bataller R, Sancho-Bru P, Gines P, Lora JM, Al-Garawi A, Sole M, Colmenero J, Nicolas JM, Jimenez W, Weich N, Gutierrez-Ramos JC, Arroyo V and Rodes J 2003 Activated human hepatic stellate cells express the renin-angiotensin system and synthesize angiotensin II *Gastroenterology* 125 **1** 117–25

Bataller R, Schwabe RF, Choi YH, Yang L, Paik YH, Lindquist J, Qian T, Schoonhoven R, Hagedorn CH, Lemasters JJ and Brenner DA 2003 NADPH oxidase signal transduces angiotensin II in hepatic stellate cells and is critical in hepatic fibrosis *J Clin Invest* 112 **9** 1383–94

Benter IF, Ferrario CM, Morris M and Diz DI 1995 Antihypertensive actions of angiotensin-(1-7) in spontaneously hypertensive rats *Am J Physiol* 269 **1 Pt 2** H313–9

Bosch J, Arroyo V, Betriu A, Mas A, Carrilho F, Rivera F, Navarro-Lopez F and Rodes J 1980 Hepatic hemodynamics and the renin-angiotensin-aldosterone system in cirrhosis *Gastroenterology* 78 **1** 92–9

Brasier AR, Li J and Copland A 1994 Transcription factors modulating angiotensinogen gene expression in hepatocytes *Kidney Int* 46 **6** 1564–6

Brosnihan KB, Li P and Ferrario CM 1996 Angiotensin-(1-7) dilates canine coronary arteries through kinins and nitric oxide *Hypertension* 27 **3 Pt 2** 523–8

Burrell LM, Johnston CI, Tikellis C and Cooper ME 2004 ACE2, a new regulator of the renin-angiotensin system *Trends Endocrinol Metab* 15 **4** 166–9

Cassiman D and Roskams T 2002 Beauty is in the eye of the beholder: emerging concepts and pitfalls in hepatic stellate cell research *J Hepatol* 37 **4** 527–35

Castro CH, Santos RA, Ferreira AJ, Bader M, Alenina N and Almeida AP 2005 Evidence for a functional interaction of the angiotensin-(1-7) receptor Mas with AT1 and AT2 receptors in the mouse heart *Hypertension* 46 **4** 937–42

Collister JP and Hendel MD 2003 The role of Ang (1-7) in mediating the chronic hypotensive effects of losartan in normal rats *J Renin Angiotensin Aldosterone Syst* 4 **3** 176–9

Corpechot C, Barbu V, Wendum D, Kinnman N, Rey C, Poupon R, Housset C and Rosmorduc O 2002 Hypoxia-induced VEGF and collagen I expressions are associated with angiogenesis and fibrogenesis in experimental cirrhosis *Hepatology* 35 **5** 1010–21

Croquet V, Moal F, Veal N, Wang J, Oberti F, Roux J, Vuillemin E, Gallois Y, Douay O, Chappard D and Cales P 2002 Hemodynamic and antifibrotic effects of losartan in rats with liver fibrosis and/or portal hypertension *J Hepatol* 37 **6** 773–80

Donoghue M, Hsieh F, Baronas E, Godbout K, Gosselin M, Stagliano N, Donovan M, Woolf B, Robison K, Jeyaseelan R, Breitbart RE and Acton S 2000 A novel angiotensin-converting enzyme-related carboxypeptidase (ACE2) converts angiotensin I to angiotensin 1-9 *Circ Res* 87 **5** E1–9

Enomoto N, Ikejima K, Bradford BU, Rivera CA, Kono H, Goto M, Yamashina S, Schemmer P, Kitamura T, Oide H, Takei Y, Hirose M, Shimizu H, Miyazaki A, Brenner DA, Sato N and Thurman RG 2000 Role of Kupffer cells and gut-derived endotoxins in alcoholic liver injury *J Gastroenterol Hepatol* 15 Suppl D20–5

Fernandes L, Fortes ZB, Nigro D, Tostes RC, Santos RA and Catelli De Carvalho MH 2001 Potentiation of bradykinin by angiotensin-(1-7) on arterioles of spontaneously hypertensive rats studied in vivo *Hypertension* 37 **2 Part 2** 703–9

Ferrario CM 2003 Commentary on Tikellis et al: There is more to discover about angiotensin-converting enzyme *Hypertension* 41 **3** 390–1

Ferreira AJ, Santos RA and Almeida AP 2001 Angiotensin-(1-7): cardioprotective effect in myocardial ischemia/reperfusion *Hypertension* 38 **3 Pt 2** 665–8

Ferreira AJ, Santos RA and Almeida AP 2002 Angiotensin-(1-7) improves the post-ischemic function in isolated perfused rat hearts *Braz J Med Biol Res* 35 **9** 1083–90

Freeman EJ, Chisolm GM, Ferrario CM and Tallant EA 1996 Angiotensin-(1-7) inhibits vascular smooth muscle cell growth *Hypertension* 28 **1** 104–8

Friedman SL, Maher JJ and Bissell DM 2000 Mechanisms and therapy of hepatic fibrosis: report of the AASLD Single Topic Basic Research Conference *Hepatology* 32 **6** 1403–8

Gorelik G, Carbini LA and Scicli AG 1998 Angiotensin 1-7 induces bradykinin-mediated relaxation in porcine coronary artery *J Pharmacol Exp Ther* 286 **1** 403–10

Grobe JL, Mecca AP, Lingis M, Shenoy V, Bolton TA, Machado JM, Speth RC, Raizada MK and Katovich M 2006 Prevention of Angiotensin II-Induced Cardiac Remodeling by Angiotensin-(1-7) *Am J Physiol Heart Circ Physiol*

Grobe JL, Mecca AP, Mao H and Katovich MJ 2006 Chronic angiotensin-(1-7) prevents cardiac fibrosis in DOCA-salt model of hypertension *Am J Physiol Heart Circ Physiol* 290 **6** H2417–23

Hamming I, Timens W, Bulthuis ML, Lely AT, Navis GJ and van Goor H 2004 Tissue distribution of ACE 2 protein, the functional receptor for SARS coronavirus. A first step in understanding SARS pathogenesis *J Pathol* 203 **2** 631–7

Harmer D, Gilbert M, Borman R and Clark KL 2002 Quantitative mRNA expression profiling of ACE 2, a novel homologue of angiotensin converting enzyme *FEBS Lett* 532 **1-2** 107–10

Herath CB, Warner FJ, Lubel JS, Dean R, Lew RA, Smith AI, Burrell LM and Angus PW 2006 The balance between hepatic ACE2 and ACE determines plasma levels of vasodilator peptide angiotensin (1-7) in experimental biliary fibrosis *Journal of Gastroenterology and Hepatology* 21 **Suppl. 4** A325

Ikura Y, Ohsawa M, Shirai N, Sugama Y, Fukushima H, Suekane T, Hirayama M, Ehara S, Naruko T and Ueda M 2005 Expression of angiotensin II type 1 receptor in human cirrhotic livers: Its relation to fibrosis and portal hypertension *Hepatol Res* 32 **2** 107–16

Iwata M, Cowling RT, Gurantz D, Moore C, Zhang S, Yuan JX and Greenberg BH 2005 Angiotensin-(1-7) binds to specific receptors on cardiac fibroblasts to initiate antifibrotic and antitrophic effects *Am J Physiol Heart Circ Physiol* 289 **6** H2356–63

Iyer SN, Ferrario CM and Chappell MC 1998 Angiotensin-(1-7) contributes to the antihypertensive effects of blockade of the renin-angiotensin system *Hypertension* 31 **1 Pt 2** 356–61

Iyer SN, Yamada K, Diz DI, Ferrario CM and Chappell MC 2000 Evidence that prostaglandins mediate the antihypertensive actions of angiotensin-(1-7) during chronic blockade of the renin-angiotensin system *J Cardiovasc Pharmacol* 36 **1** 109–17

Jamaluddin M, Meng T, Sun J, Boldogh I, Han Y and Brasier AR 2000 Angiotensin II induces nuclear factor (NF)-kappaB1 isoforms to bind the angiotensinogen gene acute-phase response element: a stimulus-specific pathway for NF-kappaB activation *Mol Endocrinol* 14 **1** 99–113

Jonsson JR, Clouston AD, Ando Y, Kelemen LI, Horn MJ, Adamson MD, Purdie DM and Powell EE 2001 Angiotensin-converting enzyme inhibition attenuates the progression of rat hepatic fibrosis *Gastroenterology* 121 **1** 148–55

Kallis Y, Alison MR and Forbes SJ 2006 Bone marrow stem cells and liver disease *Gut*

Kanno K, Tazuma S and Chayama K 2003 AT1A-deficient mice show less severe progression of liver fibrosis induced by CCl(4) *Biochem Biophys Res Commun* 308 **1** 177–83

Kanno K, Tazuma S, Nishioka T, Hyogo H and Chayama K 2005 Angiotensin II participates in hepatic inflammation and fibrosis through MCP-1 expression *Dig Dis Sci* 50 **5** 942–8

Knittel T, Mehde M, Kobold D, Saile B, Dinter C and Ramadori G 1999 Expression patterns of matrix metalloproteinases and their inhibitors in parenchymal and non-parenchymal cells of rat liver: regulation by TNF-alpha and TGF-beta1 *J Hepatol* 30 **1** 48–60

Kojima H, Tsujimoto T, Uemura M, Takaya A, Okamoto S, Ueda S, Nishio K, Miyamoto S, Kubo A, Minamino N, Kangawa K, Matsuo H and Fukui H 1998 Significance of increased plasma adrenomedullin concentration in patients with cirrhosis *J Hepatol* 28 **5** 840–6

Kono H, Rusyn I, Yin M, Gabele E, Yamashina S, Dikalova A, Kadiiska MB, Connor HD, Mason RP, Segal BH, Bradford BU, Holland SM and Thurman RG 2000 NADPH oxidase-derived free radicals are key oxidants in alcohol-induced liver disease *J Clin Invest* 106 **7** 867–72

Kostenis E, Milligan G, Christopoulos A, Sanchez-Ferrer CF, Heringer-Walther S, Sexton PM, Gembardt F, Kellett E, Martini L, Vanderheyden P, Schultheiss HP and Walther T 2005 G-protein-coupled receptor Mas is a physiological antagonist of the angiotensin II type 1 receptor *Circulation* 111 **14** 1806–13

Kucharewicz I, Chabielska E, Pawlak D, Matys T, Rolkowski R and Buczko W 2000 The antithrombotic effect of angiotensin-(1-7) closely resembles that of losartan *J Renin Angiotensin Aldosterone Syst* 1 **3** 268–72

Kucharewicz I, Pawlak R, Matys T, Pawlak D and Buczko W 2002 Antithrombotic effect of captopril and losartan is mediated by angiotensin-(1-7) *Hypertension* 40 **5** 774–9

Kurikawa N, Suga M, Kuroda S, Yamada K and Ishikawa H 2003 An angiotensin II type 1 receptor antagonist, olmesartan medoxomil, improves experimental liver fibrosis by suppression of proliferation and collagen synthesis in activated hepatic stellate cells *Br J Pharmacol* 139 **6** 1085–94

Lambert DW, Yarski M, Warner FJ, Thornhill P, Parkin ET, Smith AI, Hooper NM and Turner AJ 2005 Tumor necrosis factor-alpha convertase (ADAM17) mediates regulated ectodomain shedding of the severe-acute respiratory syndrome-coronavirus (SARS-CoV) receptor, angiotensin-converting enzyme-2 (ACE2) *J Biol Chem* 280 **34** 30113–9

Leung PS and Chappell MC 2003 A local pancreatic renin-angiotensin system: endocrine and exocrine roles *Int J Biochem Cell Biol* 35 **6** 838–46

Leung PS, Suen PM, Ip SP, Yip CK, Chen G and Lai PB 2003 Expression and localization of AT1 receptors in hepatic Kupffer cells: its potential role in regulating a fibrogenic response *Regul Pept* 116 **1-3** 61–9

Lew RA, Warner FJ, Hanchapola I and Smith AI 2006 Characterization of angiotensin converting enzyme-2 (ACE2) in human urine *International Journal Of Peptide Research And Therapeutics* 12 **3** 283–289

Li P, Chappell MC, Ferrario CM and Brosnihan KB 1997 Angiotensin-(1-7) augments bradykinin-induced vasodilation by competing with ACE and releasing nitric oxide *Hypertension* 29 **1 Pt 2** 394–400

Li W, Moore MJ, Vasilieva N, Sui J, Wong SK, Berne MA, Somasundaran M, Sullivan JL, Luzuriaga K, Greenough TC, Choe H and Farzan M 2003 Angiotensin-converting enzyme 2 is a functional receptor for the SARS coronavirus *Nature* 426 **6965** 450–4

Li X, Meng Y, Yang XS, Zhang ZS, Wu PS and Zou JL 2004 [Perindopril attenuates the progression of CCl4-inducing rat hepatic fibrosis] *Zhonghua Gan Zang Bing Za Zhi* 12 **1** 32–4

Li X, Meng Y, Zhang ZS, Yang XS and Wu PS 2003 [Effect of ACE-I and AT-1 receptor blocker on the progression of CCl(4)-inducing rat hepatic fibrogenesis] *Zhonghua Yi Xue Za Zhi* 83 **14** 1241–5

Lodato F, Mazzella G, Festi D, Azzaroli F, Colecchia A and Roda E 2006 Hepatocellular carcinoma prevention: A worldwide emergence between the opulence of developed countries and the economic constraints of developing nations *World J Gastroenterol* 12 **45** 7239–49

Lubel JS, Herath CB, Warner FJ, Jia ZY, Burrell LM and Angus PW 2006 Upregulation of the ACE2/Ang(1-7)/Mas receptor axis in the bile duct ligation (BDL) model of hepatic fibrosis does not affect hepatic sinusoidal resistance *Journal of Gastroenterology and Hepatology* 21 **Suppl 4** A332

Marra F, DeFranco R, Grappone C, Milani S, Pastacaldi S, Pinzani M, Romanelli RG, Laffi G and Gentilini P 1998 Increased expression of monocyte chemotactic protein-1 during active hepatic fibrogenesis: correlation with monocyte infiltration *Am J Pathol* 152 **2** 423–30

McAllister-Lucas LM, Ruland J, Siu K, Jin X, Gu S, Kim DS, Kuffa P, Kohrt D, Mak TW, Nunez G and Lucas PC 2006 CARMA3/Bcl10/MALT1-dependent NF-{kappa}B activation mediates angiotensin II-responsive inflammatory signaling in nonimmune cells *Proc Natl Acad Sci U S A*

Miyoshi M, Nagata K, Imoto T, Goto O, Ishida A and Watanabe T 2003 ANG II is involved in the LPS-induced production of proinflammatory cytokines in dehydrated rats *Am J Physiol Regul Integr Comp Physiol* 284 **4** R1092–7

Morris BJ, Iwamoto HS and Reid IA 1979 Localization of angiotensinogen in rat liver by immunocytochemistry *Endocrinology* 105 **3** 796–800

Nabeshima Y, Tazuma S, Kanno K, Hyogo H, Iwai M, Horiuchi M and Chayama K 2006 Anti-fibrogenic function of angiotensin II type 2 receptor in CCl4-induced liver fibrosis *Biochem Biophys Res Commun* 346 **3** 658–64

Nakamoto H, Ferrario CM, Fuller SB, Robaczewski DL, Winicov E and Dean RH 1995 Angiotensin-(1-7) and nitric oxide interaction in renovascular hypertension *Hypertension* 25 **4 Pt 2** 796–802

Ocaranza MP, Godoy I, Jalil JE, Varas M, Collantes P, Pinto M, Roman M, Ramirez C, Copaja M, Diaz-Araya G, Castro P and Lavandero S 2006 Enalapril attenuates downregulation of Angiotensin-converting enzyme 2 in the late phase of ventricular dysfunction in myocardial infarcted rat *Hypertension* 48 **4** 572–8

Ohishi T, Saito H, Tsusaka K, Toda K, Inagaki H, Hamada Y, Kumagai N, Atsukawa K and Ishii H 2001 Anti-fibrogenic effect of an angiotensin converting enzyme inhibitor on chronic carbon tetrachloride-induced hepatic fibrosis in rats *Hepatol Res* 21 **2** 147–158

Paizis G, Cooper ME, Schembri JM, Tikellis C, Burrell LM and Angus PW 2002 Up-regulation of components of the renin-angiotensin system in the bile duct-ligated rat liver *Gastroenterology* 123 **5** 1667–76

Paizis G, Gilbert RE, Cooper ME, Murthi P, Schembri JM, Wu LL, Rumble JR, Kelly DJ, Tikellis C, Cox A, Smallwood RA and Angus PW 2001 Effect of angiotensin II type 1 receptor blockade on experimental hepatic fibrogenesis *J Hepatol* 35 **3** 376–85

Paizis G, Tikellis C, Cooper ME, Schembri JM, Lew RA, Smith AI, Shaw T, Warner FJ, Zuilli A, Burrell LM and Angus PW 2005 Chronic liver injury in rats and humans upregulates the novel enzyme angiotensin converting enzyme 2 *Gut* 54 **12** 1790–6

Pereira RM, Dos Santos RA, Teixeira MM, Leite VH, Costa LP, da Costa Dias FL, Barcelos LS, Collares GB and Simoes ESAC 2006 The renin-angiotensin system in a rat model of hepatic fibrosis: Evidence for a protective role of Angiotensin-(1-7) *J Hepatol*

Ramalho LN, Ramalho FS, Zucoloto S, Castro-e-Silva Junior O, Correa FM, Elias Junior J and Magalhaes JF 2002 Effect of losartan, an angiotensin II antagonist, on secondary biliary cirrhosis *Hepatogastroenterology* 49 **48** 1499–502

Ramos SG, Montenegro AP, Goissis G and Rossi MA 1994 Captopril reduces collagen and mast cell and eosinophil accumulation in pig serum-induced rat liver fibrosis *Pathol Int* 44 **9** 655–61

Rice GI, Jones AL, Grant PJ, Carter AM, Turner AJ and Hooper NM 2006 Circulating activities of angiotensin-converting enzyme, its homolog, angiotensin-converting enzyme 2, and neprilysin in a family study *Hypertension* 48 **5** 914–20

Rice GI, Thomas DA, Grant PJ, Turner AJ and Hooper NM 2004 Evaluation of angiotensin-converting enzyme (ACE), its homologue ACE2 and neprilysin in angiotensin peptide metabolism *Biochem J* 383 **Pt 1** 45–51

Richoux JP, Cordonnier JL, Bouhnik J, Clauser E, Corvol P, Menard J and Grignon G 1983 Immunocytochemical localization of angiotensinogen in rat liver and kidney *Cell Tissue Res* 233 **2** 439–51

Rimola A, Londono MC, Guevara G, Bruguera M, Navasa M, Forns X, Garcia-Retortillo M, Garcia-Valdecasas JC and Rodes J 2004 Beneficial effect of angiotensin-blocking agents on graft fibrosis in hepatitis C recurrence after liver transplantation *Transplantation* 78 **5** 686–91

Rincon-Sanchez AR, Covarrubias A, Rivas-Estilla AM, Pedraza-Chaverri J, Cruz C, Islas-Carbajal MC, Panduro A, Estanes A and Armendariz-Borunda J 2005 PGE2 alleviates kidney and liver damage, decreases plasma renin activity and acute phase response in cirrhotic rats with acute liver damage *Exp Toxicol Pathol* 56 **4-5** 291–303

Rivera-Huizar S, Rincon-Sanchez AR, Covarrubias-Pinedo A, Islas-Carbajal MC, Gabriel-Ortiz G, Pedraza-Chaverri J, Alvarez-Rodriguez A, Meza-Garcia E and Armendariz-Borunda J 2006 Renal dysfunction as a consequence of acute liver damage by bile duct ligation in cirrhotic rats *Exp Toxicol Pathol* 58 **2-3** 185–95

Ron D, Brasier AR and Habener JF 1990 Transcriptional regulation of hepatic angiotensinogen gene expression by the acute-phase response *Mol Cell Endocrinol* 74 **3** C97–104

Russo FP, Alison MR, Bigger BW, Amofah E, Florou A, Amin F, Bou-Gharios G, Jeffery R, Iredale JP and Forbes SJ 2006 The bone marrow functionally contributes to liver fibrosis *Gastroenterology* 130 **6** 1807–21

Sakata T, Takenaga N, Endoh T, Wada O and Matsuki K 1991 Diagnostic significance of serum angiotensin-converting enzyme activity in biochemical tests with special reference of chronic liver diseases *Jpn J Med* 30 **5** 402–7

Santos RA, Simoes e Silva AC, Maric C, Silva DM, Machado RP, de Buhr I, Heringer-Walther S, Pinheiro SV, Lopes MT, Bader M, Mendes EP, Lemos VS, Campagnole-Santos MJ, Schultheiss HP, Speth R and Walther T 2003 Angiotensin-(1-7) is an endogenous ligand for the G protein-coupled receptor Mas *Proc Natl Acad Sci U S A* 100 **14** 8258–63

Sasaki K, Taniguchi M, Miyoshi M, Goto O, Sato K and Watanabe T 2005 Are transcription factors NF-kappaB and AP-1 involved in the ANG II-stimulated production of proinflammatory cytokines induced by LPS in dehydrated rats? *Am J Physiol Regul Integr Comp Physiol* 289 **6** R1599–608

Sawa H 1990 [Angiotensinogen: gene expression and protein localization in human tissues] *Hokkaido Igaku Zasshi* 65 **2** 189–99

Schiavone MT, Santos RA, Brosnihan KB, Khosla MC and Ferrario CM 1988 Release of vasopressin from the rat hypothalamo-neurohypophysial system by angiotensin-(1-7) heptapeptide *Proc Natl Acad Sci U S A* 85 **11** 4095–8

Schuppan D, Ruehl M, Somasundaram R and Hahn EG 2001 Matrix as a modulator of hepatic fibroge-nesis *Semin Liver Dis* 21 **3** 351–72

Sewnath ME, van der Poll T, van Noorden CJ, ten Kate FJ and Gouma DJ 2004 Cholestatic interleukin-6-deficient mice succumb to endotoxin-induced liver injury and pulmonary inflammation *Am J Respir Crit Care Med* 169 **3** 413–20

Silva DM, Vianna HR, Cortes SF, Campagnole-Santos MJ, Santos RA and Lemos VS 2006 Evidence for a new angiotensin-(1-7) receptor subtype in the aorta of Sprague-Dawley rats *Peptides*

Strawn WB, Ferrario CM and Tallant EA 1999 Angiotensin-(1-7) reduces smooth muscle growth after vascular injury *Hypertension* 33 **1 Pt 2** 207–11

Tallant EA, Ferrario CM and Gallagher PE 2005 Angiotensin-(1-7) inhibits growth of cardiac myocytes through activation of the mas receptor *Am J Physiol Heart Circ Physiol* 289 **4** H1560–6

Thomas MC and Tikellis C 2005 ACE2; an ACE up the Sleeve *Current enzyme inhibition* **1** 51–63

Tigerstedt R BP 1898 Niere und Kreislauf *Skand Arch Physiol.* **8** 223–271

Timmermans PB, Benfield P, Chiu AT, Herblin WF, Wong PC and Smith RD 1992 Angiotensin II receptors and functional correlates *Am J Hypertens* 5 **12 Pt 2** 221S–235S

Timmermans PB, Chiu AT, Herblin WF, Wong PC and Smith RD 1992 Angiotensin II receptor subtypes *Am J Hypertens* 5 **6 Pt 1** 406–10

Tipnis SR, Hooper NM, Hyde R, Karran E, Christie G and Turner AJ 2000 A human homolog of angiotensin-converting enzyme. Cloning and functional expression as a captopril-insensitive carboxypeptidase *J Biol Chem* 275 **43** 33238–43

Toblli JE, Ferder L, Stella I, Angerosa M and Inserra F 2002 Enalapril prevents fatty liver in nephrotic rats *J Nephrol* 15 **4** 358–67

Tuncer I, Ozbek H, Ugras S and Bayram I 2003 Anti-fibrogenic effects of captopril and candesartan cilexetil on the hepatic fibrosis development in rat. The effect of AT1-R blocker on the hepatic fibrosis *Exp Toxicol Pathol* 55 **2-3** 159–66

Turner AJ 2003 Exploring the structure and function of zinc metallopeptidases: old enzymes and new discoveries *Biochem Soc Trans* 31 **Pt 3** 723–7

Ueda S, Masumori-Maemoto S, Wada A, Ishii M, Brosnihan KB and Umemura S 2001 Angiotensin(1-7) potentiates bradykinin-induced vasodilatation in man *J Hypertens* 19 **11** 2001–9

Vickers C, Hales P, Kaushik V, Dick L, Gavin J, Tang J, Godbout K, Parsons T, Baronas E, Hsieh F, Acton S, Patane M, Nichols A and Tummino P 2002 Hydrolysis of biological peptides by human angiotensin-converting enzyme-related carboxypeptidase *J Biol Chem* 277 **17** 14838–43

Vlachogiannakos J, Tang AK, Patch D and Burroughs AK 2001 Angiotensin converting enzyme inhibitors and angiotensin II antagonists as therapy in chronic liver disease *Gut* 49 **2** 303–8

von Bohlen und Halbach O 2003 Angiotensin IV in the central nervous system *Cell Tissue Res* 311 **1** 1–9

Walters PE, Gaspari TA and Widdop RE 2005 Angiotensin-(1-7) acts as a vasodepressor agent via angiotensin II type 2 receptors in conscious rats *Hypertension* 45 **5** 960–6

Wang XZ, Zhang LJ, Li D, Huang YH, Chen ZX and Li B 2003 Effects of transmitters and interleukin-10 on rat hepatic fibrosis induced by CCl4 *World J Gastroenterol* 9 **3** 539–43

Warner FJ, Lew RA, Smith AI, Lambert DW, Hooper NM and Turner AJ 2005 Angiotensin-converting enzyme 2 (ACE2), but not ACE, is preferentially localized to the apical surface of polarized kidney cells *J Biol Chem* 280 **47** 39353–62

Warner FJ, Smith AI, Hooper NM and Turner AJ 2004 Angiotensin-converting enzyme-2: a molecular and cellular perspective *Cell Mol Life Sci* 61 **21** 2704–13

Wei H, Li D, Lu H, Zhan Y, Wang Z, Huang X, Pan Q and Xu Q 2000 Effects of angiotensin II receptor blockade on hepatic fibrosis in rats *Zhonghua Gan Zang Bing Za Zhi* 8 **5** 302–4

Wei HS, Lu HM, Li DG, Zhan YT, Wang ZR, Huang X, Cheng JL and Xu QF 2000 The regulatory role of AT 1 receptor on activated HSCs in hepatic fibrogenesis:effects of RAS inhibitors on hepatic fibrosis induced by CCl(4) *World J Gastroenterol* 6 **6** 824–828

Wei YH, Jun L and Qiang CJ 2004 Effect of losartan, an angiotensin II antagonist, on hepatic fibrosis induced by CCl4 in rats *Dig Dis Sci* 49 **10** 1589–94

Whalen R, Rockey DC, Friedman SL and Boyer TD 1999 Activation of rat hepatic stellate cells leads to loss of glutathione S-transferases and their enzymatic activity against products of oxidative stress *Hepatology* 30 **4** 927–33

Yang L, Bataller R, Dulyx J, Coffman TM, Gines P, Rippe RA and Brenner DA 2005 Attenuated hepatic inflammation and fibrosis in angiotensin type 1a receptor deficient mice *J Hepatol* 43 **2** 317–23

Yokohama S, Tokusashi Y, Nakamura K, Tamaki Y, Okamoto S, Okada M, Aso K, Hasegawa T, Aoshima M, Miyokawa N, Haneda M and Yoneda M 2006 Inhibitory effect of angiotensin II receptor antagonist on hepatic stellate cell activation in non-alcoholic steatohepatitis *World J Gastroenterol* 12 **2** 322–6

Yokohama S, Yoneda M, Haneda M, Okamoto S, Okada M, Aso K, Hasegawa T, Tokusashi Y, Miyokawa N and Nakamura K 2004 Therapeutic efficacy of an angiotensin II receptor antagonist in patients with nonalcoholic steatohepatitis *Hepatology* 40 **5** 1222–5

Yoshiji H, Kuriyama S and Fukui H 2002 Angiotensin-I-converting enzyme inhibitors may be an alternative anti-angiogenic strategy in the treatment of liver fibrosis and hepatocellular carcinoma. Possible role of vascular endothelial growth factor *Tumour Biol* 23 **6** 348–56

Yoshiji H, Kuriyama S, Kawata M, Yoshii J, Ikenaka Y, Noguchi R, Nakatani T, Tsujinoue H and Fukui H 2001 The angiotensin-I-converting enzyme inhibitor perindopril suppresses tumor growth and angiogenesis: possible role of the vascular endothelial growth factor *Clin Cancer Res* 7 **4** 1073–8

Yoshiji H, Kuriyama S, Yoshii J, Ikenaka Y, Noguchi R, Nakatani T, Tsujinoue H and Fukui H 2001 Angiotensin-II type 1 receptor interaction is a major regulator for liver fibrosis development in rats *Hepatology* 34 **4 Pt 1** 745–50

Yoshiji H, Kuriyama S, Yoshii J, Ikenaka Y, Noguchi R, Yanase K, Namisaki T, Yamazaki M, Tsujinoue H, Imazu H and Fukui H 2003 Angiotensin-II induces the tissue inhibitor of metalloproteinases-1 through the protein kinase-C signaling pathway in rat liver fibrosis development *Hepatol Res* 27 **1** 51–56

Yoshiji H, Noguchi R and Fukui H 2005 Combined effect of an ACE inhibitor, perindopril, and interferon on liver fibrosis markers in patients with chronic hepatitis C *J Gastroenterol* 40 **2** 215–6

Yoshiji H, Noguchi R, Kuriyama S, Yoshii J and Ikenaka Y 2005 Combination of interferon and angiotensin-converting enzyme inhibitor, perindopril, suppresses liver carcinogenesis and angiogenesis in mice *Oncol Rep* 13 **3** 491–5

Yoshiji H, Yoshii J, Ikenaka Y, Noguchi R, Tsujinoue H, Nakatani T, Imazu H, Yanase K, Kuriyama S and Fukui H 2002 Inhibition of renin-angiotensin system attenuates liver enzyme-altered preneoplastic lesions and fibrosis development in rats *J Hepatol* 37 **1** 22–30

Yoshiji H, Yoshii J, Ikenaka Y, Noguchi R, Yanase K, Tsujinoue H, Imazu H and Fukui H 2002 Suppression of the renin-angiotensin system attenuates vascular endothelial growth factor-mediated tumor development and angiogenesis in murine hepatocellular carcinoma cells *Int J Oncol* 20 **6** 1227–31

Zhang X, Yu WP, Gao L, Wei KB, Ju JL and Xu JZ 2004 Effects of lipopolysaccharides stimulated Kupffer cells on activation of rat hepatic stellate cells *World J Gastroenterol* 10 **4** 610–3

Zhang Y, Yang X, Wu P, Xu L, Liao G and Yang G 2003 Expression of angiotensin II type 1 receptor in rat hepatic stellate cells and its effects on cell growth and collagen production *Horm Res* 60 **3** 105–10

Zhang YJ, Yang XS, Wu PS, Li X, Zhang XF, Chen XQ and Yu ZX 2003 Effects of angiotensin II and losartan on the growth and proliferation of hepatic stellate cells *Di Yi Jun Yi Da Xue Xue Bao* 23 **3** 219–21, 227

Zisman LS, Keller RS, Weaver B, Lin Q, Speth R, Bristow MR and Canver CC 2003 Increased angiotensin-(1-7)-forming activity in failing human heart ventricles: evidence for upregulation of the angiotensin-converting enzyme Homologue ACE2 *Circulation* 108 **14** 1707–12

Zisman LS, Meixell GE, Bristow MR and Canver CC 2003 Angiotensin-(1-7) formation in the intact human heart: in vivo dependence on angiotensin II as substrate *Circulation* 108 **14** 1679–81

CHAPTER 7

THE RENIN-ANGIOTENSIN SYSTEM
IN THE BREAST

GAVIN P. VINSON, STEWART BARKER,
JOHN R. PUDDEFOOT, AND MASSOUMEH TAHMASEBI

School of Biological and Chemical Sciences, Queen Mary University of London, Mile End Road, London E1 4NS, United Kingdom

1.   INTRODUCTION

The relationship between the endocrine system and cancer, it can be fairly said, was first identified in the breast, and has since been most extensively studied in this tissue. The early demonstration that breast cancer cell growth was regulated by oestrogen, and proof of the beneficial effects of surgical removal of the sources of oestrogen, led to the development of anti-oestrogen drugs, exemplified by tamoxifen, and more recently, the aromatase inhibitors, that have been remarkably successful (Barnes *et al* 2004; Howell *et al* 2004; Jones *et al* 2004).

It is this success, perhaps, that has overshadowed the substantial (and long estab-lished) evidence that regulation of breast tissue, and particularly breast epithelial tissue growth and function, is multifactorial, and many hormones and growth factors are involved (Haagensen 1986; Dickson *et al* 1992; Hansen *et al* 2000; Tucker 2000; Pollard 2001; Goffin *et al* 2002; Singer *et al* 2003; Lamote *et al* 2004; Nicolini *et al* 2006; see also Wysolmerski and van Houten, 2002). This particularly comes to the fore when tumours that are non-responsive to tamoxifen, or do not contain oestrogen receptors, are studied. In these, growth factors and their receptors have been targeted for drug development, and this in turn reflects the fairly long-held recognition that several of the proto-oncogenes have functions connected with the growth factors, their receptors, or the intracellular signalling mechanisms that they activate (Ross *et al* 2004; Bianco *et al* 2005; Hynes *et al* 2005; Pal *et al* 2005; Zhang *et al* 2005). Yet there remain still further possibilities.

The renin-angiotensin system (RAS, Fig. 1) has received most attention in relation to its functions in the circulation, in which the generation of the most prominent active hormone, angiotensin II, is associated with the regulation of aldosterone

135

Po Sing Leung (ed.), Frontiers in Research of the Renin-Angiotensin System on Human Disease, 135–153.
© 2007 *Springer.*

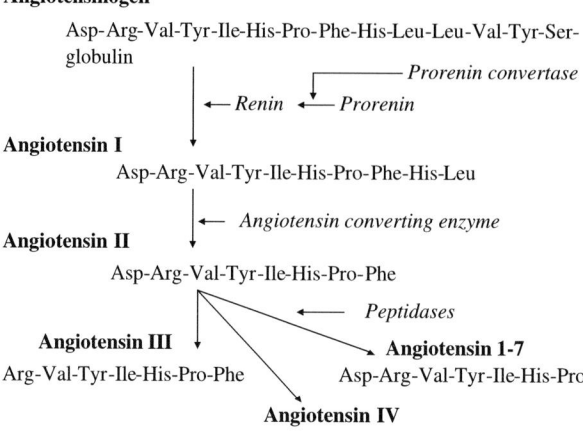

Angiotensinogen

Asp-Arg-Val-Tyr-Ile-His-Pro-Phe-His-Leu-Leu-Val-Tyr-Ser-
globulin

Prorenin convertase

← *Renin*   ← *Prorenin*

Angiotensin I

Asp-Arg-Val-Tyr-Ile-His-Pro-Phe-His-Leu

← *Angiotensin converting enzyme*

Angiotensin II

Asp-Arg-Val-Tyr-Ile-His-Pro-Phe

← *Peptidases*

Angiotensin III   **Angiotensin 1-7**

Arg-Val-Tyr-Ile-His-Pro-Phe   Asp-Arg-Val-Tyr-Ile-His-Pro

Angiotensin IV

Val-Tyr-Ile-His-Pro-Phe

Figure 1. The renin-angiotensin system (cf. Peach 1977; Stroth et al 1999)

secretion, salt and water metabolism and blood pressure (Mulrow 1999; Kaschina *et al* 2003). In recent years, attention has also focused on the evidence for widespread local tissue RASs (Vinson *et al* 1997; Mulrow 1999; Tahmasebi *et al* 1999; Li *et al* 2004), including in the breast (Tahmasebi *et al* 1998; Tahmasebi *et al* 2006), and see below.

It was with the development of antibodies to the angiotensin II receptors that the relevance of the RAS became apparent, because, though ligand binding assays had previously demonstrated the widespread distribution of these receptors in many tissues, it was immunocytochemistry that first showed that it is in secretory epithelia, including in the breast, that they are most abundant. Reflection on the well known functions of angiotensin II suggests several ways in which it may be crucial to epithelial function.

These include water and electrolyte transport and secretion (Lees *et al* 1993; Leung *et al* 1997; Mahmood *et al* 2002; Norris *et al* 1991; Quan *et al* 1996; Wang *et al* 1996; Wong *et al* 1990), ciliary beat activity (Saridogan *et al* 1996), and, at least by extrapolation from its actions in other tissue types, tissue modelling through regulation of mitosis and apoptosis, not only in the heart and vasculature (Schorb *et al* 1995; Linz *et al* 1989; Weber *et al* 1991; Motz *et al* 1992; Johnston 1992; Booz *et al* 1995; Kaschina *et al* 2003), but also in the adrenal cortex (Natarajan *et al* 1992; Quan *et al* 1996; Vinson *et al* 1998), kidney (Wolf *et al* 1993), and possibly skeletal muscle and connective tissue as well (Millan *et al* 1989).

The relevance to dysplasia and carcinoma is immediately obvious, and here the most important of these properties of angiotensin are those concerned with regulation of mitosis and of apoptosis. It was quickly established that several different types of cancer, including breast cancer, also express angiotensin receptors (Marsigliante *et al* 1996; Inwang *et al* 1997; Kucerova *et al* 1998; De Paepe *et al* 2001; Fujimoto *et al* 2001; Suganuma *et al* 2005; Uemura *et al* 2005b).

2.   RECEPTORS AND SIGNALLING

Angiotensin II exerts most of its activities through two G-protein coupled receptors, designated AT_1 and AT_2. This is also true of angiotensin III and angiotensin 1-7, though it is thought that angiotensin IV (the hexapeptide, angiotensin 3-8; Fig. 1) also interacts with a specific receptor, designated AT_4 (Hall *et al* 1995; Jarvis *et al* 1992; Chai *et al* 2004; Haulica *et al* 2005). In rodents, there are also two variants of the AT_1 receptor, designated AT_{1a} and AT_{1b}, which have 95% homology and share signalling pathways (Smith *et al* 1994; Clauser *et al* 1996; Martin *et al* 1995), though with different promoter regions. Such AT_1 subtypes do not exist in man (de Gasparo *et al* 2000). Signalling pathways for the AT_1 and AT_2 angiotensin receptors have been extensively studied (Figs. 2, 3). The AT_1 receptor is known to signal primarily through linkage to Gq/11, leading thus to increased intracellular calcium, IP_3 and diacylglycerol mediated cellular events, and also to tyrosine kinase linked pathways, including ERK1 and ERK2 activation. The AT_2 receptor, in contrast, appears in general to oppose the actions of AT_1 receptor activation on phospholipase activation and downstream phosphorylation of signalling molecules such as the ERKs, and this is associated with increased phosphatase activity (de Gasparo *et al* 2000; de Gasparo 2002; Kaschina *et al* 2003). The key point here in relation to cancer is, initially at least, that events mediated through the AT_1 receptor promote mitosis and cell proliferation, whereas AT_2 receptor activation leads to apoptosis (Horiuchi *et al* 1997; Horiuchi *et al* 1999a; Horiuchi *et al* 1999b; Bedecs *et al* 1997; de Gasparo *et al* 2000; de Gasparo 2002; Dinh *et al*

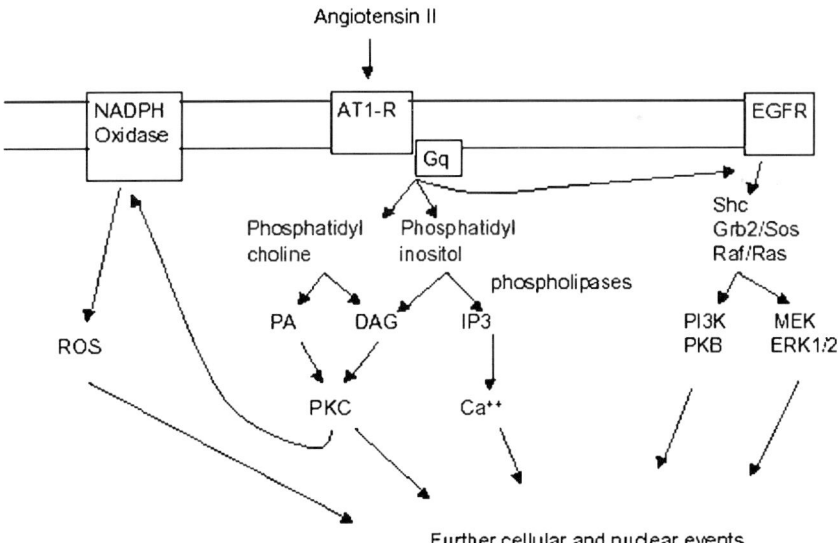

Figure 2. Signalling pathways for the AT_1 receptor (cf. Stroth et al 1999; de Gasparo et al 2000; Berry et al 2001; Hunyady and Catt 2006)

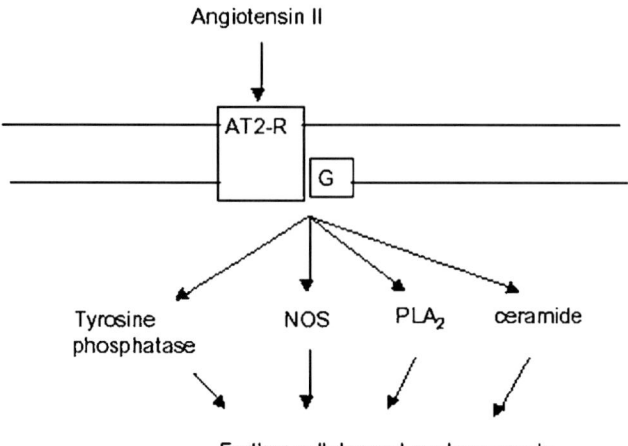

Figure 3. Signalling pathways for the AT$_2$ receptor (cf. Stroth et al 1999; de Gasparo et al 2000; Berry et al 2001)

2001; Gross *et al* 2004; Kaschina *et al* 2003; Yamada *et al* 1996; Hunyady and Catt 2006). The situation is complex, AT$_1$ and AT$_2$ receptors are not invariably antagonistic (D'Amore *et al* 2005), and more recently it appears that both receptors can mediate apoptotic events at least in some tissues (Diep *et al* 2002; Suzuki *et al* 2002; Li *et al* 2003b) though not all (Weidekamm *et al* 2002; Yamada *et al* 1998).

The possible relationship between angiotensin signalling via the AT$_1$ receptor and cancer becomes clearer in the light of the many studies on the cross talk between AT$_1$ and the tyrosine kinase receptors, including EGF receptors. Tyrosine kinase activation by AT$_1$ receptor interactions has been shown for several signalling molecules, including the JAK/STAT pathway and MAPK (Booz *et al* 1995; Griendling *et al* 1997), and in this case the AT$_1$ receptor is known to interact directly with JAK2, which in turn links to JAK1 (Ali *et al* 2000; Hunyady and Catt 2006). This pathway is independent of AT$_1$ mediated increases in intracellular calcium (Doan *et al* 2001), and is thus an important intrinsic action of the AT$_1$ receptor. Further evidence for transactivation of EGF receptors via the AT$_1$ receptor has demonstrated Akt/PKB/PIP kinase activation (Greco *et al* 2003; Lin *et al* 2003; Shah *et al* 2004; Chiu *et al* 2005; Olivares-Reyes *et al* 2005; Yang *et al* 2005), with inhibition via the AT$_2$ receptor (De Paolis *et al* 2002). Another AT$_1$ receptor signalling pathway is the activation of reactive oxygen species generation (Ushio-Fukai *et al* 1999; Griendling *et al* 2000; Hunyady and Catt 2006). In a further intriguing development, the non-genomic actions of oestrogens in breast cancer cells, which occur whether or not the cells express oestrogen receptors, has been found to depend on the presence of AT$_1$R (Lim *et al* 2006).

3. ANGIOTENSIN IN CANCER

An early study suggested that long term use of angiotensin converting enzyme (ACE) inhibitors in patients may limit the development of cancer (Lever *et al* 1998), but this has been questioned (Meier *et al* 2000; Li *et al* 2003a; Gonzalez-Perez *et al* 2004; Ronquist *et al* 2004), and no evidence was found in breast cancer specifically for any effect of a range of antihypertensive drugs, including ACE inhibitors and angiotensin II antagonists (Fryzek *et al* 2006). Indeed, despite its possibly unwelcome actions on tumours, angiotensin II has actually been used acutely in cancer to enable better accessibility of chemotherapeutic drugs to the tumour, through its vasoconstrictive actions (Noguchi *et al* 1988; Yamaue *et al* 1990; Goldberg *et al* 1990; Anderson *et al* 1991).

Given the upregulation of the AT_1 receptor reported in various hyperplastic and cancer tissues (De Paepe *et al* 2001), (though not according to all reports (Dinh *et al* 2002)), and also of MAPK (Sivaraman *et al* 1997) it is clear that angiotensin should not be dismissed as merely a peripheral player in the natural history of cancer (Deshayes *et al* 2005). In fact, in experimental conditions, ACE inhibitors have been found to limit several different types of tumour cell growth, including breast cells, in vitro (Chen *et al* 1991; Reddy *et al* 1995; Small *et al* 1997), and also in animal models in vivo, though here the response is often attributed to their anti-angiogenic effects (Volpert *et al* 1996; Yoshiji *et al* 2004). Similarly, AT_1 receptor antagonists are also effective anti-cancer agents in vitro (Rivera *et al* 2001) and in animal models in vivo (Fujimoto *et al* 2001; Fujita *et al* 2002). Indeed, AT_1 receptor blockers have also been used in patients with prostate cancer, who showed decreased prostate specific antigen and improved performance, though previously refractory to endocrine therapy (Uemura *et al* 2005a). It is worth noting, however, that the concentrations of the drugs used in the experimental studies are high compared with those used for anti-hypertensive therapy. For example, candesartan inhibited ovarian tumour growth in mice by $\sim 50\%$ at doses of 10–100mg/kg/day (Suganuma *et al* 2005), compared with the usual anti-hypertensive dose range in adult humans of up to perhaps 0.2 mg/kg/day. Losartan inhibited glioma tumours in vivo by 39% to 79% at a dose range of 40–80mg/kg/day (Rivera *et al* 2001), whereas a more usual dose in hypertensive patients would be up to 1.5mg/kg/day. It is perhaps not surprising that in general it has been difficult to detect any anti cancer activity of these drugs in patients undergoing treatment for cardiovascular indications.

Angiogenesis and neovascularisation are also important components of tumour growth and metastasis. Angiotensin II is directly involved in stimulating this process. This may be an additional contribution made by angiotensin II but which is distinct from other direct actions of angiotensin II on tumour cells. Studies relating to several other non-breast cancers have demonstrated a role for angiotensin II through induction of vascular endothelial growth factor (VEGF). This action occurs via the AT_1 receptor. In AT_1 receptor null mice implanted with S-180 murine sarcoma cells, tumour-associated angiogenesis is reduced, along with VEGF expression (Fujita *et al* 2005). It is also a feature confined to the stromal tissue, and newly formed endothelial cells, and may involve protein kinase C and activating protein-1 (AP-1) dependent signalling pathways. Fujita and colleagues also showed how the AT_1 receptor is involved in tumour metastasis in a lung carcinoma model (Fujita *et al* 2002). Both of these studies found that the effects of angiotensin II could be inhibited using the AT_1 receptor blocker, candesartan cilexetil. Similarly, in an *in vivo* model of head and neck cancer, the ACE inhibitor perindopril was found to inhibit tumour growth, and associated neovascularisation, along with VEGF expression, although no direct cytotoxic effects on the tumour cells was observed (Yasumatsu *et al* 2004). Studies of angiotensin II in angiogenesis have thus far been concerned with non-breast cancers, however, it may be worthwhile stating that certain polymorphisms in either the ACE or AT_1 receptor genes are associated with a reduced risk of developing breast cancer (Koh *et al* 2005).

Extracellular matrix remodelling is an important process in normal development of the mammary gland which undergoes many changes, including ductal development, lactation and involution (see Fig. 4). This process of tissue remodelling requires the breakdown (and subsequent resynthesis) of extracellular matrix components, which is effected by secretion of the zinc-dependent matrix metalloproteinases (MMPs) which act upon the basement membrane. Disruption of the matrix also invariably occurs during mammary tumour growth and and invasion (Ambili *et al* 1998; Rudolph-Owen *et al* 1998), and MMPs have been found to be expressed in the myoepithelial cells of both normal and hyperplastic breast tissue. It is thought that they are regulated by cellular oncogenes and thus play a role in

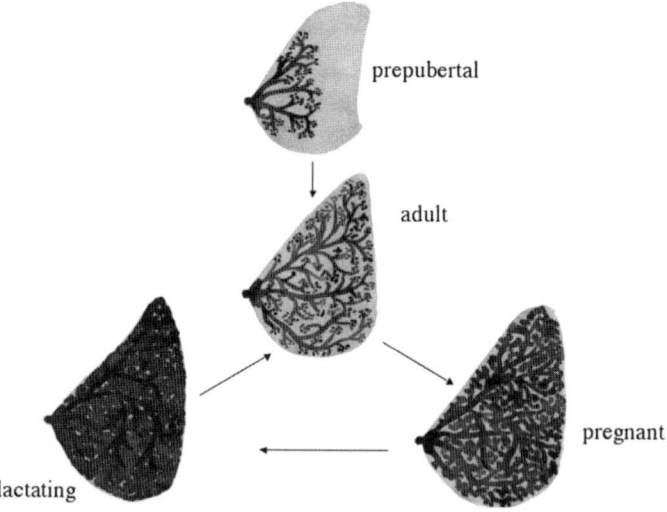

Figure 4. The breast cycle: note particularly extensive duct and gland development during pregnancy and lactaction, followed by apoptotic involution when lactation ceases. (cf. Wiseman et al 2002; Boutinaud et al 2004; Green et al 2004). Drawing by Bronwen Vinson

breast tumour growth and metastasis, and an increased level of active MMP2 has been observed in invasive breast cancers. In addition, high levels of MMPs have been found to correlate with poor outcome in breast cancer patients (Duffy *et al* 2000).

The basement membrane is vital for survival of epithelial cells and loss of contact results in a specialised form of apoptosis. Collagen IV is an important component in the basement membrane and both its expression and degradation must be balanced during normal tissue development. Thus proteolysis, or any disparity in its production, can lead to pathological changes in breast tissue. In many organs, including heart (Galis *et al* 2002), lung (Karakiulakis *et al* 2006) and kidney (Gack *et al* 1994), tissue remodelling is known to be controlled through the direct or indirect actions of angiotensin II either by altering the level of collagen expression (Ford *et al* 1999) or changes in MMP activity (Dzau 2001) - indeed pathological changes occurring in these tissues, such as ventricular hypertrophy or diabetic nephropathy, can be controlled by using either ACE inhibitors or AT_1-receptor blockers (Petrovic *et al* 2005; Porteri *et al* 2005; Reinhardt *et al* 2002; Sakata *et al* 2004; Sun *et al* 2006). The presence of a localised RAS in breast tissue suggests that angiotensin II is likely to exercise a similar control here, particularly since there is co-expression of components of the RAS and MMPs in the myoepithelial cells lining the breast ducts and lobules (see below).

There are also seemingly reciprocal, hence complex, relationships between angiotensin II, angiotensin receptors, oestrogens and ER. Angiotensin II treatment reduces ER and increases PR in ductal carcinoma cells in vitro (Small *et al* 1997), in turn oestrogen may upregulate angiotensinogen in rat and human tissues (Gordon *et al* 1992; Klett *et al* 1993; Fischer *et al* 2002), and also the AT_2 receptor in rat ovary and human myometrium (Mancina *et al* 1996; Pucell *et al* 1987). In contrast, the AT_1 receptor is downregulated by oestrogen in some tissues (Seltzer *et al* 1992; Kisley *et al* 1999; Fischer *et al* 2002), as are renin and ACE (Fischer *et al* 2002): the oestrogen/progesterone ratio is inversely proportional to prorenin in bovine follicular fluid (Mukhopadhyay *et al* 1991). Furthermore, overall RAS activity is highest when circulating oestrogen is high, and angiotensin II and plasma renin activity (PRA) are increased by oestrogen treatment in sheep (Magness *et al* 1993) but are highest during the luteal phase of the menstrual cycle in women (Sealey *et al* 1994; Chapman *et al* 1997; Chidambaram *et al* 2002).

From the abundance of evidence suggesting direct actions of angiotensin II on cancer cell growth, and in addition, because of its clear interactions with the well studied hormone and growth factor mediators, it is time to consider the possibility that angiotensin's role is crucial in cancer.

4.   THE RENIN-ANGIOTENSIN SYSTEM IN THE BREAST

What is the source of angiotensin II available to breast or other carcinomas? In recent years, attention has also focused on the evidence for local tissue RASs, particularly in the adrenal (Gupta *et al* 1995; Mulrow 1998; Vinson *et al* 1998), gonads and reproductive tract (Hagemann *et al* 1994; Li *et al* 2004; Nielsen *et al* 1995; Vinson *et al* 1997; Ganong 1995) kidney (Phillips *et al* 1993; Zimmerman *et al* 1997); heart (Okura *et al* 1992; Bader 2002; Dean *et al* 2006), brain, pituitary (Vila-Porcile *et al* 1998; McKinley *et al* 2003; Dean *et al* 2006) and pancreas (Tahmasebi *et al* 1999; Leung *et al* 2001; Leung *et al* 2005). It seems likely that the multiple roles of angiotensin II in these various tissues are sustained by its local generation, adjacent to its sites of action.

Early evidence showed (pro)renin gene transcription in normal and abnormal breast tissue using in situ hybridisation (Tahmasebi *et al* 1998). In normal breast ducts, transcription was seen in myoepithelial cells and in fibroblasts, but none was found in the secretory epithelium. In cancer, overall (pro)renin transcription was seemingly reduced with the loss of myoepithelial cells, and it also became more sporadic in fibroblasts (Fig. 5).

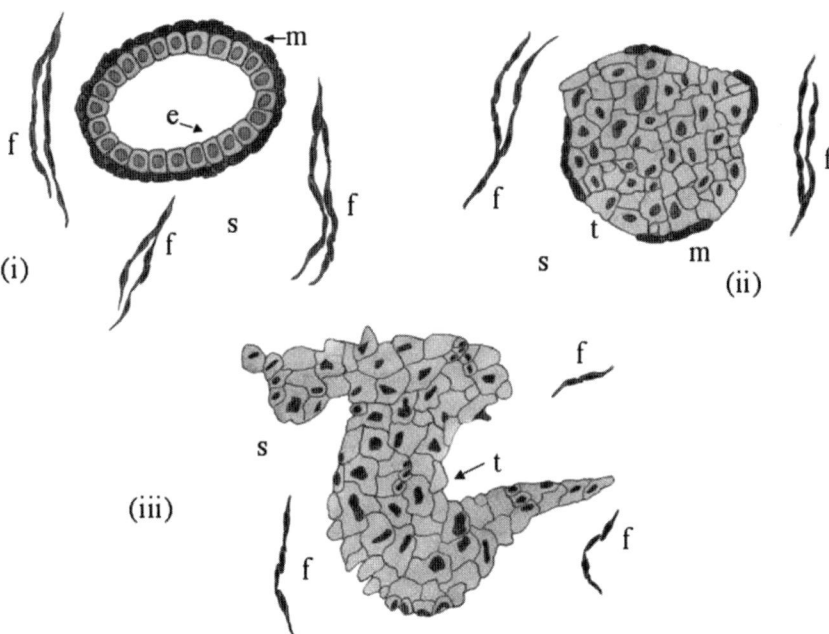

Figure 5. Angiotensin II receptors, and ACE are both present in epithelial cells and in cancer cells. Sites of (pro)renin mRNA transcription (dark shading) are shown in (i) normal breast ducts, (ii) intraductal carcinoma in situ and (iii) invasive carcinoma. The myoepithelial source of (pro)renin transcription is lost as cancer develops. Since in normal tissue this lies in close proximity to the epithelium, the configuration strongly suggests that angiotensin II can be produced at its epithelial site of action. This tightly linked system is lost in cancer, suggesting that the AT_1 and AT_2 receptor-containing carcinoma eventually becomes deprived of its source of angiotensin II. From (Tahmasebi et al 1998; Tahmasebi et al 2006). e = epithelium, m = myoepithelium, f = fibroblast, t = tumour, s = stroma. Drawing by Bronwen Vinson

In other studies, evidence for transcription of mRNA coding for RAS components was sought using quantitative RT-PCR. Angiotensinogen mRNA was shown to be present, though in low amounts compared with the liver, and (pro)renin mRNA was present though lower than in the kidney. This is perhaps unsurprising, since liver and kidney are usually considered to be the major sources of these components (Mulrow 1999) (Kaschina *et al* 2003). However, confirming the previously reported in situ hybridisation data (Tahmasebi *et al* 1998), there was significantly less (pro)renin mRNA in carcinoma than in normal tissue. Finally, the quantification of ACE mRNA showed that expression was present in carcinoma, though again in lower amounts than in normal tissue (Tahmasebi *et al* 2006).

In contrast to these data on the presence of mRNA, immunocytochemistry revealed that, in most samples of normal breast tissue, (pro)renin was in present in abundance in myoepithelial cells, though it was absent from connective tissues surrounding the ducts, unlike its mRNA. Somewhat different patterns were seen in cancer, and while the distribution seen in normal tissue was broadly reflected in ductal and in lobular carcinoma in situ, varying staining patterns were seen in fibroadenoma, and in infiltrating ductal carcinoma in which the antigen was weakly and sporadically present in epithelial cells, but also more strikingly, in fibroblasts as well. Abundance of (pro)renin also varied according to the stage of malignancy, suggesting that its expression varied inversely with tumour grading. Thus (pro)renin staining was still present in fibroblasts in advanced cancer, though at relatively low intensity.

Together with previous data on the distribution of (pro)renin mRNA, which in normal tissue was detected mostly in fibroblasts and myoepithelium, the data suggest that (pro)renin, is formed in the fibroblasts (and myoepithelium) and is transported from these sites of synthesis, perhaps to myoepithelium (though the myoepithelium is also a source), and possibly even to the epithelium, though this is rarely visible. In cancer, though, (pro)renin mRNA and protein are both found in fibroblasts. This suggests that the link between fibroblasts, myoepithelium and epithelium are essential for any such transfer to occur. Together with the progressive loss overall of both (pro)renin mRNA and protein, such physical disruption suggests that the system for local angiotensin II generation is greatly impaired in cancer (Fig. 5).

The localisation of ACE is especially important to the concept of a local RAS supplying purely local requirements for angiotensin II, and, tellingly, it was found to be located in the ductal epithelium in normal breast tissue, and also in fibroadenoma and carcinoma (Tahmasebi *et al* 2006). It supports the view that angiotensin II in breast tissue is not necessarily derived from the circulation and may originate from a local source. Most importantly, it suggests that angiotensin II is produced directly in the epithelium, the site at which it acts. Clearly it may be formed from angiotensin I provided by renin activity in the myoepithelium. This reveals a tightly organised RAS that is geared to the production of angiotensin II in the breast duct epithelium alone, and it is the apparently close coupling of (pro)renin and ACE expression with the epithelial site of angiotensin II action that is so compelling. Since angiotensin II has numerous functions in epithelial and other tissues, including

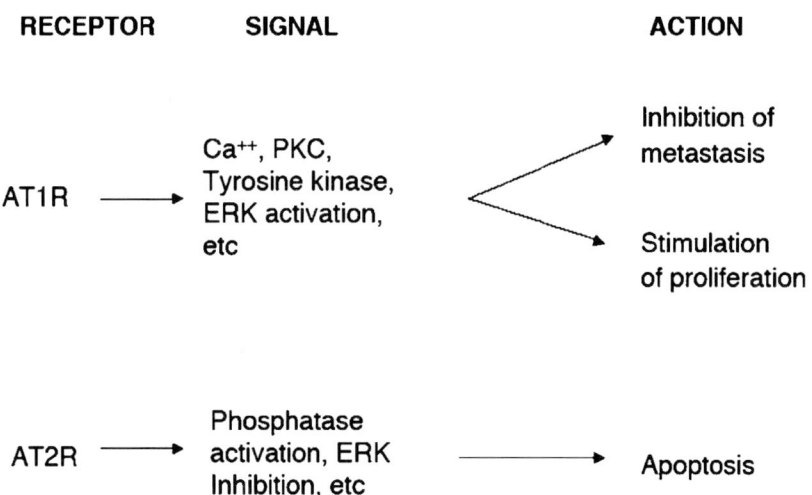

Figure 6. Possible actions of angiotensin in cancer. Note that angiotensin II may stimulate both cell proliferation (via the AT$_1$ receptor) and apoptosis (via the AT$_2$ receptor). However, signalling via the AT$_1$ receptor may also inhibit cell adhesion to, and migration through the extracellular matrix, processes that are associated with metastasis. Simply blocking the AT$_1$ receptor could thus conceivably bring both beneficial and damaging responses, through limiting proliferation, but promoting metastasis at the same time. Clearly, loss of angiotensin II generation in cancer (cf Fig. 5) could also bring both of these consequences

the regulation of mitosis and tissue differentiation (Fig. 6), the observation that (pro)renin transcription apparently fails in invasive carcinoma, crucially suggests that here angiotensin II is not available to maintain these functions. This has profound implications for our understanding of cancer. We conclude that the local RAS may be important for the regulation of epithelial function in the breast. Such regulation is lost as the renin producing fibroblasts and myoepithelium are physically separated from the bulk of the proliferating cells. The characteristic invasiveness of malignant cells may reflect this loss of RAS control.

5. CANCER RELATED FUNCTIONS OF ANGIOTENSIN II IN THE BREAST

Other studies describe the actions of angiotensin II on breast cells. Primary among these is the stimulation of cell proliferation in cancer cells via the AT$_1$ receptor (Muscella *et al* 2002). The signalling pathways involved have been explored, and include calcium mobilisation (Greco *et al* 2002a), PKC activation (specifically through subtypes zeta (atypical form) and iota) and ERK activation (Greco *et al* 2002b; Greco *et al* 2003; Muscella *et al* 2003; Muscella *et al* 2005). There is also evidence, as in other examples of angiotensin II signalling, for cross-activation of EGF function (Greco *et al* 2003). The AT$_1$ receptor also mediates Na$^+$/K$^+$ ATPase activation (Muscella *et al* 2002; Muscella *et al* 2005).

Most intriguingly, the relationship with other cancer related functions has shown that angiotensin II also has beneficial as well as damaging actions. Using the MCF-7 and T47D breast cancer cell lines in in-vitro assays, angiotensin II has been shown to inhibit expression of the specific integrin subtypes $\alpha 3$ and $\beta 1$, and also to inhibit cancer cell adhesion to cell matrix proteins, and cell invasion. These effects too are mediated via the AT_1 receptor (Puddefoot et al 2006).

In breast cancer, in other words, angiotensin II action on the AT_1 receptor may have both damaging effects, through the stimulation of cell proliferation, and beneficial actions, through inhibiting cell adhesion to, and migration through, components of the extracellular matrix, processes that are associated with metastasis (see Fig. 6). Because of this duality of action, it is clear to see that simple suppression of angiotensin II formation, or inhibition of angiotensin II binding to AT_1 receptors, may not be wholly beneficial or appropriate therapies (cf. ref (Magy et al 2005)). This may also contribute to the inconclusive results that have been obtained in patients (see above), despite the clear actions of angiotensin II on tumour cells in vitro, and in laboratory animals.

To understand the significance of these complex events, it is useful to consider the physiology of the normal breast. In development, complexity of the ductal system begins to appear at the time of puberty, and it reaches a stable state in the nulliparous adult female. However, in pregnancy, the ductal system proliferates further, and this development continues so as to form the highly secretory gland of lactation.

When lactation ceases, the breast ducts involute, and regain the non-pregnant condition (Wiseman et al 2002; Boutinaud et al 2004; Green et al 2004). Thus in normal physiology breast duct cells undergo periods of proliferation, and others of apoptotic involution (Fig. 4). The situation is complex, and it appears that the propensity for metaplastic change varies at different stages of the cycle, leading to the proposition that there are at least two types of stem cell, or a hierarchy of stem cells (Villadsen 2005; Russo et al 2006). It is furthermore known that epithelial cells in general are not fully functional in the absence of the surrounding stroma which provides essential factors that stimulate its proper development and function, among which growth factors and integrins are prominent (Chrenek et al 2001; Pollard 2001; Wiseman et al 2002; Barcellos-Hoff et al 2005). On the basis of the evidence presented here, we propose that angiotensin II is also one such factor. Since angiotensin II has both proliferative and apoptotic actions, via AT_1 and AT_2 receptors, it is plausible that it is active throughout the whole breast cycle. It is easy to see how, when invasive cancer develops, the disruption of the tightly co-ordinated tissue RAS that we have described may have complex effects on tumour development, and contribute to the overall threat to health.

6. CONCLUSIONS

The tissue RAS and the local generation and action of angiotensin II are key components in the function of the normal breast epithelium. These functions may include the homeostatic regulation of gland and duct integrity throughout the breast cycle during pregnancy, lactation, and post lactation, as well as regulation of normal epithelial functions, such as electrolyte transport. Though breast cancer cells still retain angiotensin II receptors, the partial loss of the tissue RAS as cancer develops may contribute to the progress of the disease. It is therefore appropriate to consider the breast tissue RAS as an appropriate target for the development of new therapies.

REFERENCES

Ali, M.S., Sayeski, P.P., Bernstein, K.E., 2000, Jak2 acts as both a STAT1 kinase and as a molecular bridge linking STAT1 to the angiotensin II AT1 receptor. *J Biol Chem* **275**, 15586–15593.

Ambili, M., Jayasree, K., Sudhakaran, P.R., 1998, 60K gelatinase involved in mammary gland involution is regulated by beta-oestradiol. *Biochim Biophys Acta* **1403**, 219–231.

Anderson, J.H., Willmott, N., Bessent, R., Angerson, W.J., Kerr, D.J., McArdle, C.S., 1991, Regional chemotherapy for inoperable renal carcinoma: a method of targeting therapeutic microspheres to tumour. *Br.J.Cancer.* **64**, 365–368.

Bader, M., 2002, Role of the local Renin-Angiotensin system in cardiac damage: a minireview focussing on transgenic animal models. *J Mol Cell Cardiol* **34**, 1455–1462.

Barcellos-Hoff, M.H., Medina, D., 2005, New highlights on stroma-epithelial interactions in breast cancer. *Breast Cancer Res* **7**, 33–36.

Barnes, D.M., Millis, R.R., Gillett, C.E., Ryder, K., Skilton, D., Fentiman, I.S., Rubens, R.D., 2004, The interaction of oestrogen receptor status and pathological features with adjuvant treatment in relation to survival in patients with operable breast cancer: a retrospective study of 2660 patients. *Endocrine-Related Cancer* **11**, 85–96.

Bedecs, K., Elbaz, N., Sutren, M., Masson, M., Susini, C., Strosberg, A.D., Nahmias, C., 1997, Angiotensin II type 2 receptors mediate inhibition of mitogen- activated protein kinase cascade and functional activation of SHP-1 tyrosine phosphatase. *Biochem.J.* **325**, 449–454.

Berry, C., Touyz, R., Dominiczak, A.F., Webb, R.C., Johns, D.G., 2001, Angiotensin receptors: signaling, vascular pathophysiology, and interactions with ceramide. *Am J Physiol* **281**, H2337–H2365.

Bianco, R., Daniele, G., Ciardiello, F., Tortora, G., 2005, Monoclonal antibodies targeting the epidermal growth factor receptor. *Current Drug Targets* **6**, 275–287.

Booz, G.W., Baker, K.M., 1995, Molecular signalling mechanisms controlling growth and function of cardiac fibroblasts. *Cardiovasc Res* **30**, 537–543.

Boutinaud, M., Guinard-Flament, J., Jammes, H., 2004, The number and activity of mammary epithelial cells, determining factors for milk production. *Reprod Nutr Develop* **44**, 499–508.

Chai, S.Y., Fernando, R., Peck, G., Ye, S.Y., Mendelsohn, F.A., Jenkins, T.A., Albiston, A.L., 2004, The angiotensin IV/AT4 receptor. *Cell Mol Life Sci* **61**, 2728–2737.

Chapman, A.B., Zamudio, S., Woodmansee, W., Merouani, A., Osorio, F., Johnson, A., Moore, L.G., Dahms, T., Coffin, C., Abraham, W.T., Schrier, R.W., 1997, Systemic and renal hemodynamic changes in the luteal phase of the menstrual cycle mimic early pregnancy. *Am J Physiol* **42**, F777–F782.

Chen, L., Re, R.N., Prakash, O., Mondal, D., 1991, Angiotensin-converting enzyme-inhibition reduces neuroblastoma cell- growth rate. *Proc Soc Exp Biol Med* **196**, 280–283.

Chidambaram, M., Duncan, J.A., Lai, V.S., Cattran, D.C., Floras, J.S., Scholey, J.W., Miller, J.A., 2002, Variation in the renin angiotensin system throughout the normal menstrual cycle. *J Am Soc Nephrol* **13**, 446–452.

Chiu, T., Santiskulvong, C., Rozengurt, E., 2005, EGF receptor transactivation mediates ANG II-stimulated mitogenesis in intestinal epithelial cells through the PI3-kinase/Akt/mTOR/p70S6K1 signaling pathway. *Am J Physiol* **288**, G182–194.

Chrenek, M.A., Wong, P., Weaver, V.M., 2001, Tumour-stromal interactions. Integrins and cell adhesions as modulators of mammary cell survival and transformation. *Breast.Cancer Res.* **3**, 224–229.

Clauser, E., Curnow, K.M., Davies, E., Conchon, S., Teutsch, B., Vianello, B., Monnot, C., Corvol, P., 1996, Angiotensin II receptors: protein and gene structures, expression and potential pathological involvements. *Eur J Endocrinol* **134**, 403–411.

D'Amore, A., Black, M.J., Thomas, W.G., 2005, The Angiotensin II type 2 receptor causes constitutive growth of cardiomyocytes and does not antagonize angiotensin II type 1 receptor - Mediated hypertrophy. *Hypertension* **46**, 1347–1354.

de Gasparo, M., Catt, K.J., Inagami, T., Wright, J.W., Unger, T., 2000, International union of pharmacology. XXIII. The angiotensin II receptors. *Pharmacol Rev* **52**, 415–472.

de Gasparo, M., 2002, AT(1) and AT(2) angiotensin II receptors: Key features. *Drugs* **62**, 1–10.

De Paepe, B., Verstraeten, V.L., De Potter, C.R., Vakaet, L.A., Bullock, G.R., 2001, Growth stimulatory angiotensin II type-1 receptor is upregulated in breast hyperplasia and in situ carcinoma but not in invasive carcinoma. *Histochem.Cell Biol.* **116**, 247–254.

De Paolis, P., Porcellini, A., Savoia, C., Lombardi, A., Gigante, B., Frati, G., Rubattu, S., Musumeci, B., Volpe, M., 2002, Functional cross-talk between angiotensin II and epidermal growth factor receptors in NIH3T3 fibroblasts. *J Hypertens* **20**, 693–699.

Dean, S.A., Tan, J., White, R., O'Brien E, R., Leenen, F.H., 2006, Regulation of components of the brain and cardiac renin-angiotensin systems by 17β-estradiol following myocardial infarction in female rats. *Am J Physiol* **291**, R155–62

Deshayes, F., Nahmias, C., 2005, Angiotensin receptors: a new role in cancer? *Trends in Endocy Metab* **16**, 293–299.

Dickson, R.B., Johnson, M.D., Bano, M., Shi, E., Kurebayashi, J., Ziff, B., Martinezlacaci, I., Amundadottir, L.T., Lippman, M.E., 1992, Growth-Factors in Breast-Cancer - Mitogenesis to Transformation. *J steroid Biochem Mol Biol* **43**, 69–78.

Diep, Q.N., El Mabrouk, M., Yue, P., Schiffrin, E.L., 2002, Effect of AT(1) receptor blockade on cardiac apoptosis in angiotensin II-induced hypertension. *Am J Physiol* **282**, H1635–H1641.

Dinh, D.T., Frauman, A.G., Johnston, C.I., Fabiani, M.E., 2001, Angiotensin receptors: distribution, signalling and function. *Clin.Sci.(Lond).* **100**, 481–492.

Dinh, D.T., Frauman, A.G., Somers, G.R., Ohishi, M., Zhou, J., Casley, D.J., Johnston, C.I., Fabiani, M.E., 2002, Evidence for activation of the renin-angiotensin system in the human prostate: increased angiotensin II and reduced AT(1) receptor expression in benign prostatic hyperplasia. *J.Pathol.* **196**, 213–229.

Doan, T.N., Ali, M.S., Bernstein, K.E., 2001, Tyrosine kinase activation by the angiotensin II receptor in the absence of calcium signaling. *J Biol Chem* **276**, 20954–20958.

Duffy, M.J., Maguire, T.M., Hill, A., McDermott, E., O'Higgins, N., 2000, Metalloproteinases: role in breast carcinogenesis, invasion and metastasis. *Breast Cancer Res* **2**, 252–257.

Dzau, V.J., 2001, Theodore Cooper Lecture: Tissue angiotensin and pathobiology of vascular disease: a unifying hypothesis. *Hypertension* **37**, 1047–1052.

Fischer, M., Baessler, A., Schunkert, H., 2002, Renin angiotensin system and gender differences in the cardiovascular system. *Cardiovasc Res* **53**, 672–677.

Ford, C.M., Li, S., Pickering, J.G., 1999, Angiotensin II stimulates collagen synthesis in human vascular smooth muscle cells. Involvement of the AT(1) receptor, transforming growth factor-beta, and tyrosine phosphorylation. *Arterioscler Thromb Vasc Biol* **19**, 1843–1851.

Fryzek, J.P., Poulsen, A.H., Lipworth, L., Pedersen, L., Norgaard, M., McLaughlin, J.K., Friis, S., 2006, A cohort study of antihypertensive medication use and breast cancer among Danish women. *Breast Cancer Res Treatment* **97**, 231–236.

Fujimoto, Y., Sasaki, T., Tsuchida, A., Chayama, K., 2001, Angiotensin II type 1 receptor expression in human pancreatic cancer and growth inhibition by angiotensin II type 1 receptor antagonist. *Febs Letters* **495**, 197–200.

Fujita, M., Hayashi, I., Yamashina, S., Itoman, M., Majima, M., 2002, Blockade of angiotensin AT1a receptor signaling reduces tumor growth, angiogenesis, and metastasis. *Biochem. Biophys. Res. Commun.* **294**, 441–447.

Fujita, M., Hayashi, I., Yamashina, S., Fukamizu, A., Itoman, M., Majima, M., 2005, Angiotensin type 1a receptor signaling-dependent induction of vascular endothelial growth factor in stroma is relevant to tumor-associated angiogenesis and tumor growth. *Carcinogenesis* **26**, 271–279.

Gack, S., Vallon, R., Schaper, J., Ruther, U., Angel, P., 1994, Phenotypic alterations in fos-transgenic mice correlate with changes in Fos/Jun-dependent collagenase type I expression. Regulation of mouse metalloproteinases by carcinogens, tumor promoters, cAMP, and Fos oncoprotein. *J Biol Chem* **269**, 10363–10369.

Galis, Z.S., Khatri, J.J., 2002, Matrix metalloproteinases in vascular remodeling and atherogenesis: the good, the bad, and the ugly. *Circ Res* **90**, 251–262.

Ganong, W.F., 1995, Reproduction and the renin-angiotensin system. *Neurosci Biobehav Rev* **19**, 241–250.

Goffin, V., Binart, N., Touraine, P., Kelly, P.A., 2002, Prolactin: The new biology of an old hormone. *Ann Rev Physiol* **64**, 47–67.

Goldberg, J.A., Kerr, D.J., Wilmott, N., McKillop, J.H., McArdle, C.S., 1990, Regional chemotherapy for colorectal liver metastases: a phase II evaluation of targeted hepatic arterial 5-fluorouracil for colorectal liver metastases. *Br.J.Surg.* **77**, 1238–1240.

Gonzalez-Perez, A., Ronquist, G., Rodriguez, L.A.G., 2004, Breast cancer incidence and use of antihypertensive medication in women. *Pharmacoepidem Drug Safety* **13**, 581–585.

Gordon, M.S., Chin, W.W., Shupnik, M.A., 1992, Regulation of Angiotensinogen Gene-Expression by Estrogen. *J Hypertens* **10**, 361–366.

Greco, S., Elia, M.G., Muscella, A., Storelli, C., Marsigliante, S., 2002a, AT1 angiotensin II receptor mediates intracellular calcium mobilization in normal and cancerous breast cells in primary culture. *Cell Calcium* **32**, 1–10.

Greco, S., Muscella, A., Elia, M.G., Salvatore, P., Storelli, C., Marsigliante, S., 2002b, Activation of angiotensin II type I receptor promotes protein kinase C translocation and cell proliferation in human cultured breast epithelial cells. *J. Endocrinol.* **174**, 205–214.

Greco, S., Muscella, A., Elia, M.G., Salvatore, P., Storelli, C., Mazzotta, A., Manca, C., Marsigliante, S., 2003, Angiotensin II activates extracellular signal regulated kinases via protein kinase C and epidermal growth factor receptor in breast cancer cells. *J. Cell. Physiol.* **196**, 370–377.

Green, K.A., Streuli, C.H., 2004, Apoptosis regulation in the mammary gland. *Cell Mol Life Sci* **61**, 1867–1883.

Griendling, K.K., UshioFukai, M., Lassegue, B., Alexander, R.W., 1997, Angiotensin II signaling in vascular smooth muscle - new concepts. *Hypertension* **29**, 366–373.

Griendling, K.K., Sorescu, D., Ushio-Fukai, M., 2000, NAD(P)H oxidase - role in cardiovascular biology and disease. *Circulation res* **86**, 494–501.

Gross, V., Obst, M., Luft, F.C., 2004, Insights into angiotensin II receptor function through AT2 receptor knockout mice. *Acta Physiol Scand* **181**, 487–494.

Gupta, P., Francosaenz, R., Mulrow, P.J., 1995, Locally generated angiotensin-II in the adrenal-gland regulates basal, corticotropin-stimulated, and potassium-stimulated aldosterone secretion. *Hypertension* **25**, 443–448.

Haagensen, C., 1986, Diseases of the breast. Saunders, Philadelphia.

Hagemann, A., Nielsen, A.H., Poulsen, K., 1994, The uteroplacental renin-angiotensin system - a review. *Exp clin endocr* **102**, 252–261.

Hall, K.L., Venkateswaran, S., Hanesworth, J.M., Schelling, M.E., Harding, J.W., 1995, Characterization of a functional angiotensin-IV receptor on coronary microvascular endothelial-cells. *Reg Peptides* **58**, 107–115.

Hansen, R.K., Bissell, M.J., 2000, Tissue architecture and breast cancer: the role of extracellular matrix and steroid hormones. *Endocrine-Related Cancer* **7**, 95–113.

Haulica, I., Bild, W., Serban, D.N., 2005, Angiotensin peptides and their pleiotropic actions. *J Renin Angiotensin Aldosterone Syst* **6**, 121–131.

Horiuchi, M., Hayashida, W., Kambe, T., Yamada, T., Dzau, V.J., 1997, Angiotensin type 2 receptor dephosphorylates bcl-2 by activating mitogen-activated protein kinase phosphatase-1 and induces apoptosis. *J Biol Chem* **272**, 19022–19026.

Horiuchi, M., Hamai, M., Cui, T.X., Iwai, H., Minokoshi, Y., 1999a, Cross talk between angiotensin II type 1 and type 2 receptors: Cellular mechanism of angiotensin type 2 receptor-mediated cell growth inhibition. *Hypertension Res Clin Exp* **22**, 67–74.

Horiuchi, M., Lehtonen, J.Y.A., Daviet, L., 1999b, Signaling mechanism of the AT2 angiotensin II receptor: Crosstalk between AT1 and AT2 receptors in cell growth. *Trends in Endocrinology and Metabolism* **10**, 391–396.

Howell, A., Dowsett, M., 2004, Endocrinology and hormone therapy in breast cancer - Aromatase inhibitors versus antioestrogens. *Breast Cancer Res* **6**, 269–274.

Hunyady, L., Catt, K.J., 2006, Pleiotropic AT(1) receptor signaling pathways mediating physiological and pathogenic actions of angiotensin II. *Mol Endocr* **20**, 953–970.

Hynes, N.E., Lane, H.A., 2005, ERBB receptors and cancer: The complexity of targeted inhibitors. *Nature Rev Cancer* **5**, 341–354.

Inwang, E.R., Puddefoot, J.R., Brown, C.L., Goode, A.W., Marsigliante, S., Ho, M.M., Payne, J.G., Vinson, G.P., 1997, Angiotensin II type 1 receptor expression in human breast tissues. *Br.J.Cancer* **75**, 1279–1283.

Jarvis, M.F., Gessner, G.W., Ly, C.Q., 1992, The angiotensin hexapeptide 3–8 fragment potently inhibits [^{125}I]angiotensin II binding to non-AT$_1$ or -AT$_2$ recognition sites in bovine adrenal cortex. *Eur J Pharm* **219**, 319–322.

Johnston, C.I., 1992, Franz Volhard Lecture. Renin-angiotensin system: a dual tissue and hormonal system for cardiovascular control. *J.Hypertens.Suppl.* **10**, S13–S26.

Jones, K.L., Buzdar, A.U., 2004, A review of adjuvant hormonal therapy in breast cancer. *Endocrine-Related Cancer* **11**, 391–406.

Karakiulakis, G., Papakonstantinou, E., Aletras, A.J., Tamm, M., Roth, M., 2006, Cell type specific effect of hypoxia and PDGF-BB on extracellular matrix turnover and its consequences for lung remodelling. *J Biol Chem*

Kaschina, E., Unger, T., 2003, Angiotensin AT1/AT2 receptors: Regulation, signalling and function. *Blood Press* **12**, 70–88.

Kisley, L.R., Sakai, R.R., Fluharty, S.J., 1999, Estrogen decreases hypothalamic angiotensin II AT(1) receptor binding and mRNA in the female rat. *Brain Res* **844**, 34–42.

Klett, C., Hellmann, W., Hackenthal, E., Ganten, D., 1993, Modulation of tissue angiotensinogen gene expression by glucocorticoids, estrogens, and androgens in SHR and WKY rats. *Clin.Exp.Hypertens.* **15**, 683–708.

Koh, W.P., Yuan, J.M., Van Den Berg, D., Lee, H.P., Yu, M.C., 2005, Polymorphisms in angiotensin II type 1 receptor and angiotensin I-converting enzyme genes and breast cancer risk among Chinese women in Singapore. *Carcinogenesis* **26**, 459–464.

Kucerova, D., Zelezna, B., Sloncova, E., Sovova, V., 1998, Angiotensin II receptors on colorectal carcinoma cells. *Int J Mol Med* **2**, 593–595.

Lamote, I., Meyer, E., Massart-Leen, A.M., Burvenich, C., 2004, Sex steroids and growth factors in the regulation of mammary gland proliferation, differentiation, and involution. *Steroids* **69**, 145–159.

Lees, K.R., MacFadyen, R.J., Doig, J.K., Reid, J.L., 1993, Role of angiotensin in the extravascular system. *J.Hum.Hypertens.* **7**, S 7-S 12.

Leung, P.S., Chan, H.C., Fu, L.X., Zhou, W.L., Wong, P.Y., 1997, Angiotensin II receptors, AT1 and AT2 in the rat epididymis. Immunocytochemical and electrophysiological studies. *Biochim.Biophys.Acta* **1357**, 65–72.

Leung, P.S., Carlsson, P.O., 2001, Tissue renin-angiotensin system: its expression, localization, regulation and potential role in the pancreas. *J. Mol. Endocrinol.* **26**, 155–164.

Leung, P.S., Carlsson, P.O., 2005, Pancreatic islet renin angiotensin system - Its novel roles in islet function and in diabetes mellitus. *Pancreas* **30**, 293–298.

Lever, A.F., Hole, D.J., Gillis, C.R., McCallum, I.R., McInnes, G.T., MacKinnon, P.L., Meredith, P.A., Murray, L.S., Reid, J.L., Robertson, J.W.K., 1998, Do inhibitors of angiotensin-I-converting enzyme protect against risk of cancer? *Lancet* **352**, 179–184.

Li, C.I., Malone, K.E., Weiss, N.S., Boudreau, D.M., Cushing-Haugen, K.L., Daling, J.R., 2003a, Relation between use of anti hypertensive medications and risk of breast carcinoma among women ages 65–79 years. *Cancer* **98**, 1504–1513.

Li, X.P., Rayford, H., Uhal, B.D., 2003b, Essential roles for angiotensin receptor AT1a in bleomycin-induced apoptosis and lung fibrosis in mice. *Am J Path* **163**, 2523–2530.

Li, Y.H., Jiao, L.H., Liu, R.H., Chen, X.L., Wang, H., Wang, W.H., 2004, Localization of angiotensin II in pig ovary and its effects on oocyte maturation in vitro. *Theriogenology* **61**, 447–459.

Lim, K.T., Cosgrave, N., Hill, A.D., Young, L.S., 2006, Nongenomic oestrogen signalling in oestrogen receptor negative breast cancer cells: a role for the angiotensin II receptor AT1. *Breast Cancer Res* **8**,

Lin, J.Q., Freeman, M.R., 2003, Transactivation of ErbBl and ErbB2 receptors by angiotensin II in normal human prostate stromal cells. *Prostate* **54**, 1–7.

Linz, W., Scholkens, B.A., Ganten, D., 1989, Converting enzyme inhibition specifically prevents the development and induces regression of cardiac hypertrophy in rats. *Clin.Exp.Hypertens.A.* **11**, 1325–1350.

Magness, R.R., Parker, C.R., Rosenfeld, C.R., 1993, Systemic and Uterine Responses to Chronic Infusion of Estradiol-17-Beta. *Am J Physiol* **265**, E690–E698.

Magy, L., Vincent, F., Faure, S., Messerli, F.H., Wang, J.G., Achard, J.M., Fournier, A., 2005, The renin-angiotensin systems: evolving pharmacological perspectives for cerebroprotection. *Curr Pharm Des* **11**, 3275–3291.

Mahmood, T., Djahanbakhch, O., Burleigh, D.E., Puddefoot, J.R., O'Mahony, O.A., Vinson, G.P., 2002, Effect of angiotensin II on ion transport across human Fallopian tube epithelial cells in vitro. *Reproduction* **124**, 573–579.

Mancina, R., Susini, T., Renzetti, A., Forti, G., Razzoli, E., Serio, M., Maggi, M., 1996, Sex steroid modulation of AT(2) receptors in human myometrium. *J clin Endocr Metab* **81**, 1753–1757.

Marsigliante, S., Resta, L., Muscella, A., Vinson, G.P., Marzullo, A., Storelli, C., 1996, AT1 angiotensin II receptor subtype in the human larynx and squamous laryngeal carcinoma. *Cancer Let* **110**, 19–27.

Martin, M.M., White, C.R., Li, H., Miller, P.J., Elton, T.S., 1995, A functional comparison of the rat type-1 angiotensin II receptors (AT1AR and AT1BR). *Regul Pept* **60**, 135–147.

McKinley, M.J., Albiston, A.L., Allen, A.M., Mathai, M.L., May, C.N., McAllen, R.M., Oldfield, B.J., Mendelsohn, F.A., Chai, S.Y., 2003, The brain renin-angiotensin system: location and physiological roles. *Int J Biochem Cell Biol* **35**, 901–918.

Meier, C.R., Derby, L.E., Jick, S.S., Jick, H., 2000, Angiotensin-converting enzyme inhibitors, calcium channel blockers, and breast cancer. *Arch Int Med* **160**, 349–353.

Millan, M.A., Carvallo, P., Izumi, S., Zemel, S., Catt, K.J., Aguilera, G., 1989, Novel sites of expression of functional angiotensin II receptors in the late gestation fetus. *Science* **244**, 1340–1342.

Motz, W.H., Scheler, S., Strauer, B.E., 1992, Medical repair of hypertensive left ventricular remodeling. *J.Cardiovasc.Pharmacol.* **20 Suppl 1**, S32–S36.

Mukhopadhyay, A.K., Holstein, K., Szkudlinski, M., Brunswig-Spickenheier, B., Leidenberger, F.A., 1991, The relationship between prorenin levels in follicular fluid and follicular atresia in bovine ovaries. *Endocrinology* **129**, 2367–2375.

Mulrow, P.J., 1998, Renin-angiotensin system in the adrenal. *Horm.Metab.Res.* **30**, 346–349.

Mulrow, P.J., 1999, Angiotensin II and aldosterone regulation. *Regul Pept* **80**, 27–32.

Muscella, A., Greco, S., Elia, M.G., Storelli, C., Marsigliante, S., 2002, Angiotensin II stimulation of Na+/K+ATPase activity and cell growth by calcium-independent pathway in MCF-7 breast cancer cells. *J.Endocrinol.* **173**, 315–323.

Muscella, A., Greco, S., Elia, M.G., Storelli, C., Marsigliante, S., 2003, PKC-zeta is required for angiotensin II-induced activation of ERK and synthesis of C-FOS in MCF-7 cells. *J. Cell. Physiol.* **197**, 61–68.

Muscella, A., Storelli, C., Marsigliante, S., 2005, Atypical PKC-zeta and PKC-iota mediate opposing effects on MCF-7 Na+/K+ ATPase activity. *J. Cell. Physiol.* **205**, 278–285.

Natarajan, R., Gonzales, N., Hornsby, P.J., Nadler, J., 1992, Mechanism of angiotensin II-induced proliferation in bovine adrenocortical cells. *Endocrinology.* **131**, 1174–1180.

Nicolini, A., Carpi, A., Tarro, G., 2006, Biomolecular markers of breast cancer. *Front Biosci* **11**, 1818–1843.

Nielsen, A.H., Hagemann, A., Poulson, K., 1995, The tissue renin-angiotensin system in the female reproductive tissues. In Tissue renin-angiotensin systems, pp. 253–268, Edited by A.K. Mukhopadhyay and M.K. Raizada, Plenum, New York & London.

Noguchi, S., Miyauchi, K., Nishizawa, Y., Sasaki, Y., Imaoka, S., Iwanaga, T., Koyama, H., Terasawa, T., 1988, Augmentation of anticancer effect with angiotensin II in intraarterial infusion chemotherapy for breast carcinoma. *Cancer.* **62**, 467–473.

Norris, B., Gonzalez, C., Concha, J., Palacios, S., Contreras, G., 1991, Stimulatory Effect of Angiotensin-Ii on Electrolyte Transport in Canine Tracheal Epithelium. *Genl Pharmacol* **22**, 527–531.

Okura, T., Kitami, Y., Wakamiya, R., Marumoto, K., Iwata, T., Hiwada, K., 1992, Renal and extra-renal renin gene expression in spontaneously hypertensive rats. *Blood.Press.Suppl.* **3**, 6–11.

Olivares-Reyes, J.A., Shah, B.H., Hernandez-Aranda, J., Garcia-Caballero, A., Farshori, M.P., Garcia-Sainz, J.A., Catt, K.J., 2005, Agonist-induced interactions between angiotensin AT(1) and epidermal growth factor receptors. *Mol Pharm* **68**, 356–364.

Pal, S.K., Pegram, M., 2005, Epidermal growth factor receptor and signal transduction: potential targets for anti-cancer therapy. *Anti-Cancer Drugs* **16**, 483–494.

Peach, M.T., 1977, Renin-angiotensin system: biochemistry and mechanism of action. *Physiol Rev* **57**, 313–370.

Petrovic, I., Petrovic, D., Vukovic, N., Zivanovic, B., Dragicevic, J., Vasiljevic, Z., Babic, R., 2005, Ventricular and vascular remodelling effects of the angiotensin II receptor blocker telmisartan and/or the angiotensin-converting enzyme inhibitor ramipril in hypertensive patients. *J Int Med Res* **33 Suppl 1**, 39A–49A.

Phillips, M.I., Speakman, E.A., Kimura, B., 1993, Levels of angiotensin and molecular biology of the tissue renin angiotensin systems. *Regul.Pept.* **43**, 1–20.

Pollard, J.W., 2001, Tumour-stromal interactions - Transforming growth factor-beta isoforms and hepatocyte growth factor/scatter factor in mammary gland ductal morphogenesis. *Breast Cancer Res* **3**, 230–237.

Porteri, E., Rodella, L., Rizzoni, D., Rezzani, R., Paiardi, S., Sleiman, I., De Ciuceis, C., Boari, G.E., Castellano, M., Bianchi, R., Agabiti-Rosei, E., 2005, Effects of olmesartan and enalapril at low or high doses on cardiac, renal and vascular interstitial matrix in spontaneously hypertensive rats. *Blood Press* **14**, 184–192.

Pucell, A.G., Bumpus, F.M., Husain, A., 1987, Rat ovarian angiotensin-II receptors - characterization and coupling to estrogen secretion. *J.biol.Chem.* **262**, 7076–7080.

Puddefoot, J.R., Udeozo, U.K.I., Barker, S., Vinson, G.P., 2006, The role of angiotensin II in the regulation of breast cancer cell adhesion and invasion. *Endocrine related cancer* **13**, 895–903.

Quan, A., Baum, M., 1996, Endogenous production of angiotensin-II modulates rat proximal tubule transport. *J.Clin.Invest.* **97**, 2878–2882.

Reddy, M.K., Baskaran, K., Molteni, A., 1995, Inhibitors of angiotensin-converting enzyme modulate mitosis and gene expression in pancreatic cancer cells. *Proc Soc exp Biol Med* **210**, 221–226.

Reinhardt, D., Sigusch, H.H., Hensse, J., Tyagi, S.C., Korfer, R., Figulla, H.R., 2002, Cardiac remodelling in end stage heart failure: upregulation of matrix metalloproteinase (MMP) irrespective of the underlying disease, and evidence for a direct inhibitory effect of ACE inhibitors on MMP. *Heart* **88**, 525–530.

Rivera, E., Arrieta, O., Guevara, P., Duarte-Rojo, A., Sotelo, J., 2001, AT1 receptor is present in glioma cells; its blockage reduces the growth of rat glioma. *Br. J. Cancer* **85**, 1396–1399.

Ronquist, G., Rodriguez, L.A., Ruigomez, A., Johansson, S., Wallander, M.A., Frithz, G., Svardsudd, K., 2004, Association between captopril, other antihypertensive drugs and risk of prostate cancer. *Prostate* **58**, 50–56.

Ross, J.S., Schenkein, D.P., Pietrusko, R., Rolfe, M., Linette, G.P., Stec, J., Stagliano, N.E., Ginsburg, G.S., Symmans, W.F., Pusztai, L., Hortobagyi, G.N., 2004, Targeted therapies for cancer 2004. *Am J clin Pathol* **122**, 598–609.

Rudolph-Owen, L.A., Matrisian, L.M., 1998, Matrix metalloproteinases in remodeling of the normal and neoplastic mammary gland. *J Mammary Gland Biol Neoplasia* **3**, 177–189.

Russo, J., Balogh, G.A., Chen, J.Q., Fernandez, S.V., Fernbaugh, R., Heulings, R., Mailo, D.A., Moral, R., Russo, P.A., Sheriff, F., Vanegas, J.E., Wang, R., Russo, I.H., 2006, The concept of stem cell in the mammary gland and its implication in morphogenesis, cancer and prevention. *Front Biosci* **11**, 151–172.

Sakata, Y., Yamamoto, K., Mano, T., Nishikawa, N., Yoshida, J., Hori, M., Miwa, T., Masuyama, T., 2004, Activation of matrix metalloproteinases precedes left ventricular remodeling in hypertensive heart failure rats: its inhibition as a primary effect of Angiotensin-converting enzyme inhibitor. *Circulation* **109**, 2143–2149.

Saridogan, E., Djahanbakhch, O., Puddefoot, J.R., Demetroulis, C., Collingwood, K., Mehta, J.G., Vinson, G.P., 1996, Angiotensin II receptors and angiotensin II stimulation of ciliary activity in human fallopian tube. *J.Clin.Endocrinol.Metab.* **81**, 2719–2725.

Schorb, W., Conrad, K.M., Singer, H.A., Dostal, D.E., Baker, K.M., 1995, Angiotensin-II is a potent stimulator of MAP-kinase activity in neonatal rat cardiac fibroblasts. *J mol cell Cardiol* **27**, 1151–1160.

Sealey, J.E., Itskovitzeldor, J., Rubattu, S., James, G.D., August, P., Thaler, I., Levron, J., Laragh, J.H., 1994, Estradiol-Related and Progesterone-Related Increases in the Renin-Aldosterone System - Studies During Ovarian Stimulation and Early-Pregnancy. *J clin Endocr Metab* **79**, 258–264.

Seltzer, A., Pinto, J.E.B., Viglione, P.N., Correa, F.M.A., Libertun, C., Tsutsumi, K., Steele, M.K., Saavedra, J.M., 1992, Estrogens Regulate Angiotensin-Converting Enzyme and Angiotensin Receptors in Female Rat Anterior-Pituitary. *Neuroendocrinology* **55**, 460–467.

Shah, B.H., Yesilkaya, A., Olivares-Reyes, J.A., Chen, H.D., Hunyady, L., Catt, K.J., 2004, Differential pathways of angiotensin II-induced extracellularly regulated kinase 1/2 phosphorylation in specific cell types: Role of heparin-binding epidermal growth factor. *Mol Endocr* **18**, 2035–2048.

Singer, C.F., Hudelist, G., Galid, A., Kubista, E., 2003, Pharmacological modulation of local feedback mechanisms as a therapeutic approach in breast cancer treatment. *Drugs of Today* **39**, 917–926.

Sivaraman, V.S., Wang, H.Y., Nuovo, G.J., Malbon, C.C., 1997, Hyperexpression of mitogen-activated protein kinase in human breast cancer. *J.Clin.Invest.* **99**, 1478–1483.

Small, W., Jr., Molteni, A., Kim, Y.T., Taylor, J.M., Chen, Z., Ward, W.F., 1997, Captopril modulates hormone concentration and inhibits proliferation of human mammary ductal carcinoma cells in culture. *Breast.Cancer Res.Treat.* **44**, 217–224.

Smith, R.D., Timmermans, P.B., 1994, Human angiotensin receptor subtypes. *Curr Opin Nephrol Hypertens* **3**, 112–122.

Stroth, U., Unger, T., 1999, The renin-angiotensin system and its receptors. *J Cardiovasc Pharmacol* **33** **Suppl 1**, S21–28; discussion S41–23.

Suganuma, T., Ino, K., Shibata, K., Kajiyama, H., Nagasaka, T., Mizutani, S., Kikkawa, F., 2005, Functional expression of the angiotensin II type 1 receptor in human ovarian carcinoma cells and its blockade therapy resulting in suppression of tumor invasion, angiogenesis, and peritoneal dissemination. *Clin. Cancer Res.* **11**, 2686–2694.

Sun, S.Z., Wang, Y., Li, Q., Tian, Y.J., Liu, M.H., Yu, Y.H., 2006, Effects of benazepril on renal function and kidney expression of matrix metalloproteinase-2 and tissue inhibitor of metalloproteinase-2 in diabetic rats. *Chin Med J (Engl)* **119**, 814–821.

Suzuki, J., Iwai, M., Nakagami, H., Wu, L., Chen, R., Sugaya, T., Hamada, M., Hiwada, K., Horiuchi, M., 2002, Role of angiotensin II-regulated apoptosis through distinct AT(1) and AT(2) receptors in neointimal formation. *Circulation* **106**, 847–853.

Tahmasebi, M., Puddefoot, J.R., Inwang, E.R., Goode, A.W., Carpenter, R., Vinson, G.P., 1998, Transcription of the prorenin gene in normal and diseased breast. *Eur.J.Cancer* **34**, 1777–1782.

Tahmasebi, M., Puddefoot, J.R., Inwang, E.R., Vinson, G.P., 1999, The tissue renin-angiotensin system in human pancreas. *J. Endocrinol.* **161**, 317–322.

Tahmasebi, M., Barker, S., Puddefoot, J.R., Vinson, G.P., 2006, Localisation of renin-angiotensin system (RAS) components in breast. *Br J Cancer* **95**, 67–74.

Tucker, H.A., 2000, Hormones, mammary growth, and lactation: a 41-year perspective. *J Dairy Sci* **83**, 874–884.

Uemura, H., Ishiguro, H., Nagashima, Y., Sasaki, T., Nakaigawa, N., Hasumi, H., Kato, S., Kubota, Y., 2005a, Antiproliferative activity of angiotensin II receptor blocker through cross-talk between stromal and epithelial prostate cancer cells. *Mol cancer Therapeut* **4**, 1699–1709.

Uemura, H., Nakaigawa, N., Ishiguro, H., Kubota, Y., 2005b, Antiproliferative efficacy of angiotensin II receptor blockers in prostate cancer. *Curr. Cancer Drug Targets* **5**, 307–323.

Ushio-Fukai, M., Alexander, R.W., Akers, M., Yin, Q.Q., Fujio, Y., Walsh, K., Griendling, K.K., 1999, Reactive oxygen species mediate the activation of Akt/protein kinase B by angiotensin II in vascular smooth muscle cells. *J.biol.Chem.* **274**, 22699–22704.

Vila-Porcile, E., Corvol, P., 1998, Angiotensinogen, prorenin, and renin are Co-localized in the secretory granules of all glandular cells of the rat anterior pituitary: an immunoultrastructural study. *J Histochem Cytochem* **46**, 301–311.

Villadsen, R., 2005, In search of a stem cell hierarchy in the human breast and its relevance to breast cancer evolution. *Apmis* **113**, 903–921.

Vinson, G.P., Saridogan, E., Puddefoot, J.R., Djahanbakhch, O., 1997, Tissue renin-angiotensin systems and reproduction. *Hum Reprod* **12**, 651–662.

Vinson, G.P., Ho, M.M., 1998, The adrenal renin/angiotensin system in the rat. *Hormone Metab Res* **30**, 355–359.

Volpert, O.V., Ward, W.F., Lingen, M.W., Chesler, L., Solt, D.B., Johnson, M.D., Molteni, A., Polverini, P.J., Bouck, N.P., 1996, Captopril inhibits angiogenesis and slows the growth of experimental tumors in rats. *J clin Invest* **98**, 671–679.

Wang, T., Giebisch, G., 1996, Effects of angiotensin II on electrolyte transport in the early and late distal tubule in rat kidney. *Am.J.Physiol.* **271**, F143–F149.

Weber, K.T., Brilla, C.G., Janicki, J.S., 1991, Signals for the remodeling of the cardiac interstitium in systemic hypertension. *J.Cardiovasc.Pharmacol.* **17 Suppl 2**, S14–S19.

Weidekamm, C., Hauser, P., Hansmann, C., Schwarz, C., Klingler, H., Mayer, G., Oberbauer, R., 2002, Effects of AT1 and AT2 receptor blockade on angiotensin II induced apoptosis of human renal proximal tubular epithelial cells. *Wien. Klin. Wochen.* **114**, 725–729.

Wiseman, B.S., Werb, Z., 2002, Stromal effects on mammary gland development and breast cancer. *Science* **296**, 1046–1049.

Wysolmerski J., and van Houten, N.J. (2002) http: //www.endotext.org/pregnancy/pregnancy5/pregnancy5.htm

Wolf, G., Neilson, E.G., 1993, Angiotensin II as a renal growth factor. *J Am Soc Nephrol* **3**, 1531–1540.

Wong, P.Y.D., Fu, W.O., Huang, S.J., Law, W.K., 1990, Effect of angiotensins on electrogenic anion transport in monolayer- cultures of rat epididymis. *J. Endocrinol.* **125**, 449–456.

Yamada, T., Horiuchi, M., Dzau, V.J., 1996, Angiotensin-II type-2 receptor mediates programmed cell-death. *Proc. Natl. Acad. Sci. U. S. A.* **93**, 156–160.

Yamada, T., Akishita, M., Pollman, M.J., Gibbons, G.H., Dzau, V.J., Horiuchi, M., 1998, Angiotensin II type 2 receptor mediates vascular smooth muscle cell apoptosis and antagonizes angiotensin II type 1 receptor action: An in vitro gene transfer study. *Life Sciences* **63**, PL289-PL295.

Yamaue, H., Tanimura, H., Terashita, S., Iwahashi, M., Tani, M., Tsunoda, T., Tamai, M., Mori, K., 1990, Clinical evaluation of chemotherapy under angiotensin II-induced hypertension in patients with advanced cancer. *Nippon.Geka.Hokan.* **59**, 302–309.

Yang, X., Zhu, M.J., Sreejayan, N., Ren, J., Du, M., 2005, Angiotensin II promotes smooth muscle cell proliferation and migration through release of heparin-binding epidermal growth factor and activation of EGF-receptor pathway. *Mol Cells* **20**, 263–270.

Yasumatsu, R., Nakashima, T., Masuda, M., Ito, A., Kuratomi, Y., Nakagawa, T., Komune, S., 2004, Effects of the angiotensin-I converting enzyme inhibitor perindopril on tumor growth and angiogenesis in head and neck squamous cell carcinoma cells. *J Cancer Res Clin Oncol* **130**, 567–573.

Yoshiji, H., Kuriyama, S., Noguchi, R., Fukui, H., 2004, Angiotensin-I converting enzyme inhibitors as potential anti- angiogenic agents for cancer therapy. *Curr. Cancer Drug Targets* **4**, 555–567.

Zhang, Z., Li, M., Rayburn, E.R., Hill, D.L., Zhang, R.W., Wang, H., 2005, Oncogenes as novel targets for cancer therapy - (Part I) - Growth factors and protein tyrosine kinases. *Am J Pharmacogenom* **5**, 173–190.

Zimmerman, B.G., Dunham, E.W., 1997, Tissue renin-angiotensin system: a site of drug action? *Ann Rev Pharm Tox* **37**, 53–69.

CHAPTER 8

ROLE OF LOCAL RENIN-ANGIOTENSIN SYSTEM IN THE CAROTID BODY AND IN DISEASES

MAN LUNG FUNG[1] AND PO SING LEUNG[2]

[1]*Department of Physiology, University of Hong Kong, Pokfulam, Hong Kong*
[2]*Department of Physiology, Chinese University of Hong Kong, Shatin, Hong Kong*

1.   INTRODUCTION

The carotid bodies are a pair of small organs bilaterally located at the bifurcation of the carotid artery. The organ is highly vascularized and perfused by arterial blood supply from the carotid artery. Peripheral chemoreceptors of the carotid body play a major role in the sensory chemotransduction of chemical changes in the arterial blood, which is essential to the rapid adjustment of cardiovascular and respiratory activities via the chemoreflex pathways. Under hypoxemic conditions with a fall of arterial oxygen tension below 50 mm Hg, this causes an exponential rise in the activity of the carotid sinus nerve of the carotid body. The increase in chemoreceptor afferent activities excites the neurons in the nucleus tractus solitarius, which is the primary relaying nucleus in the medulla. Activation of the chemoreflex results in the elevation of central drives and efferent nerve activities, which increases ventilation, cardiac performance and redistribution of blood flow for the physiological compensation matching metabolic needs (Marshall 1994).

Type-I glomus cells are the major cell type in the carotid body. These cells play a major role in sensory chemotransduction because these cells are closely apposed to nerve endings formed in group clusters or glomeruli (Gonzalez *et al* 1994). These glomic clusters are encapsulated by glial-like (type-II) cells; however, they are not as numerous as the type-I glomus cells. In addition, it is generally believed that type-I glomus cells are the chemosensitive cells in the carotid body, because these cells respond to various physiological stimuli such as hypoxia and hypercapnic acidosis. Upon activation of the chemical stimulus, type-I glomus cells depolarize causing a rise in intracellular calcium, which is essential for signaling the vesicular secretion of catecholamines and other putative neurotransmitters such as

155

Po Sing Leung (ed.), Frontiers in Research of the Renin-Angiotensin System on Human Disease, 155–177.
© 2007 *Springer.*

acetylcholine and ATP from the chemosensitive cells (Gonzalez *et al* 1994; Lahiri *et al* 2006). This in turn elevates the excitability of the nerve endings that cause an increase in the activity of the carotid sinus nerve of the carotid body.

The carotid body is a highly vascularized organ with blood perfusion exceeding the needs of local tissue metabolism. Thus, changes in arterial oxygen tension or pH, circulating hormones and locally produced substances from the vessels and tissues acting as autocrines or paracrines can readily diffuse to the chemosensory components of the carotid body. In fact, mounting evidence suggests that vasoactive peptides can regulate the excitability of the carotid chemoreceptors. For example, studies have shown that angiotensin II modulates carotid afferent discharge of the carotid sinus nerve in the isolated carotid body superfused in vitro, thus demonstrating an effect directly on the carotid chemoreceptor, but not from the vascular and hemodynamic effect of angiotensin II (Allen 1998; Leung *et al* 2000). In addition, a high density of angiotensin II receptors was detected in the carotid body with *in vitro* autoradiography (Allen 1998). These findings provide initial evidence for a functional role of angiotensin II receptors in the carotid body and raise a number of questions on: (i) the expression and regulation of angiotensin II receptors in the carotid body under physiological or pathophysiological conditions and (ii) the physiological or pathophysiological significance of alterations of the carotid chemoreceptor activity by angiotensin II.

Research studies have shown the influence of the renin-angiotensin system (RAS) on numerous tissues and organs. The RAS is mainly a blood-borne hormone system that regulates blood pressure and fluid homeostasis (Peach 1977; Reid *et al* 1978). In addition, the local RAS is primarily of autocrine or paracrine origin and caters to specific organ and tissue needs through actions that are complementary to, or differ from, the circulating RAS (Campbell 1987; Leung 2004). Interestingly, our recent data have demonstrated a functional expression of RAS in the carotid body, wherein this may play a physiological role in the regulation of autonomic responses to changes in arterial chemical content. Hence, it has been reported that angiotensin II as well as other vasoactive substances can directly alter the excitability of the carotid chemoreceptor (Lahiri *et al* 2001; Fung 2003; Fung and Tipoe 2003; Leung *et al* 2003; Tipoe *et al* 2006). Although these findings support a physiological role for RAS in the carotid body, the significance and clinical implication have yet to be clearly defined.

Moreover, chronic exposure to moderate hypoxia (chronic hypoxia) modifies the level of gene expression in the carotid body including an upregulation of the expression of AT_1 receptors associated with increased sensitivity of the chemoreceptor to angiotensin II (Leung *et al* 2000; Fung *et al* 2002). In chronic hypoxia, alterations of the carotid body are closely linked to structural remodeling including increased vasculature, hypertrophy and hyperplasia of the glomus cells (Dhillon *et al* 1984; McGregor *et al* 1984; Bee *et al* 1986), as well as functional modifications such as neurochemical synthesis and release of catecholamines (Hanbauer *et al* 1981; Pequignot *et al* 1987; Czyzyk-Krzeska *et al* 1992; Millhorn *et al* 1993). Furthermore, carotid afferent activities are also known to play a role in the natriuresis and diuresis that occur during hypoxia (Honig 1989). Therefore, the extent and the cellular and molecular mechanisms that mediate the effect of chronic hypoxia on the RAS in the carotid body as a physiological response to hypoxia and the significant role in salt and water homeostasis are of great interest. Hence, the focus of research studies has been on several facets. These are: (i) the cellular and molecular mechanisms underlying the carotid responses to angiotensin II; (ii) the expression of essential components of the RAS in the carotid body; (iii) the physiological changes upon activation of the RAS in the carotid body at both cellular and organ levels, and (iv) alterations of the carotid chemoreceptor response to acute hypoxia in humans or animals in chronic hypoxia (Bisgard 2000; Lahiri *et al* 2001; Lahiri and Forster 2003) or in diseases associated with hypoxemia. Combining data from the recent literature and unpublished observations from our own laboratories, this chapter aims to summarize the findings on the expression of RAS in the carotid body and its modulation by hypoxia. Changes of the RAS in the carotid body and its clinical implications during hypoxia will also be discussed.

2.   ROLES OF CHEMOREFLEX AND RENIN-ANGIOTENSIN SYSTEM IN HYPOXIA AND DISEASES

2.1.   Physiological Responses to Hypoxia via Chemoreflex

The peripheral chemoreflex forms the feedback part of the respiratory regulator for the ventilatory response to carbon dioxide and hypoxia. Physiologically, the peripheral chemoreceptors are important for: (i) an exponential increase in ventilation during hypoxia; (ii) an increase in the sensitivity of the ventilatory response to arterial levels of carbon dioxide when the oxygen level alters from hyperoxic to hypoxic (Duffin 1990; Duffin and Mahamed 2003). In addition, changes in the activity of the peripheral chemoreflex can account for the ventilatory alterations in hypoxia reported by experimental studies and described by models of chemoreflex behaviour during exposures to hypoxia of various durations (Duffin and Mahamed 2003). The first synapse of the afferent terminals of the carotid chemoreceptor is in the medial aspect of the commissural nucleus tractus solitarii (Donoghue *et al* 1984; Donoghue *et al* 1985; Mifflin 1992; Zhang and Mifflin 1993) where neurons are activated or inhibited for the efferent control of the respiratory network (Lawson *et al* 1989). In addition to respiratory control, activation of the chemoreflex induces an increase in arterial pressure, bradycardia and tachypnea in awake animals (Haibara *et al* 1995). The cardiovascular responses to chemoreflex activiation are mediated by the sympathetic activity for a pressor response. The bradycardic response is mediated by parasympathoexcitation and is independent to the changes in arterial pressure and ventilation (Marshall 1994).

2.2.   Autonomic Control by Central RAS

Angiotensin II modulates autonomic control of the cardiovascular system via AT_1 receptors that are localized in several brain regions involved in the baroreflex including the nucleus tractus solitarii, the dorsal motor nucleus of vagus, the rostral and caudal ventrolateral medulla and intermediolateral cell column of the spinal cord. In the nucleus tractus solitarii these presynaptic receptors could mediate the known baroreflex inhibitory action of angiotensin II by blockade of neurotransmitter release. Also, AT_1 receptors are largely expressed in the rostral ventrolateral medulla. Angiotensin II applied locally to the rostral ventrolateral medulla produces sympathetically mediated pressor responses (Allen *et al* 1988; Allen *et al* 1999). Indeed, blockade of the AT_1 receptor with losartan can significantly reduce the central and peripheral sympathetic nerve activity in neurogenic hypertension in rats (Ye *et al* 2002b).

Recently, a local RAS has been described in the CNS. Hence, angiotensinogen, renin, angiotensin-converting enzyme, and aminopeptidases are expressed in the brain. AT_1, AT_2 and AT_4 receptors are also localized to brain regions in addition to the regions for baroreflex control. AT_1 receptors are also found in the hypothalamic paraventricular and supraoptic nuclei, the lamina terminalis, lateral parabrachial nucleus, all of which are known to play roles in the central regulation of body fluid and electrolyte balance. Interestingly, angiotensinogen is synthesised predominantly in astrocytes, and angiotensin II is localized in neurons as a neurotransmitter although the processes of local synthesis is unknown (McKinley *et al* 2003). AT_1 receptor antagonists or angiotensinogen antisense oligonucleotides administered centrally decrease sympathetic activity and arterial blood pressure, and disrupt water drinking and sodium appetite, vasopressin secretion, sodium excretion, renin release and thermoregulation under physiological or pathophysiological conditions. Hence, the central RAS is important in the neural regulation of cardiovascular function, osmoregulation and thermoregulation (McKinley *et al* 2003).

2.3.   Regulation of RAS in Diseases with Hypoxia

The RAS plays important roles in the development of diseases including hypertension, renal diseases, ischemic heart disease, cardiac hypertrophy and heart failure. It has been shown that angiotensin receptor blockers have protective properties against tissue injuries induced by ischemia/hypoxia reperfusion. For example, in hypertensive type II diabetic rats with nephropathy, the AT_1 receptor antagonist olmesartan significantly reduces proteinuria and prevents glomerular and tubulointerstitial damage related to oxidative stress, in addition to lowering blood pressure (Izuhara *et al* 2005). Furthermore, hypoxia and angiotensin II are the major stimuli of vascular endothelial growth factor (VEGF), which is a potent angiogenic cytokine and also contributes to the atherogenic process. Patients with obstructive sleep apnea have significantly increased levels of serum angiotensin II, VEGF and VEGF mRNA expression in their leukocytes. Also, it was found that angiotensin II stimulates VEGF expression in the peripheral blood mononuclear cell and that VEGF mRNA and protein expression is decreased by olmesartan. Thus, activation of the AT_1 receptor pathway plays a role in the pathogenesis of obstructive sleep apnea (Takahashi *et al* 2005).

Moreover, it has been reported that angiotensin-converting enzyme and angiotensin II have a role in the pulmonary hypertension and vascular remodeling induced by hypoxia (Zakheim *et al* 1975; Morrell *et al* 1995; Morrell *et al* 1999). In chronically hypoxic rats, olmesartan significantly decreases the pathological development of hypoxic cor pulmonale (Nakamoto *et al* 2005). However, the AT_1 receptor antagonist losartan (at 50 mg) did not lead to a significant improvement in pulmonary hypertension in a double-blind study with forty patients with chronic obstructive pulmonary disease (Morrell *et al* 2005). In another randomized trial, the effect of the angiotensin receptor blocker irbesartan given over four months was evaluated in sixty patients with chronic obstructive pulmonary disease. Although irbesartan did not significantly change the respiratory muscle strength or spirometric results, it did lead to a significant decrease in haematocrit in the irbesaran but not the placebo group. This raises the possibility that angiotensin II receptor blockade can produce beneficial effects in chronic obstructive pulmonary disease patients with the decrease in haematocrit (Andreas *et al* 2006). The effect of RAS blockade in diseases associated with hypoxia needs more clinical trial studies in future.

3.   EXPRESSION AND FUNCTION OF RAS IN THE CAROTID BODY

3.1.   Expression of Angiotensin Receptors in the Carotid Body

The current understanding of the carotid chemoreceptor responses to angiotensin II has been mainly focused on the excitatory response of the biphasic effect. Angiotensin II induces a brief inhibition followed by a major excitation of the afferent nerve discharge in the *ex vivo* carotid body when superfused by a bicarbonate buffer (Allen 1998; Leung *et al* 2000). At concentrations from physiological to pharmacological levels, angiotensin II dose-dependently increases the baseline activity of the carotid sinus nerve by about two folds when a threshold concentration of 0.1 nM at the physiological level of plasma angiotensin II is reached (Allen 1998; Leung *et al* 2000). Losartan abolishes both the inhibitory and excitatory effects of angiotensin II on the carotid afferent activity, suggesting the ligand binding is mediated by the AT_1 receptors. The physiological significance of this finding is that the circulating levels of angiotensin II can alter the basal discharging activity of the carotid chemoreceptors, and possibly activation of the chemoreflex without significant decreases in the arterial oxygen level. In addition, systemic hypoxia increases the plasma angiotensin II levels in chronically hypoxic animals (Zakheim *et al* 1976) and this could be an alternative pathway for regulating the carotid chemoreceptor response to hypoxia. Besides the circulating angiotensin II, the discussion in Section 3.2 will show that the presence of local RAS in the carotid body could provide a much higher level of angiotensin II in the local tissue, which could be a major source of angiotensin II for a more prominent effect on the carotid chemoreceptor activity.

The fact that the carotid body is innervated by sympathetic and parasympathetic efferent nerves (Gonzalez *et al* 1994) raises the possibility that the effect of

angiotensin II is on the autonomic nerve endings instead of the carotid chemoreceptors, thereby modifying both the release of norepinephrine and the afferent
activity. However, evidence suggests that angiotensin II exerts its effect directly
on the chemosensitive cells in the carotid body. Hence, it has been shown that
angiotensin II increases intracellular calcium levels in glomus cells freshly dissociated from rat carotid bodies (Fung *et al* 2001a). Moreover, the intracellular calcium
response can be blocked by pretreatment with losartan but not by PD-123319, an
antagonist for AT_2 receptors. This suggests that the effect is mediated by AT_1
receptors located in the glomus cells. In fact, AT_1-immunostaining is localized in
lobules of the carotid body, strongly supporting that AT_1 receptors are expressed
in the glomus cells that are clustered in glomeruli (Fung *et al* 2001a). Indeed,
these findings are consistent with an autoradiographic study, which shows that
neither sympathetic nor afferent denervation of the carotid body reduce the AT_1
receptor-ligand bindings (Allen 1998). Thus, evidence supports that AT_1 receptors
in the chemosensitive cell mediate the effects of angiotensin II on the carotid
chemoreceptor.

Intriguingly, immunohistochemical localization of AT_1-immunoreactivity is
found in some but not all lobules of the parenchyma, suggesting the expression
of AT_1 receptors is not uniform within the carotid body (Fung *et al* 2001a). The
physiological significance of this heterogeneity is not known, but this observation
is in agreement with functional studies that show only about 40% of glomus cells
are responsive to angiotensin II with an elevation of the intracellular calcium
level (Fung *et al* 2001a). In addition, AT_1 receptors are co-localized with cells
containing the enzyme tyrosine hydroxylase, which is important for the synthesis
of catecholamines for sensory transduction in the glomus cells (Fung *et al* 2002).
These findings further support the idea that AT_1 receptors are largely located in
the chemosensitive cells of the carotid body. Upon ligand activation of the AT_1
receptors, this triggers an elevation of intracellular calcium level and a secretory
response from the glomus cell for increasing the afferent activity of the chemoreceptors.

The AT_1 receptor has been cloned (Murphy *et al* 1991; Sasaki *et al* 1991), and
found to be a member of the seven-transmembrane-spanning, G-protein-coupled
receptor family (de Gasparo *et al* 2000). In adrenal glomerulosa cells, angiotensin
II binding of the AT_1 receptor stimulates the phospholipase C pathway in the
plasma membrane and leads to the formation of 1,2-diacylglycerol and inositol-
1,4,5-triphosphate (IP_3). This, in turn, mobilizes the endoplasmic calcium to store
and elevate intracellular calcium (Balla *et al* 1989; Balla *et al* 1991; Balla *et al*
1998). Studies have speculated that similar intracellular pathways can mediate
the effect of angiotensin II on the glomus cells. In this context, it is known that
endothelin-1 increases the cyclic AMP and IP_3 levels in the carotid body and the
intracellular calcium in the glomus cells via the ET_A receptor (Chen *et al* 2000;
Chen *et al* 2002a; Chen *et al* 2002b). These receptors also belong to the G-protein
coupling receptor family. The intracellular signaling components that are present
in the carotid body are likely to be activated by angiotensin II. Nevertheless, the

details of the intracellular signaling pathways, which mediate the activation of AT_1 receptors in the glomus cells, await further study.

In the rat, there are two subtypes of AT_1 receptors, namely AT_{1a} and AT_{1b} that play distinct roles and are transcriptionally expressed in the carotid body (Leung et al 2000; Fung et al 2002). Studies have demonstrated that the AT_{1a} receptor is the major subtype involved in the effect of angiotensin II on the carotid chemoreceptors, whereas AT_{1b} may play a limited role especially in the early maturational stages of the rat. In adults, chronic hypoxia enhances both AT_{1a} and AT_{1b} expression and the carotid chemoreceptor responses to angiotensin II, thus allowing the receptors to mediate the effect of angiotensin II on the carotid chemoreceptors (Leung et al 2000). However, in early maturation, the up-regulation is manifested only in the AT_{1a} subtype while the AT_{1b} subtype is down regulated by hypoxia in the rat pups in chronic hypoxia (Fung et al 2002). Apparently, this differential regulation of AT_1 receptors suggests that the AT_{1a} receptor is the major subtype responsible for the enhancement of the angiotensin II sensitivity (Fung et al 2002). The details of the developmental difference and the expression regulation by hypoxia will be further discussed in Section 4.1.

In addition to the AT_1 receptor, an AT_2 receptor has also been cloned as a unique class of seven-transmembrane receptor (Mukoyama et al 1993). Even though it has been shown that activation of the AT_2 receptor has various effects on vasodilation, apoptosis, cell differentiation and antiproliferation in a cell specific manner (Carey 2005; Steckelings et al 2005; Wolf 2005), the biological functions of the AT_2 receptor have yet to be further elucidated. Interestingly, mRNA transcripts of the AT_2 receptor have also been detected in the carotid body (Leung et al 2000; Fung et al 2002). Although evidence suggests that the AT_1 receptor is responsible for the excitatory response of the carotid chemoreceptors, it is plausible that angiotensin II can exert its action via the mediation of AT_2 receptor on other cell types such as vascular smooth muscle cells in the carotid body. In this regards, nitric oxide (NO) is a physiological mediator upon activation of AT_2 receptors (Carey et al 2000). Endogenous NO is locally produced in the carotid body under normoxic and hypoxic conditions, and NO plays an important role as a negative modulator in regulating the carotid chemoceptor activity (Fung et al 2001b; Ye et al 2002a; Campanucci et al 2006; Yamamoto et al 2006). There may be a functional link between the AT_2 receptor and NO in the carotid body but is currently unclear. Certainly, future studies are needed to clarify the functional significance of the expression of AT_2 receptors in the carotid body.

3.2. Expression of Local RAS Components in the Carotid Body

The circulating RAS is composed of the hepatic angiotensinogen, which is hydrolyzed by the renal renin to a decapeptide called angiotensin I. This peptide is then split by an angiotensin-converting enzyme (ACE) in the lungs that yields angiotensin II. The circulating RAS exerts its physiological actions primarily via specific angiotensin II receptors (Peach and Dostal 1990; Matsusaka and Ichikawa

1997; de Gasparo *et al* 2000); however, numerous tissues and organs have intrinsic angiotensin-generating systems that cater to specific local needs through actions that add to, or differ from, the circulating RAS. Such tissue RAS can act locally as an autocrine or paracrine action in finely regulating target tissue functions, as seen in various tissues and organs (Campbell 1987; Campbell 2003; Leung and Chappell 2003; Leung 2004).

Even though there is an association between the functional expression of the AT_1 receptor and its regulation by chronic hypoxia as to be discussed in Section 4, limited information is available on the presence of an intrinsic RAS in the carotid body. In this context, the expression and localization of several key RAS components, notably angiotensinogen, which is an obligatory element for the existence for an intrinsic RAS, have been demonstrated in the rat carotid body (Lam and Leung 2002). Specifically, protein and mRNA of angiotensinogen are localized to the type-I glomus cells; however, mRNA of renin is not expressed whereas mRNA expression of ACE is present. These findings suggest that an intrinsic angiotensin-generating system is localized in the rat carotid body, possibly functioning via a locally renin-independent biosynthetic pathway. Thus, locally produced angiotensin II from the glomus cell and probably other cell types in the carotid body could act via an autocrine or paracrine manner onto the AT_1 receptor located in the nearby glomus cells.

Interestingly, recent findings have shown that ACE genotype-dependent modulation might provide a genetic influence on respiratory drive and arterial oxygen saturation in high altitude natives and in endurance performances among high-altitude mountaineers (Woods and Montgomery 2001; Woods *et al* 2002; Patel *et al* 2003; Tsianos *et al* 2005). Physiologically, it is plausible that the ventilatory response to hypoxia at altitude could be modulated by the expression of local RAS and AT_1 receptors in the carotid body, contributing to different levels of increases in pulmonary ventilation (Leung *et al* 2000). Thus, a locally generated angiotensin system in the carotid body and its local regulation by chronic hypoxia could be important for regulating the carotid chemoreceptor activity.

3.3.   Physiological Functions of RAS in the Carotid Body

The circulating RAS plays a pivotal role in the endocrine control of salt and water balance in the body (Peach 1977; Reid *et al* 1978; Matsusaka and Ichikawa 1997). Physiological stimuli, such as changes in extracellular fluid volume, osmolarity, blood volume or sodium depletion, stimulate the RAS and this results in an increase in the plasma angiotensin II level (Matsusaka and Ichikawa 1997). Angiotensin II, acting as a potent arteriolar constrictor, is the major circulating hormone for stimulating aldosterone secretion by the adrenal cortex (Balla *et al* 1991; Matsusaka and Ichikawa 1997). As discussed in Sections 3.1 and 3.2, the carotid body can directly respond to angiotensin II in the circulating blood and local tissues, thus increasing the carotid chemoreceptor activity that activates the chemoreflex for increases in ventilation, cardiac output and changes in autonomic activities. Also, the activation of the chemoreflex pathway can elevate renal sympathetic activity causing a rise in renin secretion by the juxtaglomerular cells in the kidney, which can in turn activate the RAS to increase sodium reabsorption and water intake (Honig 1989; Marshall 1994). The change in sodium and water homeostasis could result when there is an increase in hemoglobin concentration and oxygen capacity of the blood, which is essential for the physiological response to hypoxia (Raff *et al* 1984). A recent study has also shown that carotid glomectomy in the rat reduces daily water consumption and increases daily consumption of NaCl solution compared with the sham operation (Serova *et al* 2004). Intraperitoneal injection of angiotensin II does not stimulate drinking motivation in the carotid glomectomized rat, whereas it induces water and salt consumption in the sham group (Serova *et al* 2004). Thus, besides the local RAS and angiotensin II-sensitive neurons in the circumventricular organs of the brain (Simpson 1981; McKinley *et al* 1998; Ganong 2000), peripheral carotid chemoreceptors can be another physiological pathway by which angiotensin II can confer and provide feedback to regulate and adjust the autonomic output of the central nervous system. Integrating to the central response, the peripheral signal could be important in adjusting the sympathetic and parasympathetic activities for an increasing cardiorespiratory activity and for regulating the salt and water balance under normoxic and hypoxia conditions.

4.   ROLES OF RAS IN THE CAROTID BODY IN DISEASES

4.1.   Regulation of Carotid RAS by Chronic Hypoxia: Implications on Chronic Obstructive Pulmonary Diseases

The carotid body enlarges in humans and animals, that inhabit high altitudes (Arias-Stella and Valcarcel 1976). Comparable changes in the carotid body were reported in clinical conditions associated with chronic hypoxemia (Lack 1978). Thus, the carotid body undergoes hypertrophy and hyperplasia when there is chronic hypoxia due to congenital heart disease, cystic fibrosis or chronic obstructive pulmonary diseases (Lack 1977; Lack 1978; Lack *et al* 1985). These structural changes are due to increased vasculature, hypertrophy and hyperplasia of the glomus cells (Dhillon *et al* 1984; McGregor *et al* 1984; Bee *et al* 1986; Bee and Howard 1993; Tipoe and Fung 2003). Functionally, chronic hypoxia modulates the ventilatory response to acute hypoxia (Eden and Hanson 1987; Bisgard 2000; Lahiri *et al* 2000; Prabhakar and Peng 2004). Therefore, the anatomical and physiological responses of the carotid body to chronic hypoxia are of great interest to researchers because of the functional implications regarding physiological acclimatization and also their clinical relevance.

The proportion of glomus cells that responds to angiotensin II is about 80 % in rats that have had prior exposure to chronic hypoxia, and this figure about double that of the normoxic controls (Leung *et al* 2000; Fung *et al* 2001a; Fung *et al* 2002). The intracellular calcium response to angiotensin II is also enhanced by about three-fold as a result of hypoxia; however, this response can be blocked by losartan but not by an AT_2 antagonist (Leung *et al* 2000; Fung *et al* 2002). In addition, electrophysiological studies consistently demonstrate the enhancement of AT_1 receptor-mediated excitation of carotid body chemoreceptor activity (about two-fold in the hypoxic group, compared with that of the controls) (Leung *et al* 2000; Fung *et al* 2002). Thus, an increase in the AT_1 receptor sensitivity to angiotensin II supports the hypothesis that it is enhanced or influenced by hypoxia. By using double-labeling immunohistochemistry, it has been shown that there is an enhanced immunoreactivity of AT_1 receptors co-localized in lobules of glomus cells in the carotid body of chronically hypoxic rats (Fung *et al* 2002). The mRNA expression of both subtypes of the AT_1 receptor as well as the AT_2 receptor increased in the carotid body of mature rats that were exposed to chronic hypoxia (Leung *et al* 2000). These study results confirm that chronic hypoxia upregulates the transcriptional and post-transcriptional expression of AT_1 receptors in the carotid body, and that the upregulation of the expression enhances AT_1 receptor-mediated excitation of the glomus cells and carotid body afferent activity.

The AT_{1a} receptors in the carotid body of rat pups were upregulated following postnatal exposure to chronic hypoxia, whereas the AT_{1b} receptors were down-regulated at the transcriptional level. This suggests a differential regulation of the expression of AT_1 receptor subtypes by postnatal hypoxia (Fung *et al* 2002). Apparently, the effects of chronic hypoxia on the AT_1 receptors in the carotid body were dependent on maturation. It is also possible that subtypes of AT_1 receptors play differential functional roles and are regulated by different mechanisms in their expression during early development. Nevertheless, chronic hypoxemia appears to be a major factor that increases AT_{1a} receptor expression, resulting in enhancement of the angiotensin II sensitivity of the carotid chemoreceptor.

The major effects of chronic hypoxia on the RAS of the carotid body are: (i) it increases the functional expression of the AT_1 receptors, and (ii) enhances the carotid afferent activity to angiotensin II stimulation. These alterations could contribute to an elevation of cardiovascular and respiratory performance to match metabolic needs and possibly changes to the sodium and water content of the blood for the fluid homeostasis under hypoxic conditions (Honig 1989). The upregulation of the AT_1 receptors can increase the sensitivity of the carotid body to the salt and water homeostasis in hypoxia. It has been shown that the plasma angiotensin II concentration increases in the first week and then returns to a normoxic level by two weeks in chronic hypoxia (Zakheim *et al* 1976). In addition, the plasma renin activity remains unchanged during chronic hypoxia (Jain *et al* 1990). Thus, it is postulated that the enhancement of the chemoreceptor sensitivity to angiotensin II provides a chemoreflex pathway by which it recruits the carotid chemoreceptor activity for maintenance of renal sympathetic activity. This could lead to a stimulation of the renin-angiotensin-aldosterone system that increases the sodium reabsorption and water intake. Such a change could compensate for the loss of sodium and water caused by the natriuretic and diuretic effects of carotid chemoreceptor stimu-lation during the early phase of hypoxia (Honig 1989). As a result the increased carotid body sensitivity to angiotensin II could be important in enhancing the cardiorespiratory effort and the renal sympathetic tone that are crucial changes in responding to hypoxia. Moreover, the carotid chemoreceptor can become hypoxic if the blood flow is markedly decreased because of hypotension, as observed in severe hemorrhage. Such hypotension has been demonstrated to increase the discharge rate of carotid chemoreceptors (Lahiri et al 1980), and this could be due to the mediation of upregulation of the AT_1 receptor during hypoxia (Leung et al 2000; Fung et al 2002).

Chronic hypoxia is of importance in high altitude physiology and in clinical conditions such as congenital heart defects, chronic lung disease of pre-maturity and chronic obstructive pulmonary diseases (Forth and Montgomery 2003; Prabhakar and Peng 2004). Given that the presence of RAS in the carotid body and the augmentation of angiotensin II sensitivity in the chemoreceptors, these mechanisms may play roles in the hypertrophy and hyperplasia of the glomus cells and in the angiogenesis of the vasculature in the carotid body. This could occur via the well-known mitogenic effect of angiotensin II on vascular cells. In addition, the mechanisms may modulate the chemoreceptor excitability for the adaptive changes in the carotid body during hypoxia. Hypoxia modulates the ventilatory response (Bisgard 2000; Lahiri et al 2000; Lahiri et al 2002) so that chemosensitivity may be determined a balance between the excitatory and inhibitory components in the carotid body (Bisgard 2000; Prabhakar 2001). Thus the excitatory effect of angiotensin II on the glomus cell may increase the chemosensitivity of the carotid body and may counteract the blunting effect of chronic hypoxia, although details of the molecular and cellular mechanisms underlying the functional modulation require further studies.

4.2. Regulation of Carotid RAS by Intermittent Hypoxia: Implications on Sleep-disordered Breathing

Chronic exposure to episodic hypoxia (intermittent hypoxia) associated with recurrent apneas is encountered more often in life and is allied with many patho-physiological conditions such as sleep-disordered breathing, obstructive sleep apnea and hypertension (Lesske et al 1997; Fletcher 2001). Chronic hypoxia in contrast, as it occurs in those living at high-altitude, does not result in such adverse effects and is eventually adapted to by the physiological systems (Prabhakar and Kumar 2004). Recently, a growing amount of evidence suggests that the carotid body also plays a significant role in the pathogenic events associated with intermittent hypoxia (Prabhakar et al 2001; Iturriaga et al 2005; Prabhakar et al 2005). Studies have shown an augmentation of the hypoxic sensory response in animals exposed to intermittent hypoxia (Peng and Prabhakar 2004; Peng et al 2004; Rey et al 2004). In addition, intermittent hypoxia causes increases in arterial blood pressure (Fletcher et al 1992a; Fletcher et al 1992b), sympathetic activity (Greenberg et al 1999; Fletcher 2003), blood level of catecholamines (Bao et al 1997), long term facilitation (LTF) of the respiratory motor activity (Ling et al 2001; McGuire et al 2004) and the ventilatory response to hypoxia (Katayama et al 2001; Rey et al 2004;

Katayama *et al* 2005). Importantly, Fletcher et al. (1992a) reported that denervation of the carotid body eliminates the elevated blood pressure response to intermittent hypoxia, suggesting an important role is played by carotid chemoreceptor activity in the pathogenic events induced by intermittent hypoxia. The long-term effects of intermittent hypoxia on the carotid body involve the increased generation of reactive oxygen species (ROS) because intermittent hypoxia resembles ischemia-reperfusion. The fact that scavengers of ROS attenuate the hypoxic sensitivity and the magnitude of LTF induced by intermittent hypoxia suggests an essential role of ROS in the alterations in the carotid body function in intermittent hypoxia (Prabhakar and Kumar 2004).

The plasma angiotensin II level increases during hypoxic conditions (Zakheim *et al* 1976) and peripheral infusion of angiotensin II stimulates ventilation (Potter and McCloskey 1979; Ohtake and Jennings 1993; Ohtake *et al* 1993). The activation of AT_1 receptors in the carotid body has a role in the hypoxic response and leads to the activation of chemoreflex and sympathetic activity as well as functional changes in the hypoxic sensory response during chronic hypoxia (Leung *et al* 2000). It has been shown that losartan attenuates the hypertension induced by intermittent hypoxia, indicating an involvement of the RAS in the pathogenesis during intermittent hypoxia (Fletcher *et al* 1999). Accordingly, ongoing studies are to examine the hypothesis that the RAS in the carotid body plays an important role in the functional modulation of the carotid chemoreceptor activity in intermittent hypoxia. It has been speculated that the generation of ROS and its by-products in the carotid body associated with intermittent hypoxia may contribute to the response of the carotid body to intermittent hypoxia.

Our recent unpublished results from immunohistochemical studies demonstrate that AT_1 receptors are mainly observed in glomic clusters of the carotid body in rats exposed to intermittent hypoxia (Fig. 1). The expression of the AT_1 receptor is markedly elevated in the carotid body of the rat exposed to intermittent hypoxia for three days and the level of expression reaches a plateau on day 7 in intermittent hypoxia, compared with a moderate level of the increase in the carotid body of chronically hypoxic rats (Fig. 1). Also, intracellular calcium response to exogenous angiotensin II is enhanced in the fura-2 loaded dissociated glomus cells from the 3-day group with intermittent hypoxia when compared with the normoxic controls (Fig. 2). These data suggest that an upregulation of the expression of AT_1 receptors may play a role in the enhancement of excitability in the carotid chemoreceptor in responding to intermittent hypoxia.

Levels of oxidative stress in the carotid body are studied with an immunohisto-chemical method using specific antibody against nitrotyrosine and ELISA for the detection of total 8-isoprostane in the serum. Results show that levels of nitroty-rosine are significantly elevated in the 7-day group with intermittent hypoxia. The expression level of nitrotyrosine returns to normoxic levels by day 14, whereas the expression of nitrotyrosine is mild in the chronic hypoxia and normoxic controls throughout the time course (Fig. 3). In addition, levels of 8-isoprostance are elevated in the 7-day group with intermittent hypoxia and it returns to normoxic levels by day

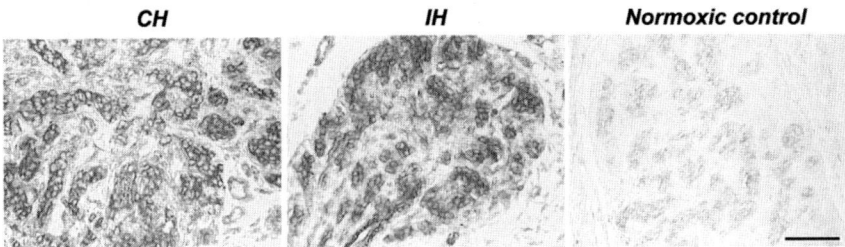

Figure 1. Immunohistochemical localization of AT_1 receptors in the carotid body of rats exposed to 7-day chronic hypoxia (CH, 10% inspired oxygen 24 hour/day) or intermittent hypoxia (IH, cyclic between air and 5% O_2 per minute, 8 hour/day), comparing with that of the normoxic control. Calibration bar is 40 μm

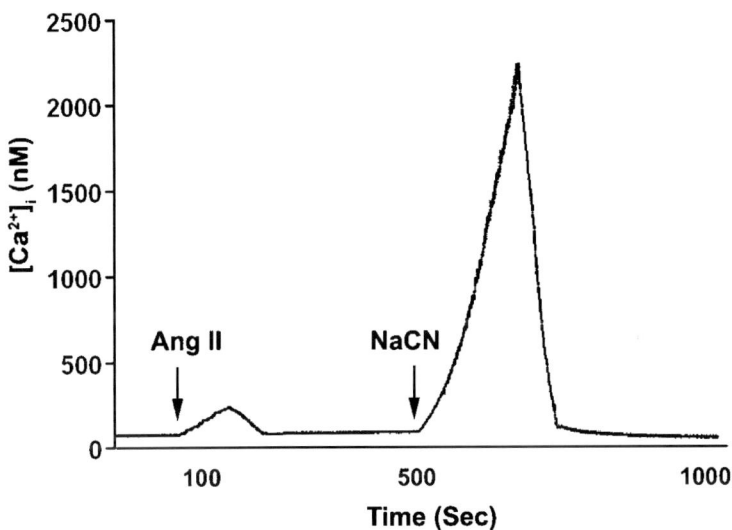

Figure 2. Angiotensin II increased the cytosolic calcium ($[Ca^{2+}]_i$) level in dissociated type-I glomus cells from the carotid bodies of rats exposed to 3-day intermittent hypoxia. The $[Ca^{2+}]_i$ level was measured in fura-2-loaded glomus cells by spectrofluorimetry. The cells were perfused with HEPES-Ringer at 0.5 ml/min at room temperature ($\sim$ 22°C). Fluorescent signals were obtained at 340 and 380 nm excitation wavelengths and the ratio of the fluorescence intensity [R(340/380)] was used to estimate $[Ca^{2+}]_i$ was calculated by using the equation: $[Ca^{2+}]_i = K_d[(R_0-R_{min})/(R_{max}-R_0)]\beta$ where R_0 is the fluorescence ratio, R_{min} the ratio at zero Ca^{2+}, R_{max} ratio at saturated Ca^{2+}, K_d the dissociation constant for fura-2 (334 nM) and β the ratio of fluorescence intensity (at 380 nm) at zero Ca^{2+} to that at saturated Ca^{2+}. Concentration dependence was determined by the $[Ca^{2+}]_i$ response to AngII at 100 nM. Acute hypoxia was inducted by NaCN (2 mM, in bolus) to confirm the chemosensitivity of the type-I cells

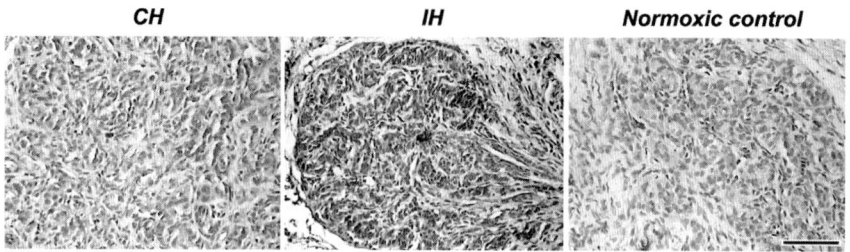

Figure 3. Immunohischemical localization of nitrotyrosine in the carotid body of rats exposed to 7-day chronic hypoxia (CH, 10% inspired oxygen 24 hour/day) or intermittent hypoxia (IH, cyclic between air and 5% O$_2$ per minute, 8 hour/day), comparing with that of the normoxic control. Calibration bar is 40 μm

14. Also, the levels of 8-isoprostane are mild in the chronic hypoxia and normoxic controls throughout the time course. These data suggest that there is a significant level of oxidative stress in the carotid body during the first week of intermittent hypoxia.

The aforementioned results demonstrate that (i) both the AT$_1$ receptors and nitrotyrosine are localized in lobules of type-I glomus cells in the rat carotid body, along with an upregulation of their expressions during intermittent hypoxia; (ii) angiotensin II increases intracellular calcium levels in the chemosensitive cells of the carotid body of rats exposed to intermittent hypoxia, and (iii) both the nitrotyrosine and 8-isoprostane levels are elevated within the first week of intermittent hypoxia, whereas mild expression of which are observed in chronic hypoxia and normoxic controls throughout the time course. Taken together, these preliminary findings support the hypothesis that an upregulation of AT$_1$ receptor expression plays a functional role in the enhancement of the excitability of the carotid body during intermittent hypoxia when there is a significant increase in the level of oxidative stress during an early time course.

As in the discussion in previous Sections, activation of the AT$_1$ receptor can increase the excitability of the carotid chemoreceptors. In chronically hypoxic rats, the intracellular calcium response of glomus cells to angiotensin II is enhanced by three-fold and the response can be blocked by losartan. Also, the carotid chemoreceptor activity is increased by two-fold in the hypoxic group (Fung *et al* 2002). These functional changes are confirmed by an increase in mRNA and protein levels of the AT$_1$ receptors in the carotid body during chronic hypoxia (Ganong 2000; Leung *et al* 2000). Thus, hypoxia is a regulatory factor that can increase the expression of AT$_1$ receptors, resulting in enhancement of the angiotensin II response of the carotid chemoreceptor. Acute and chronic episodic hypoxia recurrently stimulate the peripheral chemoreceptors as evidenced by elimination of the chronic elevated blood pressure response in episodic hypoxia-exposed rats with the denervation of the carotid body (Fletcher *et al* 1992a). The diurnal increase in blood pressure is also blocked by chemical peripheral sympathectomy (Fletcher *et al* 1992b). It is known that adrenal gland and renal sympathetic nerves participates in the chronic diurnal blood pressure elevation (Bao *et al* 1997). The sympathetic activity of these two organs may act in a complementary manner in intermittent hypoxia, possibly by the potentiation of the release of epinephrine from the adrenal gland, which binds peripheral sympathetic nervous synapses to potentiate neurotransmission and the facilitation of the release of renin by kidney (Prabhakar 2001). The facts that, losartan can attenuate the systemic hypertension induced by intermittent hypoxia as well as the increased RAS in rats exposed to intermittent hypoxia, further support the hypothesis that RAS is involved in the pathogenic processes in intermittent hypoxia (Fletcher *et al* 1999). This is further supported by our results demonstrating that AT_1 receptor expression was markedly elevated in the carotid body in intermittent hypoxia for 3, 7, 14 and 28 days. Also, intracellular calcium response to angiotensin II is enhanced in the fura-2 loaded dissociated glomus cells from 3-day rats with intermittent hypoxia, suggesting the AT_1 receptor expression is functionally significant. Thus, these data support the idea that an upregulation of the expression of AT_1 receptors can play a pathogenic role in the enhancement of the excitability of the carotid chemoreceptors during intermittent hypoxia. The data also highlight the roles played by the RAS and the carotid body in the over-activity of the sympathetic nervous system in the pathogenesis of systemic hypertension induced by intermittent hypoxia.

During reperfusion, the cellular generation of ROS increases. Increased ROS may contribute to the systemic response to intermittent hypoxia since intermittent hypoxia resembles ischemia-reperfusion (Prabhakar and Kumar 2004). Scavengers of ROS attenuates the hypoxic sensitivity and the magnitude of LTF of the carotid body induced by intermittent hypoxia, indicating that effects of intermittent hypoxia on the carotid body involve the increased generation of ROS (Prabhakar 2001; Prabhakar and Kumar 2004). Mobilization of intracellular calcium stores by the activation of the IP_3 signaling pathway promotes sensitizing effects of the carotid body to intermittent hypoxia. The IP_3 signaling pathway acted on by ROS contributes to the amplification of acute hypoxia-induced neurotransmitter release from the chemosensitive cells by intermittent hypoxia (Prabhakar 2001; Prabhakar and Kumar 2004; Prabhakar and Peng 2004). Indeed, elevated levels of 8-isoprostance and nitrotyrosine indicate an increased level of oxidative stress. In fact, our findings demonstrate that 8-isoprostance and nitrotyrosine levels are notably elevated in the 7-day group with intermittent hypoxia, but levels of 8-isoprostance and nitrotyrosine are mild in the chronic hypoxia and normoxic controls, suggesting an involvement of oxidative stress in the pathogenesis.

In summary, the upregulation of the AT_1 receptor expression and the intracellular calcium response to angiotensin II suggest that the RAS in the carotid body plays an important role in the modulation of carotid chemoreceptor activity during intermittent hypoxia. Together with an increase in the generation of ROS and oxidative stress during an early time course of intermittent hypoxia, these may play important pathogenic roles in the altered oxygen chemosensitivity of the carotid body during intermittent hypoxia.

4.3.   An Involvement of Carotid RAS in Heart Failure

Heart failure is strongly associated with sleep-disordered breathing with central or obstructive sleep apnea. The deleterious effects of sleep-disordered breathing on the failing heart have been reported and potential mechanisms by which treatment of sleep-disordered breathing may result in improved cardiac performance and long-term outcomes. Recent evidence also shows that cardiac dysfunction may contribute to sleep-disordered breathing. In fact, data supports the role of cardiac function in certain forms of central sleep apnea, although the relationship with obstructive sleep apnea remains to be firmly established (Caples *et al* 2005). Sympatho-excitation is a hallmark of the chronic heart failure (CHF) state. Recent studies suggest that the sympatho-excitation is mediated by a reduction in sensory input from cardiopulmonary and arterial baroreceptors, which is important in the initiation of the sympatho-excitatory state. In addition, the sustained increase in sympathetic nerve activity in CHF may involve angiotensin II and NO. Hence, blockade of AT_1 receptors in combination with NO donation reduces sympathetic nerve activities in animals with CHF, while NO donation alone has no effect on sympathetic nerve activities. Also, animals with CHF exhibit a downregulation in central gene expression for the neuronal isoform of nitric oxide synthase (nNOS). Thus, data suggest that the sympatho-excitatory state that is typical of CHF is, in part, due to changes in angiotensin II and NO (Zucker and Liu 2000; Zucker *et al* 2001; Zucker *et al* 2004).

Angiotensin II plays an important role in the enhanced chemoreflex function that occurs in CHF. Recent studies have been shown that angiotensin II enhances the hypoxic chemosensitivity of the carotid body in CHF rabbits (Li *et al* 2006). In this study, renal sympathetic nerve activity (RSNA) in response to graded hypoxia was measured before and after intravenous administration of angiotensin II or AT_1 receptor antagonist L-158809 in conscious sham and pacing-induced CHF rabbits. Li and colleagues also investigate the effects of angiotensin II and L-158809 on the carotid chemoreceptor activity in perfused preparations of the carotid body from sham and CHF rabbits. Interestingly, they found that angiotensin II enhanced hypoxia-induced RSNA increases in sham rabbits but not in CHF rabbits. However, L-158809 attenuates hypoxia-induced responses in RSNA in CHF rabbits but not in sham rabbits. Results also show that the mRNA and protein expression of AT_1 receptor in the carotid body from CHF rabbits are greater than that in sham rabbits. The carotid chemoreceptor afferent activities during normoxia and graded hypoxia are increased in CHF rabbits compared with sham rabbits. In addition, angiotensin II increases the response of carotid chemoreceptors to hypoxia in sham rabbits but not in CHF rabbits. Also, L-158809 decreases the chemoreceptor responses to hypoxia in CHF rabbits but not in sham rabbits. They suggest that elevation of angiotensin II and the upregulation of AT_1 receptor in the carotid body contribute to the increased carotid chemoreceptor activity and enhanced peripheral chemoreflex function in CHF (Li *et al* 2006).

In another study, Li and colleagues show that angiotensin II can exert its effect on the potassium channels in the type-I glomus cell (Li and Schultz 2006). Specifically, using the conventional whole-cell patch clamp technique, the sensitivity of

Ca^{2+}-independent, voltage-gated K^+ (Kv) channels to hypoxia was examined in the glomus cells from CHF rabbits. They found that Kv currents under normoxic conditions are blunted in the glomus cells from CHF rabbits compared with sham rabbits. Also, the inhibition of IK and the decrease of resting membrane potential induced by hypoxia are greater in CHF versus sham glomus cells. Interestingly, angiotensin II (0.1 nM) has no effect on Kv currents in normoxia, but at this concentration angiotensin II increases the sensitivity of Kv currents and resting membrane potential to hypoxia in sham glomus cells. In CHF glomus cells, L-158809 alone has no effect on Kv currents at normoxia, but it reduces the sensitivity of Kv currents and resting membrane potential to hypoxia. Angiotensin II (> 1 nM) dose-dependently reduces IK under normoxic conditions in sham and CHF glomus cells. Moreover, expression studies demonstrate a down-expression of Kv3.4 but not Kv4.3 channels in CHF glomus cells. They concluded that (i) angiotensin II-AT_1 receptor signaling pathway increases the sensitivity of Kv channels to hypoxia in the glomus cells from CHF rabbits; (ii) high concentrations of angiotensin II can directly inhibit Kv currents in the glomus cells from sham and CHF rabbits; (iii) decrease in Kv3.4 channel protein expression in the carotid body may contribute to the suppression of Kv currents and enhanced sensitivity of Kv currents to hypoxia in CHF (Li and Schultz 2006).

5. CONCLUSIONS

In addition to the circulating RAS and the local RAS in the brain for the endocrine and cardiovascular control, recent results obtained from expression studies and functional analyses suggest that the AT_1 receptor regulates the excitability of the carotid chemoreceptor. Hence, angiotensin II elevates the intracellular calcium level of glomus cells and the carotid afferent activity that activates the chemoreflex pathway. This could be a peripheral control important for integrating the physiological response to hypoxia and the maintenance of salt and water balance.

The RAS expressed in the carotid body is regulated by hypoxia. Hence, chronic hypoxia is associated with an enhanced sensitivity of chemoreceptor activities to angiotensin II via an upregulation of AT_1 receptor expression. In addition, postnatal hypoxia increases AT_{1a} receptor expression in the rat carotid body, suggesting an involvement of AT_{1a} subtype in the functional changes. This modulation may be important for the adaptation of the carotid body functions in the hypoxic ventilatory response, for the purpose of enhancing the cardiorespiratory response and adjusting electrolyte and water homeostasis during the stress of chronic hypoxia.

Furthermore, a local expression of RAS in the carotid body and its upregulation are relevant to the pathogenesis of diseases including sleep-disordered breathing and heart failure. Increases in AT_1 receptor expression could be significant in the enhancement of carotid chemoreceptor response to hypoxia, leading to a sympatho-excitation that is central to the endothelial dysfunction and heart failure during the course of pathogenesis. Certainly, future studies toward this direction warrant a better understanding of the physiological role of RAS in the peripheral chemoreceptor and its pathogenic roles in the diseases associated with hypoxemia.

ACKNOWLEDGEMENTS

The authors wish to thank the support from the Research Grants Council of Hong Kong, Competitive Earmarked Research Grants: HKU 7184/01M, HKU 7510/06M (MLF) and CUHK 4075/00M, CUHK 4116/01M (PSL), and by the University of Hong Kong and the Chinese University of Hong Kong.

REFERENCES

Allen AM, 1998, Angiotensin AT1 receptor-mediated excitation of rat carotid body chemoreceptor afferent activity. *J Physiol.* **510**: 773–781.

Allen AM, MacGregor DP, McKinley MJ, Mendelsohn FA, 1999, Angiotensin II receptors in the human brain. *Regul Pept.* **79**: 1–7.

Allen AM, McKinley MJ, Oldfield BJ, Dampney RA, Mendelsohn FA, 1988, Angiotensin II receptor binding and the baroreflex pathway. *Clin Exp Hypertens A.* **10 Suppl 1**: 63–78.

Andreas S, Herrmann-Lingen C, Raupach T, Luthje L, Fabricius JA, Hruska N, Korber W, Buchner B, Criee CP, Hasenfuss G, Calverley P, 2006, Angiotensin II blockers in obstructive pulmonary disease: a randomised controlled trial. *Eur Respir J.* **27**: 972–979.

Arias-Stella J, Valcarcel J, 1976, Chief cell hyperplasia in the human carotid body at high altitudes; physiologic and pathologic significance. *Hum Pathol.* **7**: 361–373.

Balla T, Baukal AJ, Eng S, Catt KJ, 1991, Angiotensin II receptor subtypes and biological responses in the adrenal cortex and medulla. *Mol Pharmacol.* **40**: 401–406.

Balla T, Baukal AJ, Hunyady L, Catt KJ, 1989, Agonist-induced regulation of inositol tetrakisphosphate isomers and inositol pentakisphosphate in adrenal glomerulosa cells. *J Biol Chem.* **264**: 13605–13611.

Balla T, Varnai P, Tian Y, Smith RD, 1998, Signaling events activated by angiotensin II receptors: what goes before and after the calcium signals. *Endocr Res.* **24**: 335–344.

Bao G, Metreveli N, Li R, Taylor A, Fletcher EC, 1997, Blood pressure response to chronic episodic hypoxia: role of the sympathetic nervous system. *J Appl Physiol.* **83**: 95–101.

Bee D, Howard P, 1993, The carotid body: a review of its anatomy, physiology and clinical importance. *Monaldi Arch Chest Dis.* **48**: 48–53.

Bee D, Pallot DJ, Barer GR, 1986, Division of type I and endothelial cells in the hypoxic rat carotid body. *Acta Anat (Basel).* **126**: 226–229.

Bisgard GE, 2000, Carotid body mechanisms in acclimatization to hypoxia. *Respir Physiol.* **121**: 237–246.

Campanucci VA, Zhang M, Vollmer C, Nurse CA, 2006, Expression of multiple P2X receptors by glossopharyngeal neurons projecting to rat carotid body O2-chemoreceptors: role in nitric oxide-mediated efferent inhibition. *J Neurosci.* **26**: 9482–9493.

Campbell DJ, 1987, Tissue renin-angiotensin system: sites of angiotensin formation. *J Cardiovasc Pharmacol.* **10 Suppl 7**: S1–8.

Campbell DJ, 2003, The renin-angiotensin and the kallikrein-kinin systems. *Int J Biochem Cell Biol.* **35**: 784–791.

Caples SM, Wolk R, Somers VK, 2005, Influence of cardiac function and failure on sleep-disordered breathing: evidence for a causative role. *J Appl Physiol.* **99**: 2433–2439.

Carey RM, 2005, Update on the role of the AT2 receptor. *Curr Opin Nephrol Hypertens.* **14**: 67–71.

Carey RM, Jin X, Wang Z, Siragy HM, 2000, Nitric oxide: a physiological mediator of the type 2 (AT2) angiotensin receptor. *Acta Physiol Scand.* **168**: 65–71.

Chen J, He L, Dinger B, Fidone S, 2000, Cellular mechanisms involved in rabbit carotid body excitation elicited by endothelin peptides. *Respir Physiol.* **121**: 13–23.

Chen J, He L, Dinger B, Stensaas L, Fidone S, 2002a, Role of endothelin and endothelin A-type receptor in adaptation of the carotid body to chronic hypoxia. *Am J Physiol Lung Cell Mol Physiol.* **282**: L1314–1323.

Chen Y, Tipoe GL, Liong E, Leung S, Lam SY, Iwase R, Tjong YW, Fung ML, 2002b, Chronic hypoxia enhances endothelin-1-induced intracellular calcium elevation in rat carotid body chemoreceptors and up-regulates ETA receptor expression. *Pflugers Arch.* **443**: 565–573.

Czyzyk-Krzeska MF, Bayliss DA, Lawson EE, Millhorn DE, 1992, Regulation of tyrosine hydroxylase gene expression in the rat carotid body by hypoxia. *J Neurochem.* **58**: 1538–1546.

de Gasparo M, Catt KJ, Inagami T, Wright JW, Unger T, 2000, International union of pharmacology. XXIII. The angiotensin II receptors. *Pharmacol Rev.* **52**: 415–472.

Dhillon DP, Barer GR, Walsh M, 1984, The enlarged carotid body of the chronically hypoxic and chronically hypoxic and hypercapnic rat: a morphometric analysis. *Q J Exp Physiol.* **69**: 301–317.

Donoghue S, Felder RB, Gilbey MP, Jordan D, Spyer KM, 1985, Post-synaptic activity evoked in the nucleus tractus solitarius by carotid sinus and aortic nerve afferents in the cat. *J Physiol.* **360**: 261–273.

Donoghue S, Felder RB, Jordan D, Spyer KM, 1984, The central projections of carotid baroreceptors and chemoreceptors in the cat: a neurophysiological study. *J Physiol.* **347**: 397–409.

Duffin J, 1990, The chemoreflex control of breathing and its measurement. *Can J Anaesth.* **37**: 933–942.

Duffin J, Mahamed S, 2003, Adaptation in the respiratory control system. *Can J Physiol Pharmacol.* **81**: 765–773.

Eden GJ, Hanson MA, 1987, Effects of chronic hypoxia from birth on the ventilatory response to acute hypoxia in the newborn rat. *J Physiol.* **392**: 11–19.

Fletcher EC, 2001, Invited review: Physiological consequences of intermittent hypoxia: systemic blood pressure. *J Appl Physiol.* **90**: 1600–1605.

Fletcher EC, 2003, Sympathetic over activity in the etiology of hypertension of obstructive sleep apnea. *Sleep.* **26**: 15–19.

Fletcher EC, Bao G, Li R, 1999, Renin activity and blood pressure in response to chronic episodic hypoxia. *Hypertension.* **34**: 309–314.

Fletcher EC, Lesske J, Behm R, Miller CC, 3rd, Stauss H, Unger T, 1992a, Carotid chemoreceptors, systemic blood pressure, and chronic episodic hypoxia mimicking sleep apnea. *J Appl Physiol.* **72**: 1978–1984.

Fletcher EC, Lesske J, Qian W, Miller CC, 3rd, Unger T, 1992b, Repetitive, episodic hypoxia causes diurnal elevation of blood pressure in rats. *Hypertension.* **19**: 555–561.

Forth R, Montgomery H, 2003, ACE in COPD: a therapeutic target? *Thorax.* **58**: 556–558.

Fung ML, 2003, Hypoxia-inducible factor-1: a molecular hint of physiological changes in the carotid body during long-term hypoxemia? *Curr Drug Targets Cardiovasc Haematol Disord.* **3**: 254–259.

Fung ML, Lam SY, Chen Y, Dong X, Leung PS, 2001a, Functional expression of angiotensin II receptors in type-I cells of the rat carotid body. *Pflugers Arch.* **441**: 474–480.

Fung ML, Lam SY, Dong X, Chen Y, Leung PS, 2002, Postnatal hypoxemia increases angiotensin II sensitivity and up-regulates AT1a angiotensin receptors in rat carotid body chemoreceptors. *J Endocrinol.* **173**: 305–313.

Fung ML, Tipoe GL, 2003, Role of HIF-1 in physiological adaptation of the carotid body during chronic hypoxia. *Adv Exp Med Biol.* **536**: 593–601.

Fung ML, Ye JS, Fung PC, 2001b, Acute hypoxia elevates nitric oxide generation in rat carotid body in vitro. *Pflugers Arch.* **442**: 903–909.

Ganong WF, 2000, Circumventricular organs: definition and role in the regulation of endocrine and autonomic function. *Clin Exp Pharmacol Physiol.* **27**: 422–427.

Gonzalez C, Almaraz L, Obeso A, Rigual R, 1994, Carotid body chemoreceptors: from natural stimuli to sensory discharges. *Physiol Rev.* **74**: 829–898.

Greenberg HE, Sica A, Batson D, Scharf SM, 1999, Chronic intermittent hypoxia increases sympathetic responsiveness to hypoxia and hypercapnia. *J Appl Physiol.* **86**: 298–305.

Haibara AS, Colombari E, Chianca DA, Jr., Bonagamba LG, Machado BH, 1995, NMDA receptors in NTS are involved in bradycardic but not in pressor response of chemoreflex. *Am J Physiol.* **269**: H1421–1427.

Hanbauer I, Karoum F, Hellstrom S, Lahiri S, 1981, Effects of hypoxia lasting up to one month on the catecholamine content in rat carotid body. *Neuroscience*. **6**: 81–86.

Honig A, 1989, Peripheral arterial chemoreceptors and reflex control of sodium and water homeostasis. *Am J Physiol*. **257**: R1282–1302.

Iturriaga R, Rey S, Del Rio R, 2005, Cardiovascular and ventilatory acclimatization induced by chronic intermittent hypoxia: a role for the carotid body in the pathophysiology of sleep apnea. *Biol Res*. **38**: 335–340.

Izuhara Y, Nangaku M, Inagi R, Tominaga N, Aizawa T, Kurokawa K, van Ypersele de Strihou C, Miyata T, 2005, Renoprotective properties of angiotensin receptor blockers beyond blood pressure lowering. *J Am Soc Nephrol*. **16**: 3631–3641.

Jain S, Wilke WL, Tucker A, 1990, Age-dependent effects of chronic hypoxia on renin-angiotensin and urinary excretions. *J Appl Physiol*. **69**: 141–146.

Katayama K, Sato K, Matsuo H, Hotta N, Sun Z, Ishida K, Iwasaki K, Miyamura M, 2005, Changes in ventilatory responses to hypercapnia and hypoxia after intermittent hypoxia in humans. *Respir Physiol Neurobiol*. **146**: 55–65.

Katayama K, Sato Y, Morotome Y, Shima N, Ishida K, Mori S, Miyamura M, 2001, Intermittent hypoxia increases ventilation and Sa(O2) during hypoxic exercise and hypoxic chemosensitivity. *J Appl Physiol*. **90**: 1431–1440.

Lack EE, 1977, Carotid body hypertrophy in patients with cystic fibrosis and cyanotic congenital heart disease. *Hum Pathol*. **8**: 39–51.

Lack EE, 1978, Hyperplasia of vagal and carotid body paraganglia in patients with chronic hypoxemia. *Am J Pathol*. **91**: 497–516.

Lack EE, Perez-Atayde AR, Young JB, 1985, Carotid body hyperplasia in cystic fibrosis and cyanotic heart disease. A combined morphometric, ultrastructural, and biochemical study. *Am J Pathol*. **119**: 301–314.

Lahiri S, Di Giulio C, Roy A, 2002, Lessons from chronic intermittent and sustained hypoxia at high altitudes. *Respir Physiol Neurobiol*. **130**: 223–233.

Lahiri S, Forster RE, 2nd, 2003, CO2/H(+) sensing: peripheral and central chemoreception. *Int J Biochem Cell Biol*. **35**: 1413–1435.

Lahiri S, Nishino T, Mokashi A, Mulligan E, 1980, Relative responses of aortic body and carotid body chemoreceptors to hypotension. *J Appl Physiol*. **48**: 781–788.

Lahiri S, Roy A, Baby SM, Hoshi T, Semenza GL, Prabhakar NR, 2006, Oxygen sensing in the body. *Prog Biophys Mol Biol*. **91**: 249–286.

Lahiri S, Rozanov C, Cherniack NS, 2000, Altered structure and function of the carotid body at high altitude and associated chemoreflexes. *High Alt Med Biol*. **1**: 63–74.

Lahiri S, Rozanov C, Roy A, Storey B, Buerk DG, 2001, Regulation of oxygen sensing in peripheral arterial chemoreceptors. *Int J Biochem Cell Biol*. **33**: 755–774.

Lam SY, Leung PS, 2002, A locally generated angiotensin system in rat carotid body. *Regul Pept*. **107**: 97–103.

Lawson EE, Richter DW, Ballantyne D, Lalley PM, 1989, Peripheral chemoreceptor inputs to medullary inspiratory and postinspiratory neurons of cats. *Pflugers Arch*. **414**: 523–533.

Lesske J, Fletcher EC, Bao G, Unger T, 1997, Hypertension caused by chronic intermittent hypoxia–influence of chemoreceptors and sympathetic nervous system. *J Hypertens*. **15**: 1593–1603.

Leung PS, 2004, The peptide hormone angiotensin II: its new functions in tissues and organs. *Curr Protein Pept Sci*. **5**: 267–273.

Leung PS, Chappell MC, 2003, A local pancreatic renin-angiotensin system: endocrine and exocrine roles. *Int J Biochem Cell Biol*. **35**: 838–846.

Leung PS, Fung ML, Tam MS, 2003, Renin-angiotensin system in the carotid body. *Int J Biochem Cell Biol*. **35**: 847–854.

Leung PS, Lam SY, Fung ML, 2000, Chronic hypoxia upregulates the expression and function of AT(1) receptor in rat carotid body. *J Endocrinol*. **167**: 517–524.

Li YL, Schultz HD, 2006, Enhanced sensitivity of Kv channels to hypoxia in the rabbit carotid body in heart failure: role of angiotensin II. *J Physiol*. **575**: 215–227.

Li YL, Xia XH, Zheng H, Gao L, Li YF, Liu D, Patel KP, Wang W, Schultz HD, 2006, Angiotensin II enhances carotid body chemoreflex control of sympathetic outflow in chronic heart failure rabbits. *Cardiovasc Res.* **71**: 129–138.

Ling L, Fuller DD, Bach KB, Kinkead R, Olson EB, Jr., Mitchell GS, 2001, Chronic intermittent hypoxia elicits serotonin-dependent plasticity in the central neural control of breathing. *J Neurosci.* **21**: 5381–5388.

Marshall JM, 1994, Peripheral chemoreceptors and cardiovascular regulation. *Physiol Rev.* **74**: 543–594.

Matsusaka T, Ichikawa I, 1997, Biological functions of angiotensin and its receptors. *Annu Rev Physiol.* **59**: 395–412.

McGregor KH, Gil J, Lahiri S, 1984, A morphometric study of the carotid body in chronically hypoxic rats. *J Appl Physiol.* **57**: 1430–1438.

McGuire M, Zhang Y, White DP, Ling L, 2004, Serotonin receptor subtypes required for ventilatory long-term facilitation and its enhancement after chronic intermittent hypoxia in awake rats. *Am J Physiol Regul Integr Comp Physiol.* **286**: R334–341.

McKinley MJ, Albiston AL, Allen AM, Mathai ML, May CN, McAllen RM, Oldfield BJ, Mendelsohn FA, Chai SY, 2003, The brain renin-angiotensin system: location and physiological roles. *Int J Biochem Cell Biol.* **35**: 901–918.

McKinley MJ, Allen AM, Burns P, Colvill LM, Oldfield BJ, 1998, Interaction of circulating hormones with the brain: the roles of the subfornical organ and the organum vasculosum of the lamina terminalis. *Clin Exp Pharmacol Physiol Suppl.* **25**: S61–67.

Mifflin SW, 1992, Arterial chemoreceptor input to nucleus tractus solitarius. *Am J Physiol.* **263**: R368–375.

Millhorn DE, Czyzyk-Krzeska M, Bayliss DA, Lawson EE, 1993, Regulation of gene expression by hypoxia. *Sleep.* **16**: S44–48.

Morrell NW, Higham MA, Phillips PG, Shakur BH, Robinson PJ, Beddoes RJ, 2005, Pilot study of losartan for pulmonary hypertension in chronic obstructive pulmonary disease. *Respir Res.* **6**: 88.

Morrell NW, Morris KG, Stenmark KR, 1995, Role of angiotensin-converting enzyme and angiotensin II in development of hypoxic pulmonary hypertension. *Am J Physiol.* **269**: H1186–1194.

Morrell NW, Upton PD, Kotecha S, Huntley A, Yacoub MH, Polak JM, Wharton J, 1999, Angiotensin II activates MAPK and stimulates growth of human pulmonary artery smooth muscle via AT1 receptors. *Am J Physiol.* **277**: L440–448.

Mukoyama M, Nakajima M, Horiuchi M, Sasamura H, Pratt RE, Dzau VJ, 1993, Expression cloning of type 2 angiotensin II receptor reveals a unique class of seven-transmembrane receptors. *J Biol Chem.* **268**: 24539–24542.

Murphy TJ, Alexander RW, Griendling KK, Runge MS, Bernstein KE, 1991, Isolation of a cDNA encoding the vascular type-1 angiotensin II receptor. *Nature.* **351**: 233–236.

Nakamoto T, Harasawa H, Akimoto K, Hirata H, Kaneko H, Kaneko N, Sorimachi K, 2005, Effects of olmesartan medoxomil as an angiotensin II-receptor blocker in chronic hypoxic rats. *Eur J Pharmacol.* **528**: 43–51.

Ohtake PJ, Jennings DB, 1993, Angiotensin II stimulates respiration in awake dogs and antagonizes baroreceptor inhibition. *Respir Physiol.* **91**: 335–351.

Ohtake PJ, Walker JK, Jennings DB, 1993, Renin-angiotensin system stimulates respiration during acute hypotension but not during hypercapnia. *J Appl Physiol.* **74**: 1220–1228.

Patel S, Woods DR, Macleod NJ, Brown A, Patel KR, Montgomery HE, Peacock AJ, 2003, Angiotensin-converting enzyme genotype and the ventilatory response to exertional hypoxia. *Eur Respir J.* **22**: 755–760.

Peach MJ, 1977, Renin-angiotensin system: biochemistry and mechanisms of action. *Physiol Rev.* **57**: 313–370.

Peach MJ, Dostal DE, 1990, The angiotensin II receptor and the actions of angiotensin II. *J Cardiovasc Pharmacol.* **16 Suppl 4**: S25–30.

Peng YJ, Prabhakar NR, 2004, Effect of two paradigms of chronic intermittent hypoxia on carotid body sensory activity. *J Appl Physiol.* **96**: 1236–1242; discussion 1196.

Peng YJ, Rennison J, Prabhakar NR, 2004, Intermittent hypoxia augments carotid body and ventilatory response to hypoxia in neonatal rat pups. *J Appl Physiol.* **97**: 2020–2025.

Pequignot JM, Cottet-Emard JM, Dalmaz Y, Peyrin L, 1987, Dopamine and norepinephrine dynamics in rat carotid body during long-term hypoxia. *J Auton Nerv Syst.* **21**: 9–14.

Potter EK, McCloskey DI, 1979, Respiratory stimulation by angiotensin II. *Respir Physiol.* **36**: 367–373.

Prabhakar NR, 2001, Oxygen sensing during intermittent hypoxia: cellular and molecular mechanisms. *J Appl Physiol.* **90**: 1986–1994.

Prabhakar NR, Fields RD, Baker T, Fletcher EC, 2001, Intermittent hypoxia: cell to system. *Am J Physiol Lung Cell Mol Physiol.* **281**: L524–528.

Prabhakar NR, Kumar GK, 2004, Oxidative stress in the systemic and cellular responses to intermittent hypoxia. *Biol Chem.* **385**: 217–221.

Prabhakar NR, Peng YJ, 2004, Peripheral chemoreceptors in health and disease. *J Appl Physiol.* **96**: 359–366.

Prabhakar NR, Peng YJ, Jacono FJ, Kumar GK, Dick TE, 2005, Cardiovascular alterations by chronic intermittent hypoxia: importance of carotid body chemoreflexes. *Clin Exp Pharmacol Physiol.* **32**: 447–449.

Raff H, Shinsako J, Dallman MF, 1984, Renin and ACTH responses to hypercapnia and hypoxia after chronic carotid chemodenervation. *Am J Physiol.* **247**: R412–417.

Reid IA, Morris BJ, Ganong WF, 1978, The renin-angiotensin system. *Annu Rev Physiol.* **40**: 377–410.

Rey S, Del Rio R, Alcayaga J, Iturriaga R, 2004, Chronic intermittent hypoxia enhances cat chemosensory and ventilatory responses to hypoxia. *J Physiol.* **560**: 577–586.

Sasaki K, Yamano Y, Bardhan S, Iwai N, Murray JJ, Hasegawa M, Matsuda Y, Inagami T, 1991, Cloning and expression of a complementary DNA encoding a bovine adrenal angiotensin II type-1 receptor. *Nature.* **351**: 230–233.

Serova ON, Shevchenko LV, Elfimov AI, Kotov AV, Torshin VI, 2004, Water and salt consumption and suppression of Angiotensin-induced thirst in rats after carotid glomectomy. *Bull Exp Biol Med.* **138**: 437–439.

Simpson JB, 1981, The circumventricular organs and the central actions of angiotensin. *Neuroendocrinology.* **32**: 248–256.

Steckelings UM, Kaschina E, Unger T, 2005, The AT2 receptor–a matter of love and hate. *Peptides.* **26**: 1401–1409.

Takahashi S, Nakamura Y, Nishijima T, Sakurai S, Inoue H, 2005, Essential roles of angiotensin II in vascular endothelial growth factor expression in sleep apnea syndrome. *Respir Med.* **99**: 1125–1131.

Tipoe GL, Fung ML, 2003, Expression of HIF-1alpha, VEGF and VEGF receptors in the carotid body of chronically hypoxic rat. *Respir Physiol Neurobiol.* **138**: 143–154.

Tipoe GL, Lau TY, Nanji AA, Fung ML, 2006, Expression and functions of vasoactive substances regulated by hypoxia-inducible factor-1 in chronic hypoxemia. *Cardiovasc Hematol Agents Med Chem.* **4**: 199–218.

Tsianos G, Eleftheriou KI, Hawe E, Woolrich L, Watt M, Watt I, Peacock A, Montgomery H, Grant S, 2005, Performance at altitude and angiotensin I-converting enzyme genotype. *Eur J Appl Physiol.* **93**: 630–633.

Wolf G, 2005, Role of reactive oxygen species in angiotensin II-mediated renal growth, differentiation, and apoptosis. *Antioxid Redox Signal.* **7**: 1337–1345.

Woods DR, Montgomery HE, 2001, Angiotensin-converting enzyme and genetics at high altitude. *High Alt Med Biol.* **2**: 201–210.

Woods DR, Pollard AJ, Collier DJ, Jamshidi Y, Vassiliou V, Hawe E, Humphries SE, Montgomery HE, 2002, Insertion/deletion polymorphism of the angiotensin I-converting enzyme gene and arterial oxygen saturation at high altitude. *Am J Respir Crit Care Med.* **166**: 362–366.

Yamamoto Y, Konig P, Henrich M, Dedio J, Kummer W, 2006, Hypoxia induces production of nitric oxide and reactive oxygen species in glomus cells of rat carotid body. *Cell Tissue Res.* **325**: 3–11.

Ye JS, Tipoe GL, Fung PC, Fung ML, 2002a, Augmentation of hypoxia-induced nitric oxide generation in the rat carotid body adapted to chronic hypoxia: an involvement of constitutive and inducible nitric oxide synthases. *Pflugers Arch.* **444**: 178–185.

Ye S, Zhong H, Duong VN, Campese VM, 2002b, Losartan reduces central and peripheral sympathetic nerve activity in a rat model of neurogenic hypertension. *Hypertension*. **39**: 1101–1106.

Zakheim RM, Mattioli L, Molteni A, Mullis KB, Bartley J, 1975, Prevention of pulmonary vascular changes of chronic alveolar hypoxia by inhibition of angiotensin I-converting enzyme in the rat. *Lab Invest*. **33**: 57–61.

Zakheim RM, Molteni A, Mattioli L, Park M, 1976, Plasma angiotensin II levels in hypoxic and hypovolemic stress in unanesthetized rabbits. *J Appl Physiol*. **41**: 462–465.

Zhang W, Mifflin SW, 1993, Excitatory amino acid receptors within NTS mediate arterial chemoreceptor reflexes in rats. *Am J Physiol*. **265**: H770–773.

Zucker IH, Liu JL, 2000, Angiotensin II–nitric oxide interactions in the control of sympathetic outflow in heart failure. *Heart Fail Rev*. **5**: 27–43.

Zucker IH, Schultz HD, Li YF, Wang Y, Wang W, Patel KP, 2004, The origin of sympathetic outflow in heart failure: the roles of angiotensin II and nitric oxide. *Prog Biophys Mol Biol*. **84**: 217–232.

Zucker IH, Wang W, Pliquett RU, Liu JL, Patel KP, 2001, The regulation of sympathetic outflow in heart failure. The roles of angiotensin II, nitric oxide, and exercise training. *Ann N Y Acad Sci*. **940**: 431–443.

CHAPTER 9

BONE HOMEOSTASIS: AN EMERGING ROLE FOR THE RENIN-ANGIOTENSIN SYSTEM

C. SERNIA, H. HUANG, K. NGUYUEN, Y-H. LI, S. HSU,
M. CHEN, N. YU, AND M. FORWOOD

Department of Physiology & Pharmacology, School of Biomedical Science, University of Queensland, Brisbane, Australia

1.   INTRODUCTION

Renin and angiotensin converting enzyme (ACE) are key enzymes in the generation of Angiotensin II (AngII), the major effector hormone of the renin-angiotensin system (RAS). While the RAS is most commonly associated with cardiovascular and renal functions, it has appropriated significant roles (amongst others) in tissue repair and remodelling, in cognitive and autonomic functions, in embryonic development and in reproduction (Gard 2002; Lavoie and Sigmund 2003; Leung and Sernia, 2003). This chapter addresses a new area of regulation by the RAS: the regulation of bone homeostasis. Clinical reports on osteoporosis and on a variety of osteolytic conditions suggest a negative association between ACE activity and bone mineralization. Cell cultures of osteoblasts have been used to show that they are targets of AngII action. New data from our laboratory on the osteoblast cell line UMR-106 elaborate and elucidate the mechanisms whereby the RAS modulates bone metabolism. These studies provide a new perspective of processes relevant to common degenerative bone diseases as osteoporosis and rheumatoid arthritis. In addition, the immediate clinical relevance of this emerging area of research will be in creating awareness of the skeletal actions of current, widely prescribed antihypertensive drugs that target the RAS, such losartan and enalapril (Dendorfer *et al* 2005).

2.   THE RENIN-ANGIOTENSIN SYSTEM

The central components of RAS consist of the protein substrate angiotensinogen and two enzymes - renin (EC 3.4.23.15) and membrane-bound angiotensin-converting enzyme (EC 3.4.15.1; ACE). The sequential actions of these two enzyme generate

Po Sing Leung (ed.), Frontiers in Research of the Renin-Angiotensin System on Human Disease, 179–195.
© 2007 *Springer.*

the decapeptide angiotensin I (AngI) and the octapeptide angiotensin II (AngII), respectively; the latter being the predominant physiologically active peptide of the RAS. The actions of Ang II are mediated by the AT_1 (found in non-primates as AT_{1a} and AT_{1b} subtypes), and AT_2 receptors. Both receptors are 7-transmembrane G-protein coupled receptors sharing about 30% sequence (De Gasparo et al 2000; Thomas and Mendelsohn, 2003). The classical actions of Ang II on hydrostatic pressure and fluid and electrolyte balance are mediated by AT_1 receptors, which are abundant and widespread in the adult. While AT_2 receptor density and distribution is lower than AT_1 in the adult, it is the most abundant AT receptor in the foetus. In many respects the two AT receptors have complimentary functions: thus while AT_1 mediates vasoconstriction, apoptosis, cellular proliferation and hypertrophy, and the production of reactive oxygen species (ROS); AT_2 is vasodilatory, anti-proliferative, anti-hypertrophic and reduces ROS (Levy 2005).

The summary of the RAS given so far is shown in Fig. 1 and should be considered as describing the "core" elements of the RAS. The reality is more complex. ACE exists in a somatic and a testis-specific isoform; and a homologue, ACE2, generates angiotensin (1-7). AngII is not the only bioactive peptide. Other bioactive peptides such as angiotensin III (2-8), angiotensin IV (3-8) and angiotensin

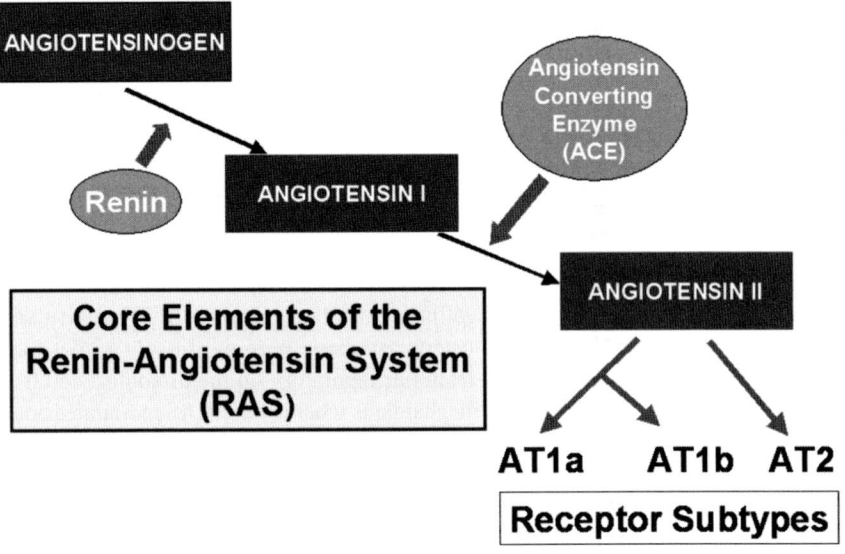

Figure 1. The core elements of the Renin-angiotensin System consist of the obligatory glycoprotein substrate Angiotensinogen (AGT), the enzymes Renin and Angiotensin Converting Enzyme (ACE), and the hydrolytic products Angiotensin I and II. Bioactive Angiotensin II exerts its actions via two receptor subtypes, AT_1 and AT_2. This enzymatic cascade occurs in the circulation as a classic hormonal system and in numerous tissues, including bone, as paracrine systems where additional, alternative enzymatic pathways lead to several bioactive peptides besides AngII. The interplay of blood-borne RAS with local angiotensin-generating systems results in an exceptional range and breadth of tissue-specific functions for the angiotensin peptides (see text for details)

(1-7), are generated by various alternate enzymatic pathways. Similarly, there is a considerable body of evidence dealing with putative AT_3, AT_4 and AT_7 receptors. These are beyond the scope of this chapter and other sources should be consulted (Engeli et al. 2003; Leung 2004; Reaux-Le Goazigo et al. 2005; Chai et al 2005; Guy et al. 2005; Miyazaki and Takai 2006).

In the classical view of the RAS, it is considered a blood-borne hormone system in which hepatic angiotensinogen circulated in plasma is sequentially cleaved by plasma renin and pulmonary membrane-bound ACE. However the widespread tissue expression of angiotensinogen, renin, ACE and other enzymes involved in alter- native pathways indicates the presence of tissue-specific angiotensin-generating systems with a capacity to function in a paracrine or autocrine manner. Local angiotensin-generating systems are numerous and varied, and have been well charac- terized. As examples, the brain, heart, ovary, testis, adrenal, pancreas and adipose tissue all have a local RAS (see reviews by Lavioe and Sigmund 2003; Leung and Sernia, 2003; Leung, 2004; Kershaw and Flier 2004; Thomas and Mendelsohn, 2004; Miaykazi and Takai, 2006; and in particular, Paul et al. 2006).

3.   THE ANGIOTENSIN-GENERATING SYSTEM IN BONE

Bone is a highly specialized tissue that requires continual cellular activity throughout life. The growth and modelling of bone that occurs during childhood and puberty gives rise to a mature skeleton that remains active via the processes of remodelling and repair that are essential for bone homeostasis. The major cells involved in bone deposition and resorption are the osteoblasts and osteoclasts, respectively. The terminal differentiation of osteoblasts produces osteocytes that remain within the bone matrix, connected by canicular channels, and bone-lining cells on the surface. These cells are resting with respect to matrix production, but are key elements of a signal detection and transduction system for bone metabolism. Osteo- cytes are the major cell type in mature calcified bone. The remaining cell type found in bone are the chondrocytes; these are responsible for epiphyseal elongation during bone growth. Remodelling is achieved by a balance of activity between osteoblasts and osteoclasts, collectively referred to as a basic multicellular unit (BMU). As a consequence of their functions, the activities of osteoblasts and osteoclasts are regulated by distinct endocrine and paracrine factors. However, a tight communication between the two cell types is essential for homeostasis to proceed smoothly. An important way in which the two cell types interact is via the RANK/RANKL/OPG "triad". This pathway consists of a receptor found on osteoclasts- the receptor activator of nuclear factor-κB (RANK)- its ligand RANKL, and osteoprotegerin (OPG), a decoy receptor for RANKL. Both RANKL and OPG are expressed by osteoblasts. Activation of RANK by its ligand RANKL increases osteoclastogenesis and osteoclast function (Yasuda et al 1998). Since OPG acts as a decoy receptor for RANKL, activation of RANK, and consequently osteclast activity, is related to the RANKL:OPG ratio and not only to the abundance of RANKL (Simonet et al 1997; Theoleyre et al 2004).

Angiotensin receptors of the AT_1 subtype have been found in human osteoblastic clonal cells and in primary cells from foetal and adult bone of uncertain cell type (Bowler *et al* 1998). The same study reported AT_2 subtype in the same cells, except for human foetal bone. AT_1 receptors have been found by various groups in primary osteoblasts harvested from calvariae and from human trabecular bone explants (Hagiwara *et al* 1998; Lamparter *et al* 1998). Figure 2 shows the expression in the rat UMR-106 cell line of both AT_{1a} and AT_{1b} receptor subtype, AT_2, angiotensinogen and, at very low abundance, of renin. The presence of ACE has not been directly tested. Its presence may however be inferred from the observation that angiotensin I stimulates bone resorption in co-cultures of osteoclasts with osteoblastic cells, and that this action can be inhibited by captopril, an ACE inhibitor (Hatton *et al* 1997). From these various data it may be concluded that the osteoblasts are potentially targets for both blood-borne and locally-generated AngII. Interestingly, ACE inhibitors have no effect on the alkaline phosphatase (ALP) activity of unstimulated osteoblasts (Nashiya and Sugimoto 2001), suggesting that it is RANKL-OPG signalling, rather than bone-forming activity, of osteoblasts that is influenced by autocrine AngII.

The balance of the current evidence limits the presence of AT receptors to osteoblasts, and, to our knowledge, there is no study that has directly and unequivocally shown AT receptors in osteoclasts. On the contrary, the data of Hatton *et al* (1997), where osteoclastic activity in response to AngII was present only in co-culture with osteoblasts, supports the view that osteoclasts do not express AT receptors.

From previous investigations in a variety of tissues, it is known that the AT_1 receptor is usually down-regulated by its ligand AngII (Bouscarel *et al.* 1988; Zhang and Sun 2006). Figure 3 shows the situation in osteoblasts to be more complex, with

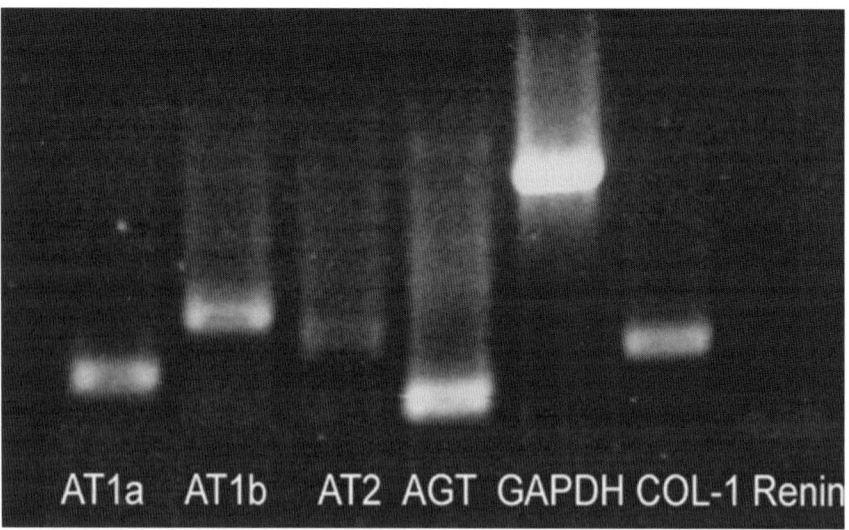

Figure 2. RT-PCR products showing the expression of components of the RAS by the rat osteoblast cell line UMR-106. From left to right: AT_{1a}, AT_{1b} and AT_2 receptors, AGT (angiotensinogen), GAPDH, Col-1 (collagen 1) and renin

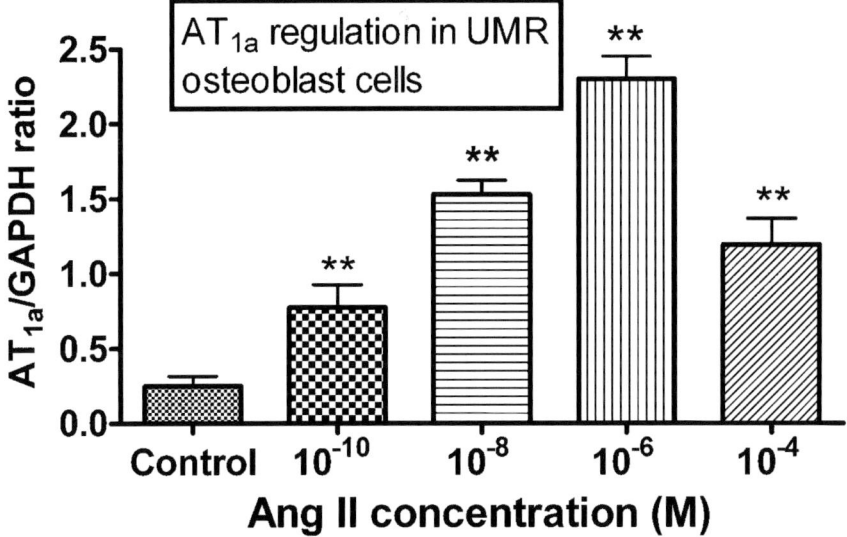

Figure 3. RT-PCR for AT_{1a} mRNA in UMR-106 cells which had been incubated in serum free medium for 24h with increasing concentrations of AngII. Data shown as mean $\pm$ s.e.m. for 4 separate experiments. Data were analysed by Anova and group means compared with control by Dunnett's t-test (**p<0.01)

stimulation of AT_{1a} occurring at lower (closer to physiological) doses, reaching a peak at 10^{-6} M, followed by a reversal, conceivably due to a down-regulation, at higher concentrations. Bimodal dose-effects of AngII are not unusual; for example, Lamparter *et al.* (1998) observed a bimodal effect in the stimulation of proliferation by AngII in human primary bone cells harvested from trabecular explants. It is noteworthy that Lamparter *et al* (1998), contrary to our data, claimed that AngII was ineffective in mature osteoblasts and cited UMR cells as being amongst this class (no data were presented).

4.   OSTEOCALCIN, ALKALINE PHOSPHATASE ACTIVITY AND COLLAGEN EXPRESSION

The differentiation of osteoblasts from mesenchymal stem cells through a series of progenitor stages to form mature matrix-secreting osteoblasts capable of miner-alization is a highly regulated process (Quarles *et al* 1992; Robling *et al.* 2006). The expression of collagen I, osteocalcin, and alkaline phosphatase (ALP) are markers of matrix-producing osteoblast phenotypes. Hagiwara *et al* (1998) found a profound decrease in osteocalcin mRNA in calvarial osteoblastc cells following AngII (10^{-7}M) treatment. The same group, and Lamparter *et al.* (1998) reported a decrease in ALP activity in rat calvarial and human adult bone cells respectively. Figure 4a shows the marked inhibition of ALP activity in UMR-106 osteoblasts treated with AngII, and the reversal of this effect in the presence of the AT_1 receptor

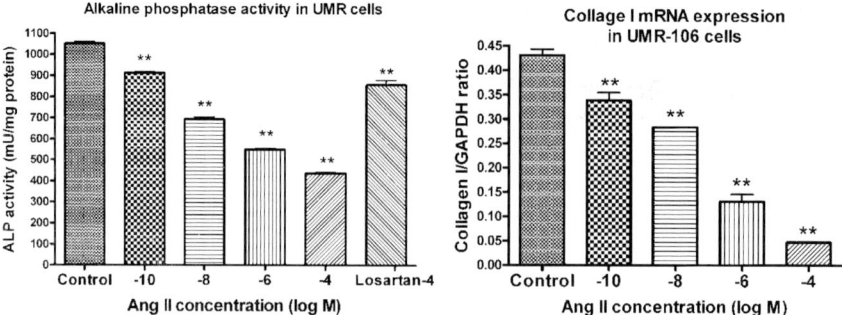

Figure 4. (a) Marked inhibition of alkaline phosphatase activity in cell lysates from osteoblasts after treatment with increasing concentrations of AngII. The AT1 receptor antagonist, Losartan prevented the decrease in ALP activity. (b) Inhibition in collagen I mRNA expression following AngII treatment for 24hours. Data shown as mean ± SEM, (N = 6). Data were analysed by Anova and group means compared with control by Dunnett's t-test (* $p < 0.05$, ** $p < 0.01$, *** $p < 0.001$)

antagonist, Losartan. Hagiwara *et al* (1998) observed a 45% fall in ALP activity of calvarial cells at 10^{-7} M AngII; a similar observation to ours.

Collagen I is the major bone matrix protein and its expression is one of the markers of osteoblast activity. Lamparter *et al* (1998) showed a 4-fold increase in procollagen synthesis, as measured by the incorporation of tritiated proline, by human bone cell cultures incubated with 10^{-7} M AngII for 48hrs. This result is in contrast to our data in Fig. 4b, which shows a >90% inhibition of collagen I mRNA in UMR-106 cells incubated with 10^{-4} M AngII for 24hrs. Differences in outcome could result from the phenotype of the cells used, as suggested by Lamparter *et al* (1998), but it is significant that the inhibition of Collagen I expression is consistent the decrease in osteocalcin and ALP activity, which in turn is consistent with the overall inhibitory role of AngII in osteoblast activity.

5.   OSTEOBLAST PROLIFERATION AND APOPTPSIS

The effect of AngII on osteoblast proliferation have been examined by the Hiruma *et al* (1997) in rat calvarial cells and Lamparter *et al* (1998) in rat calvarial and human trabecular cells. DNA synthesis and cell number increased 2–5 fold and circa 65% respectively. The involvement of mitogen-activated protein kinases (MAPKs) mediated by the AT_1 receptor was shown by Hiruma *et al* (1997). Figure 5 shows the results of incubating UMR-106 cells with Ang II and Ang IV. The bimodal effect seen with AT_{1a} receptor regulation (Fig. 2) by AngII was again found with proliferation, with a peak effect at 10^{-10} M AngII. These data are in general agreement with those of Hiruma *et al* (1997) and Lamparter *et al* (1998). When AngIV was used instead of Ang II, no effect was found, suggesting that osteoblasts lack AT_4 receptors since Ang IV has been reported to stimulate proliferation (Siesjka *et al* 2006).

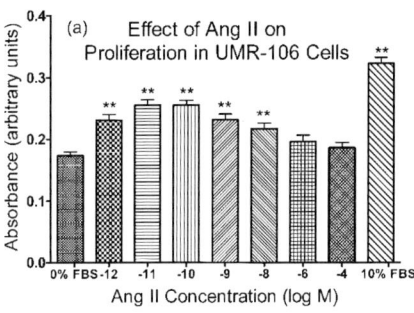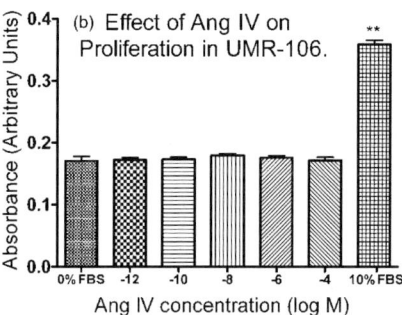

Figure 5. Proliferation of UMR-106 cells incubated for 24hrs with increasing concentration of (a) AngII and (b) Ang IV in serum-free medium (0% FBS). Incubation in normal 10% foetal bovine serum (10% FBS) was included as a positive control. An effect was observed only with AngII. Proliferation was measured by MTT [3-(4,5-dimethylthiazol-2-yl)-2,5-diphenyltetrazolium bromide] assay (Mosmann, 1983). Data are shown as mean $\pm$ SEM, (N=6). Data were analysed by Anova and group means compared with control by Dunnett's t-test (* $p < 0.05$, ** $p < 0.01$, *** $p < 0.001$)

AngII has been shown to induce senescence mediated by the AT_1 receptor, leading to an impairment of proliferation and eventual cell death (Imanishi *et al* 2004). In the differentiation and maturation of osteoblasts, the process of rapid proliferation eventually dissipates into a steady-state mature phenotype. The view that AngII is involved in this maturation process is supported by Lamparter *et al* (1998) who found that phenotypic mature osteoblastic were insensitive to the proliferative actions of AngII. Our own data, showing a proliferative bimodal dose response to AngII (Fig. 5) could be construed as the down-stream result of increasing senescence and apoptosis with increasing AngII concentrations. Figure 6 shows the results of testing this hypothesis in UMR-106 cells. At high concentrations of Ang II there was an 86% increase in apoptosis over a 24h period. Senescence was not directly tested and therefore it is possible that it is occurring at lower AngII concentrations and impairing proliferation. It is also possible that at high AngII concentrations there is significant activation of the AT_2 receptor subtype in UMR-106 cells (see Fig. 2) which is known to be anti-proliferative and to mediate apoptosis (Levy 2005; Wilms *et al.* 2005). It is clear that further probing is required before being able to accurately ascertain the role of AngII in the proliferation and maturation of osteoblasts.

6.   OSTEOBLAST MINERALIZATION

The ultimate function of the osteoblast is the mineralization of the collagen matrix. Hagiwara *et al* (1998) used calvarial cells of foetal origin to examine the effect of AngII on the formation of mineralised nodules formed by cultured cells. They observed a 55% reduction in the number of mineralised nodules after 14 days incubation with 10^{-7} M AngII.

Osteoblast UMR-106 cells incubated in the presence of special mineralization medium will show mineralization activity within 4 days. When incubated for a

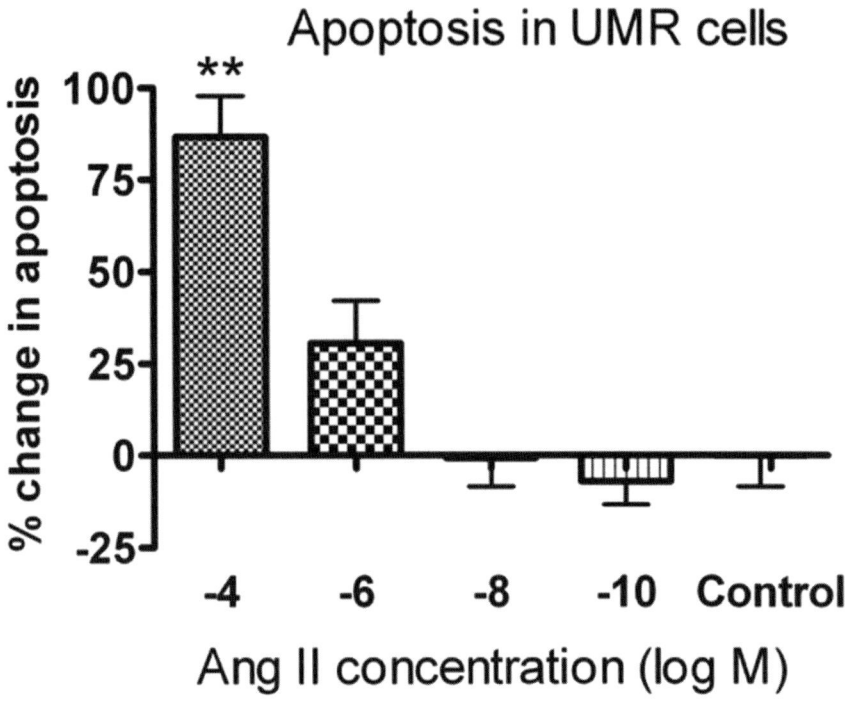

Figure 6. Increase in apoptosis in UMR-106 cells incubated for 24hrs with increasing concentrations of AngII. The incidence of cell death was determined with the chromatin-binding fluorescent dye 4' 6-diamidino-2-phenylindole (DAPI).This dye penetrates into cells with a damaged cell membrane but is excluded by live cells. The total density of cells was determined by DAPI fluorescence after cell lysis with detergent. The ratio of the two fluorometric readings is an index of apoptosis. Data were normalized to the control group were expressed as mean % changes from control. Bars represent mean ± SEM, (N = 4). Data were analysed by Anova and group means compared with control by Dunnett's t-test (* $p < 0.05$, ** $p < 0.01$, *** $p < 0.001$)

further 4 days with AngII, a dose related inhibition of mineralization could be clearly observed (Fig. 7). The effect of AngII was inhibited by the inclusion of the AT_1 receptor antagonist Losartan (data not shown), thus implicating a specific AT_1 mediated mechanism as the mode of action of AngII. These results and those of Hagiwara *et al* (1998) firmly establish AngII as a potent inhibitor of osteoblast mineralization activity.

7.   OSTEOBLAST-OSTECLAST INTERACTIONS

The osteoclast is the principal bone-resorbing cell, removing both the mineral and the organic matrix of bone. Osteoclasts are derived from a pool of non-committed monocyte-macrophage precursors which also possess the potential to differentiate into macrophages and dendritic cells. Osteoclast formation and function

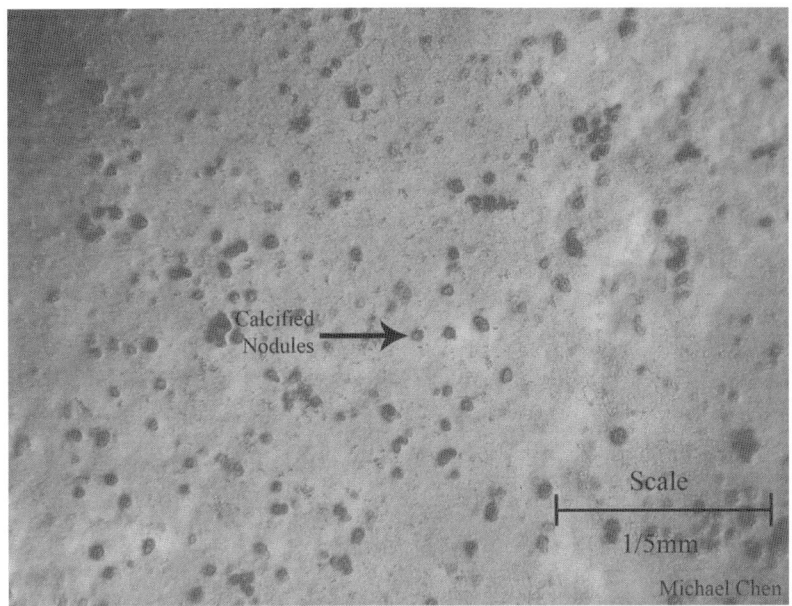

Alizarin Red Staining for Calcified Nodules

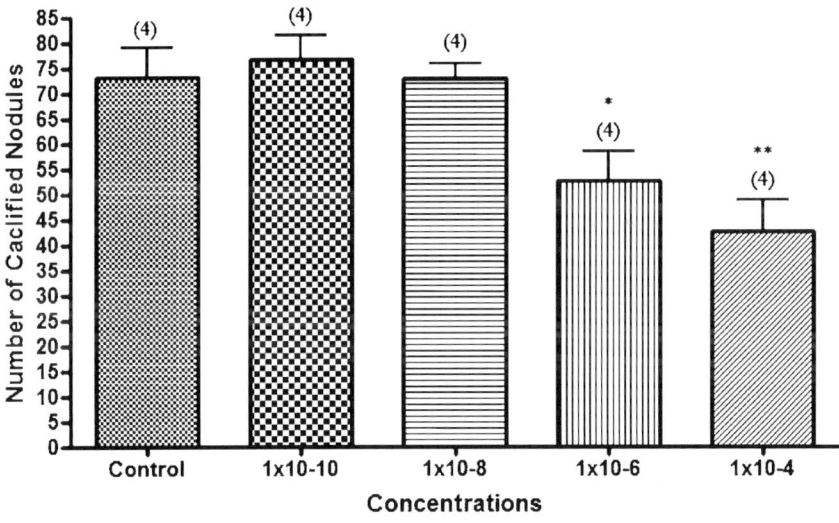

Figure 7. Mineralization activity of UMR-106 cells over a period of 8 days. Mineralization activity can be induced over a period of days by supplementation of the culture medium with 10mM β-Glycerol phosphate and 0.33mM L-Ascorbic acid 2-phosphate magnesium n-hydrate. Ang II was added after 4 days and mineralization allowed for another 4 days. Nodules of mineralized plaques are easily visualized by staining with a 2% Alizarin Red solution and the density of nodules per mm^2 counted (Uchimura et al 2003). Bars represent mean $\pm$ SEM, (N=4). Data were analysed by Anova and group means compared with control by Dunnett's t-test (* $p < 0.05$, ** $p < 0.01$, *** $p < 0.001$)

are regulated by a variety of cytokines and hormones, as well as cell-cell contact with osteoblasts (Jimi *et al.* 1996; Mundy and Elefteriou 2006). The receptor activator of nuclear factor-κB ligand (RANKL), is a tumour necrosis factor superfamily member with potent activity as a stimulator of both the formation of osteoclasts from precursor cells and bone-resorbing activity in mature osteoclasts (Yasuda *et al* 1998). RANKL is critical for the terminal differentiation of osteoclast precursor cells, as shown by the severe osteopetrosis present in RANKL-deficient mice (Blair *et al.* 2006). RANKL is expressed in marrow stromal as well as osteoblastic cells (Simonet *et al* 1997). Osteoblasts express three RANKL isoforms; two membrane-bound forms and a smaller soluble form (Theoleyre *et al.* 2006).

Osteoprotegerin (OPG) is a tumour necrosis factor receptor superfamily member secreted by various cell types, such as B lymphocytes, dendritic cells and vascular smooth muscle, as well as osteoblasts. It is a potent inhibitor of osteoclast formation by acting as a decoy receptor for RANKL, thereby decreasing RANKL avail-ability at its receptor binding site on RANK. Mice that lack OPG show severe osteoporosis, increased numbers of osteoclasts and arterial calcification (Bucay *et al* 1998) and overexpression precipitates osteopetrosis (Simonet *et al* 1997) The biologically active receptor for RANKL is RANK (receptor activator of nuclear factor-*[kappa]*B), present on osteoclast precursors and mature osteoclasts. It is an obligatory link in osteoclast formation, as no osteoclasts are detected in RANK-deficient animals (Blair *et al.* 2006; Lee and Lorenzo, 2006).

It is clear from the preceding summary that central to normal osteoclastogenesis and osteoclast function is the expression of RANKL isoforms and OPG by osteoblasts.

There is indirect published evidence to support the hypothesis that AngII interacts with OPG/RANK/RANKL. Thus, Hatton *et al* (1997) showed that AngII was ineffective in stimulating bone resorption when incubated with foetal calvarial osteoclast cells alone, but stimulated bone resorption in a mixed population of osteoblasts and osteoclasts. These results suggest that Ang II stimulates osteoclasts via some action in osteoblasts. A similar inference could be made from the report of Schurman *et al* (2004) who found a reduced calcium uptake into calvarial bone discs in the presence of 10^{-8} M AngII. Given the importance of the OPG/RANK/RANKL system, these observations raise the possibility that AngII stimulates osteoclast activity via an increase in RANKL or a decrease in OPG, or both. There is evidence that AngII mildly increases OPG mRNA in vascular smooth muscle (Zhang *et al.* 2002). However no published data on AngII and the OPG/RANK/RANKL triad are available. In a recent study by Dossing and Stern (2005) UMR-106 cells were used to show regulation of RANKL expression and secretion. Figure 8 shows data for the expression of RANKL mRNA in UMR-106 cells incubated with AngII or the cyclic AMP analogue, dibutyryl cyclic AMP, a known stimulus for RANKL expression. AngII was a potent stimulus for RANKL expression, reaching a 2.5 fold increase over control at 10^{-10} M AngII. The biphasic response typical of AngII action was observed, in contrast to linear response to cyclic AMP. These data do not reveal which RANKL isoform is involved in the AngII response and there is still no

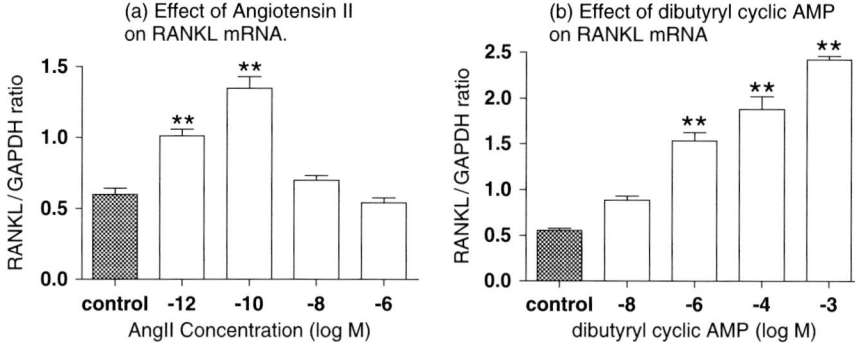

Figure 8. RT-PCR for RANKL mRNA in UMR-106 cells which had been incubated in serum free medium for 24h with increasing concentrations of AngII or dibutyryl cyclic AMP. The RT-PCR conditions were identical to those of Dossing and Stern (2005). Bars represent mean ± SEM, (N = 4). Data were analysed by Anova and group means compared with control by Dunnett's t-test (* p < 0.05, ** p < 0.01, *** p < 0.001)

information on any involvement of OPG. However, this is the first demonstration that AngII has a role in the OPG/RANK/RANKL system.

7.1.   Transforming Growth Factor-Beta (TGF-β)

While the formation of osteoclasts from monocytes is dependent on RANKL, monocytes require further co-stimulatory signals, largely from osteoblasts to undergo osteoclast differentiation. One of these signals appears to be TGF-β, a member of the TGF/activin sub-group of the TGF superfamily with a critical role in cellular differentiation. TGF-β is expressed by numerous cell types, including osteoblasts and fibroblasts; it is the most abundant growth factor in bone (Kanaan & Kanaan, 2006). Osteoblast-derived TGF-β acts directly on osteoclast precursors to prime them for RANKL-induced osteoclast formation. Without TGF-β, osteoclast formation will not occur and instead monocytes follow the macrophage differentiation pathways (Fox and Lovibon 2005; Kanaan and Kanaan 2006).

There are two studies that implicate TGF-β in the action of angII on bone. In 2000, Brown reported a study on the expression of ACE, TGF-β$_1$ and interleukin 11 in osteolytic lesions of patients with Langerhans Cell Histiocytosis. The presence of all three markers on histiocytes in proximity to osteoclasts is consistent with a stimulation of osteoclastogenesis by TGF-β$_1$ and interleukin11 released by the action of locally generated AngII. More persuasive evidence is provided by Schurman *et al* (2004), who used a bone disc bioassay to measure the uptake of calcium into bone. They found that AngII decreased calcium uptake and that antiserum to TGF-β$_1$ abolished the effect of AngII. However, until there is the direct testing of AngII action on osteoblast expression of TGF-β, this pathway of AngII-initiated osteoclastogenesis remains hypothetical.

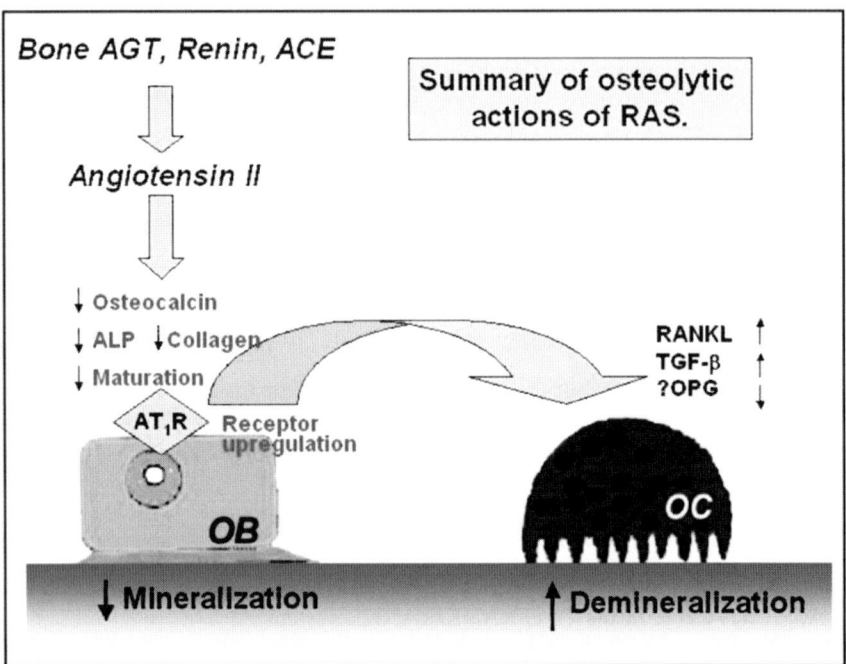

Figure 9. Summary of Proposed Actions of the bone RAS on osteoblasts (OB) and osteoclasts (OC)

8. SUMMARY OF ANGII ACTIONS

The current evidence for the actions of AngII on osteoblasts and osteoclasts is summarized in Fig. 9. The salient features are the decrease in osteoblast function via an inhibition of osteoblast maturation; inhibition of osteocalcin, alkaline phosphatase and collagen I, and finally, a decrease in mineralization. This decrease in osteoblast function, leading to a decrease in bone deposition, operates in concert with an increase in bone loss due to a stimulation of osteoclastogenesis and osteo-clast activity mediated by RANKL and TGF-β_1. Underpinning all these actions is an increase in sensitivity to local AngII mediated by an upregulation of AT$_1$ receptors. The details of these various actions of AngII are yet to be sorted, especially the osteoblast-osteoclast interactions. Nevertheless, we have the basis of a potentially powerful hormonal pathway that can deplete bone density via a simultaneous decrease in mineralization and increase in demineralization.

9. PHYSIOLOGICAL AND CLINICAL IMPORTANCE
     OF BONE RAS

The evidence required to make an assessment of the physiological importance for the RAS in bone metabolism is presently very sparse. Nevertheless, angiotensinogen knockout mice do have significantly lower body weight (Massiera *et al* 2002).

However, the skeletal system was not examined and the lower weight was attributed to changed metabolism and locomotion. Transgenic models of under- or over-expression of RAS components would be valuable in elucidating RAS involvement in bone development and homeostasis; these models should be utilized in future studies. In both humans and animals, treatment during pregnancy with ACE inhibitors such as captopril, or with AT_1 receptor antagonists, such as losartan, lead to skeletal pathologies (Buttar 1997; Mastrobattista 1997; Alwan et al. 2005; Tabacova et al. 2003; Tabacova 2005; de Leeuw 2006; Quan 2006). The most prevalent skeletal pathology is hypocalvaria, a condition where the newborn shows calvarial bones with a normal position and shape, but of smaller size. Lower incidence of anomalies in the long bones, vertebrae and ribs are also found. These foetal pathologies, especially those of membranous bones such as calvaria, have been attributed to hypoxia arising from hypotension and microvascular and renal abnormalities as a consequence of RAS inhibition. However, the existence of an active local bone RAS now gives rise to the possibility that skeletal abnormalities are due directly to the disruption of the bone RAS.

In contrast to the effects of RAS inhibition in gestation, bone abnormalities have not been observed in adult rat studies in which treatment was initiated at 12-14 weeks of age (Stimpel et al. 1995; Broulik et al. 2001). Interestingly, we have localized AGT and AT_1 receptors to chondrocytes in the epiphyseal plate of the rat tibia (Sernia et al. 2005), which implies a capacity to generate AngII locally and implicates local AngII in bone elongation. Based on these observations, we suggest that future studies on the effect of RAS inhibition on bone growth should be initiated in juveniles in the rapid growth phase.

10.   THE RAS-BONE DENSITY LINK

Clinical and epidemiological studies are revealing a link between RAS and bone density. Several studies have reported changes in bone mineral density (BMD) in hypertensive subjects. Cappuccio et al. (1999) found the rate of bone loss at the femoral neck increased with the severity of blood pressure hypertensive women and Tsuda et al. (2001) reported an inverse relationship betweenan BMD and systolic pressure. In female hypertensive patients, activation of the RAS was correlated with an increase in 24-h urinary calcium excretion, which in turn, was associated with a lower BMD (Grant et al. 1992). In post-menopausal women, plasma ACE is directly associated with bone loss (Sanada et al. 2004). An association between ACE insertion/deletion polymorphism and BMD has been reported in hypertensive women, with the highest BMD found in II and the lowest in DD polymorphism (Perez-Castrillon, Justo et al. 2003). As expected, DD patients benefited most from ACE inhibitor treatment (Perez-Castrillon, Silva et al. 2003). Most recently, case studies of postmenopausal women on ACE inhibitors reported a 7% decrease in fractures (Rejnmark et al. 2006) and an increase in BMD, which was also observed in elderly men (Lynn et al. 2006).

11.   CONCLUSIONS

While the renin-angiotensin system is accepted as having a major role in cardiovascular disease, there is emerging evidence for its involvement in bone homeostasis. We have presented the evidence supporting the existence of a local RAS with marked osteoblast inhibitory actions and probable osteoclast stimulatory actions. The physiological importance of this system in normal bone development remains to be determined but the deleterious effects of foetal inhibition of RAS and the presence of RAS in chondrocytes suggests a significant role in bone development. Clinical studies have been limited to post-menopausal hypertensive women and a greater focus on other groups, especially pubertal patients on RAS inhibitor therapy, is needed. Nevertheless, data from aged patients on RAS inhibitors already suggests a beneficial effect on BMD. Degenerative bone diseases such as osteoporosis and osteoarthritis are prevalent conditions in ageing populations; frequently co-existing with cardiovascular disease. And finally, metastases of primary tumours into bone is a common occurrence. An understanding of the bone RAS will improve the management and treatment of these conditions; possibly with the judicious use ACE inhibitors and receptor antagonists.

REFERENCES

Alwan, S., Polifka, J.E., and Friedman, J.M., 2005, Angiotensin II receptor antagonist treatment during pregnancy. *Birth Defects Res A Clin Mol Teratol.* **73**: 123–30.

Blair, J.M., Zhou, H., Seibel, M.J., and Dunstan, C.R., 2006, Mechanisms of Disease: roles of OPG, RANKL and RANK in the pathophysiology of skeletal metastasis. *Nat Clin Pract Oncol.* **3**: 41–49.

Broulik, P.D., Tesar, V., Zima, T., and Jirsa, M., 2001, Impact of antihypertensive therapy on the skeleton: effects of enalapril and AT1 receptor antagonist losartan in female rats. *Physiol Res.* **50**: 353–358.

Brown, R.E., 2000, Angiotensin-converting enzyme, transforming growth factor β_1, and interleukin 11 in the osteolytic lesions of Langerhans cell Histiocytosis. *Arch Pathol Lab Med.* **124**: 1287–1290.

Bowler, W.B., Gallagher, J.A., and Bilbe, G., 1998. G-protein coupled receptors in bone. *Front Biosci.* **1**: 769–80.

Bouscarel, B., Wilson, P.B., Blackmore, P.F., Lynch, C.J., and Exton, J.H., 1988, Agonist-induced down-regulation of the angiotensin II receptor in primary cultures of rat hepatocytes. *J Biol Chem* **263**: 14920–149204.

Bucay, S., Sarosi, J., Dunstan, CR., Morony, S.,Tarpley, J., 1998, Osteoprotegerin-deficient mice develop early-onset osteoporosis and arterial calcification. Gene Dev **12**: 1260–1268.

Buttar, H.S., 1997, An overview of the influence of ACE inhibitors on fetal-placental circulation and perinatal development. *Molec Cell Biochem.* **176**: 61–71.

Cappuccio, F.P., Meilahn, E., Zmuda, J.M., Cauley, J.A., and the Study of Osteoporotic Fractures Research Group, 1999, High blood pressure and bone mineral loss in elderly white women: A prospective study. *Lancet.* **354**: 971–975.

Chai, S.Y., Fernando, R., Peck, G., Ye, S.Y., Mendelsohn, F.A., Jenkins, T.A., and Albiston, A.L., 2004, The angiotensin IV/AT4 receptor. *Cell Mol Life Sci.* **61**: 2728–2737.

De Gasparo, M., Catt, K.J., Inagami, T., Wright, J.W., and Unger, T.H., 2000, The angiotensin II receptors. *Pharmacol Rev.* **52**: 415–472.

De Leeuw, P.W., 2006, The use of angiotensin converting enzyme (ACE) inhibitors during pregnancy clearly increases the risk of congenital malformations. *Ned Tijdschr Geneeskd.* **150**: 1605–1607.

Dendorfer, A., Dominiak, P., and Schunkert, H., 2005, ACE inhibitors and angiotensin II receptor antagonists. *Handb Exp Pharmacol.* **170**: 407–42.

Dossing, D.A., and Stern, P.H., 2005, Receptor activator of NF-kappa B ligand protein expression in UMR-106 cells is differentially regulated by parathyroid hormone and calcitriol. *J Cell Biochem.* **95**: 1029–1041.

Engeli, S., Schling, P., Gorzelniak, K., Boschmann, M., Janke, J., Ailhaud, G., Teboul, M., Massiéra, F., and Sharma, A.M., 2003, The adipose-tissue renin–angiotensin–aldosterone system: role in the metabolic syndrome? *Int J Biochem Cell Biol.* **35**: 807–825.

Fishel, R.S., Eisenberg, S., Shai, S.Y., Redden, R.A., Bernstein, K.E., and Berk, B.C., 1995, Glucocorticoids induce angiotensin-converting enzyme expression in vascular smooth muscle. *Hypertension.* **25**: 343–349.

Fox, W.F., and Lovibond, A.C., 2005, Current insights into the role of transforming growth factor-β in bone resorption. *Molec Cell Endocrinol.* **243**: 19–26.

Gard, P., 2002, The role of angiotensin II in cognition and behaviour. *Eur J Pharmacol.* **438**: 1–14.

Guy, J.L., Lamber, D.J., Warner, F.J., Hooper, N.M., and Turner, A.J., 2005, Membrane-associated zinc peptidase families: comparing ACE and ACE2. *Biochim Biophys Acta.* **1751**: 2–8.

Hagiwara, H., Hiruma, Y., Inoue, A., Yamaguchi, A., and Hirose, S., 1998, Deceleration by angiotensin II of the differentiation and bone formation of rat calvarial osteoblastic cells. *Endocrinol.* **156**: 543–50.

Hatton, R.M., Stimpel, and Chambers T.J., 1997, Angiotensin II is generated from angiotensin I by bone cells and stimulates osteoclastic bone resorption in vitro. *J Endocrinol.* **152**: 5–10.

Hiruma, Y., Inoue, A., Hirose, S., and Hagiwara, H., 1997, Angiotensin II stimulates the proliferation of osteoblast-rich populations of cells from rat calvariae. *Biochem Biophys Res Commun.* **230**: 176–8.

Imanishi, T., Hano, T., and Nishio, I., 2004, Angiotensin II accelerates endothelial progenitor cell senescence through induction of oxidative stress. *J Hypertens.* **23**: 97–104.

Jimi, E., Nakamura, I., Amano, H., Taguchi, Y., Tsurukai, T., Tamura, M., Nakahashi, N., and Suda, T., 1996, Osteoclast function is activated by osteoblastic cells through a mechanism involving cell-to-cell contact. *Endocrinology.* **137**: 2187–90.

Kanaan, R.A., and Kanaan, L.A., 2006, Transforming growth factor β1, bone connection. *Med Sci Monit.* **12**: 164–169.

Kershaw, E.E., and Flier, J., 2004, Adipose tissue as an endocrine organ. *J. Clin. Endocrinol. Metab.* **2548–2556.**

Lacey, D.L., Timms, E., Tan, H.-L., Kelley, M.J., Dunstan, C.R., Burgess, T., Elliott, R., Colombero, A., Elliott, G., Scully, S., Hsu, H., Sullivan, J., Hawkins, N., Davy, E., Capparelli, C., Eli, A., Qian, Y.-X., Kaufman, S., Sarosi, I., Shalhoub, V., Senaldi, G., Guo, J., Delaney, J., and Boyle, W. J., 1998, Osteoprotegerin ligand is a cytokine that regulates osteoclast differentiation and activation. *Cell.* **93**: 165–176.

Lamparter, S., Kling, L., Schrader, M., Ziegler, R., and Pfeilschifter, J., 1998, Effects of angiotensin II on bone cells in vitro. *J Cell Physiol.* **175**: 89–98.

Lavoie, J.L., and Sigmund, C.D., 2003, Minireview: Overview of the renin-angiotensin system—an endocrine and paracrine system. *Endocrinology* **144**: 2179–2183.

Lee, S-K., and Lorenzo, J., 2006, Cyrokine regulating osteoclast formation and function. *Curr Opin Rheumatol.* **411–418.**

Leung, P.S., 2004, The peptide hormone angiotensin II: its new functions in tissues and organs. *Curr Protein Pept Sci.* **5**: 267–273.

Leung, P.S., Sernia, C., 2003, The renin-angiotensin system and male reproduction: new functions for old hormones. *Molec Cell Endocrin.* **30**: 263–70.

Levy, B.I., 2005, How to explain the differences between renin angiotensin system modulators. *Am J Hypertens.* **134S–141S.**

Lynn, H., Kwok, T., Wong, S., Woo, J., and Leung, P.C., 2006, Angiotensin Converting enzyme use is associated with higher bone mineral density in elderly chinese. *Bone.* **38**: 584–588.

Massiera, F., Seydoux, J., Geloen, A., Quignard-Boulange, A., Turban, S., Saint-Marc, P., Fukamizu, A., Negrel, R., Ailhaud, G., and Teboul, M., 2001, Angiotensinogen-deficient mice exhibit impairment of diet-induced weight gain with alteration in adipose tissue development and increased locomotor activity. *Endocrinol.* **142**: 5220–5225.

Mastrobattista, J.M., 1997, Angiotensin converting enzyme inhibitors in pregnancy. *Semin Perinatol.* **21**: 124–134.

Miyazaki, M., and Takai, S., 2006, Tissue angiotensin II generating system by angiotensin-converting enzyme and chymase. *J Pharmacol Sci.* **100**: 391–7.

Mosmann, T., 1983, Rapid colorimetric assay for cellular growth and survival: application to proliferation and cytotoxicity assays. *J Immunol Methods.* **16**: 55–63.

Mundy, G.R., and Elefteriou, F., 2006, Boning up on ephrin signaling. *Cell.* **126**: 441–443.

Nishiya, Y., and Sugimoto, S., 2001, Effects of various antihypertensive drugs on the function of osteoblast. *Biol Pharm Bull.* **24**: 628–33

Paul, M., Poyan Mehr, A., and Kreuz, R., 2006, Physiology of local renin-angiotensin systems. *Physiol Rev.* **86**: 747–803.

Perez-Castrillon, J.L., Justo, I., Silva, J., Sanz, A., Escudero, J.C.M., Igea, R., Escudero, P., Pueyo, C., Diaz, C., Hernandez, G., and Duenas, A., 2003, Relationship between bone mineral density and angiotensin converting enzyme polymorphism in hypertensive postmenopausal women. *Am. J. Hypertens.* **233–235**.

Perez-Castrillon, J.L., Silva, J., Justo, I., Sanz, A., Martin-Luquero, M., Igea, R., Escudero, P., Pueyo, C., Diaz, C., Hernandez, G., and Duenas, A., 2003, Effect of quinapril, quinapril-hydrochlorothiazide, and enalapril on the bone mass of hypertensive subjects: Relationship with angiotensin converting enzyme polymorphisms. *Am J Hypertens.* **16**: 453–459.

Quan, A., 2006, Fetopathy associated with exposure to angiotensin converting enzyme inhibitors and angiotensin receptor antagonists. *Early Hum Dev.* **82**: 23–28.

Quarles, LD., Yohay DA, Lever LW., Caton, R., Wenstrup RJ, 1992, Distinct proliferative and differentiated stages of murine MC3T3-E1 cells in culture: an in vitro model of osteoblast development. *J Bone Miner Res.* **7**: 683–92.

Reaux-Le Goazigo, A., Iturrioz, X., Fassot, C., Claperon, C., Roques, B.P., and Llorens-Cortes, C., 2005, Role of angiotensin III in hypertension. *Curr Hypertens Rep.* **7**: 128–134.

Rejmark, L., Vestergaard , P., and Mosekilde, L., 2006. Treatment with beta-blockers, ACE inhibitors, and calcium-channel blockers is associated with a reduced fracture risk: a nationwide case-control study. *J Hypertens.* **24**: : 581–9.

Robling, A., Castillo, A.B., and Turner, C.H., 2006, Biomechanical and molecular regulation of bone remodeling. *Ann RevBiomed Eng.* **8**: 455–498.

Sanada, M., Taguchi, A., Higashi, Y., Tsuda, M., Kodama, I., Yoshizumi, M., and Ohama, K., 2004, Forearm endothelial function and bone mineral loss in postmenopausal women. *Atherosclerosis.* **176**: 387–392.

Sanchez, C.P., He, Y.-Z., Leiferman, E., and Wilsman, N., 2004, Bone elongation in rats with renal failure and mild or advanced secondary hyperparathyroidism. *Kidn Inter.* **65**: 1740–1748.

Schurman, S.J., Bergstrom, W.H., Shoemaker, L.R., and Welch, T.R., 2004, Angiotensin II reduced calcium uptake into bone. *Pediatr Nephrol.* **19**: 33–35.

Sernia, C., Li, L., and Huang, H., 2005, Localization of angiotensin receptors and angiotensinogen in the epiphyseal plate of rat tibia. ANZBMS proceedings P97.

Siejka, A., Melen-Mucha, G., Mucha, S.A., and Pawlikowski, M., 2006, Angiotensins II and IV modulate adrenocortical cell proliferation in ovariectomized rats. *J Physiol Pharmacol.* **57**: 451–456.

Simonet, WS., Lacey, DL., Dunstan, CR., Kelley M. et al. 1997. Osteoprotogerin: A novel secreted protein involved in the regulation of bone density. *Cell* **89**: 309–319.

Stimpel, M., Jee, W.S., Ma, Y., Yamamoto, N., and Chen, Y., 1995, Impact of antihypertensive therapy on postmenopausal osteoporosis: Effects of the angiotensin converting enzyme inhibitor moexipril, 17 beta-estradiol and their combination on the ovariectomy-induced cancellous bone loss in young rats. *Journal of Hypertension.* **13**: 1852–1856.

Tabacova, S., 2005, Mode of action: angiotensin-converting enzyme inhibition–developmental effects associated with exposure to ACE inhibitors. *Crit Rev Toxicol.* **35**: 747–55.

Tabacova, S., Little, R., Tsong, Y., Vega, A., and Kimmel, C.A., 2003, Adverse pregnancy outcomes associated with maternal enalapril antihypertensive treatment. *Pharmacoepidemiol and Drug Safety*.**12**: 633–646.

Theoleyre, S., Wittrant, Y., Kwan Tat, S., Fortun, Y., Redini, F., and Heymann, D., 2004. The molecular triad OPG/RANK/RANKL: involvement in the orchestration of pathophysiological bone remodeling. *Cytokine Growth Factor Rev*.**15**,457–75.

Thomas, W.G., and Mendelsohn, F.A.O., 2003, Angiotensin receptors: form and function and distribution. *Int J Biochem Cell Biol.* **35**: 774–779.

Tsuda, K., Nishio, I., and Masuyama, Y., 2001, Bone Mineral Density in Women With Essential Hypertension. *Am. J. Hypertens.* **14**: 704–707.

Uchimura, E., Machida, H., Kotobuki, N., Kihara, T., Kitamura, S., Ikeuchi, M., Hirose, M., Miyake, J., and Ohgushi, H., 2003, In-situ visualization and quantification of mineralization of cultured osteogenetic cells. *Calcif Tiss Int.* **73**: 575–583.

Wada, T., Nakashima, T., Hiroshi, N., and Penninger, J.M., 2006, RANKL-RANK signaling in osteoclastogenesis and bone disease. *Trends Molec Med.* **12**: 17–25.

Wilms, H., Rosenstiel, P., Unger, T., Deuschl, G., and Lucius, R., 2005, Neuroprotection with angiotensin receptor antagonists: a review of the evidence and potential mechanisms. *Am J Cardiovasc Drugs.* **5**: 245–53.

Wittrant, Y., Theoleyre, S., Chipoy, C., Padrines, M., Blanchard, M., Heymann, D., and Redini, F., 2004, RANKL/RANK/OPG: new therapeutic targets in bone tumours and associated osteolysis. *Biochim Biophys Acta.* **704**: 49–57.

Yasuda, H., Shima, N., Nakagawa, N., Yamaguchi, K., Kinosaki, M., Mochizuki, S.I., Tomoyasu, A., Yano, K., Goto, M., Murakami, A., Tsuda, E., Morinaga, T., Higashio, K., Udagawa, N., Takahashi, N., and Suda, T., 1998, Osteoclast differentiation factor is a ligand for osteoprotegerin osteoclastogenesis-inhibitory factor and is identical to TRANCE/RANKL. *Proc Natl Acad Sci USA.* **3597–3602.**

Zhang, J., Fu, M., Myles, D., Zhu, X., Du, J., Cao, X., and Chen, Y.E., 2002, PDGF induces osteoprotegerin expression in vascular smooth muscle cells by multiple signal pathways. *FEBS Lett.* **521**: 180–184.

Zhang, H., Sun, G.-Y., 2006, Expression and Regulation of AT_1 Receptor in Rat Lung Microvascular Endothelial Cell. *J Surg Res.* **134**: 190–197.

CHAPTER 10

THE RENIN-ANGIOTENSIN SYSTEM
AND ITS INHIBITORS IN HUMAN CANCERS

LUCIENNE JUILLERAT-JEANNERET
University Institute of Pathology, Bugnon 25, CH1011 Lausanne, Switzerland

1.   INTRODUCTION

The treatment of diseases such as cancer is challenging because these pathologies involve dysregulation of endogenous and often essential cellular processes. Human cancers evolve from various and combined genetic and epigenetic transformations in a multistep process over years, which is called cancer progression. As a consequence, human cancers are heterogeneous entities made of several different cell types: the often polyclonal cancer cells, the normal cell populations from which the disease evolved, the vascular cells, the fibroblasts and immune cells. Cancer cells differ from their normal counterparts by many properties, in particular they replicate faster. Therefore, the vast majority of clinically-used therapies for cancer capitalize on these differences in the rate of cell replication, however with only limited efficacy. The general toxicity to the whole body of current anti-cancer chemotherapeutics produces important side-effects such as sterility, loss of digestive capacities, loss of hair, defects in immune functions, etc. To reduce cytotoxicity for normal cells of the whole body sub-optimal drug concentrations must be applied, and therefore suboptimal delivery of therapeutic agents to the desired cell targets results.

Drug resistance, the appearance of reduced or absent response of cancer cells to applied chemotherapeutical drugs, is another serious therapeutic problem. Drug resistance can be divided into intrinsic drug resistance, where the application of drugs has no biological effect since the initiation of treatment, and acquired drug resistance, where a therapeutic response is observed at the initiation of chemotherapy, which disappears with time of treatment. Several drug resistance mechanisms may be involved in the resistance of cancer cells to chemotherapeutic drugs, frequently involving the simultaneous appearance of cross-resistance to a number of functionally and structurally diverse drugs, with different mechanisms of action: (i) lowering of the intracellular concentration of the drug either by blocking uptake or increasing

197

Po Sing Leung (ed.), Frontiers in Research of the Renin-Angiotensin System on Human Disease, 197–220.
© 2007 *Springer.*

efflux, mainly involving the ATP-dependent efflux multidrug resistance (MDR) protein systems, such as P-glycoprotein (Pgp), (ii) accelerated rates of drug inactivation by protein binding (*e.g.* metallothioneine and glutathione-S-transferase) and conjugation to small molecules such as glutathione, (iii) increased rates of repair pathways in response to drug damage. Therefore one of the main challenges in human cancer treatment is no longer the development of efficient drugs, but the improvement of drug selectivity and efficacy, and the overcoming of resistance mechanisms.

When the initial primary cancer nodules have reached some progression steps and size, further cancer progression requires the development of a tumor-associated vascular system, either neovascularization or co-optation of existing vessels. In many cancers tumor vasculature presents defects of vascular maturation, a loss of contractile capacity and an inadequate number of perivascular cells, resulting in increased permeability and intratumoral hydrostatic pressure, promoting further tumor proliferation, vascular dysfunction, and a poor perfusion and distribution of chemotherapeutic agents. Tumor cells are responsible for the development of this defective tumor-associated vasculature, and anti-angiogenic therapies are under evaluation to treat cancer. The molecular mechanisms underlying the defects observed in the vasculature of tumors, in particular the loss of constrictor response to vasoactive peptides resulting in poor perfusion of the tumor and increased permeability, are presently only poorly understood, however, they depend, in part, of the vascular endothelial growth factot/vascular permeability factor (VEGF/VPF) system, which is also involved in increased vascular permeability. Recent information has shown that anti-angiogenic treatments increase tumor cell mobility and tissue invasion, in particular in the brain (Lamszus *et al* 2005), suggesting that normalization of tumor vasculature would be more efficient than anti-angiogenic therapies for some cancers. These experiments have also demonstrated that in human cancers, in order to be efficient, antiangiogenic therapies must be used in combination therapies, and that distribution of the drugs to the tumor vascular tree must be enhanced, improved or induced in order to achieve efficient treatment, therefore pointing toward an important role for the systems regulating vascular functions, such as the renin-angiotensin system (RAS).

The RAS has been mainly studied as an endocrine system in the context of cardiovascular disorders, and both inhibitors for the enzymes metabolizing the precursor protein and intermediates and agonists or antagonists of their receptors have been developed for the treatment of these disorders. However, the RAS, in addition to controlling the vascular tone and fluid homeostasis, may be involved in cell growth and/or death not only in cancer, but also in fibrotic or degenerative diseases. The blood RAS comprises a circulating liver-derived precursor protein, angiotensinogen (AGT), activated by two proteases, the kidney-secreted active renin and the pulmonary endothelium-bound angiotensin converting enzyme (ACE). This proteolytic cascade produces the system-representative active peptide angiotensin II (Ang II) acting on two receptors angiotensin 1 (AT_1) and angiotensin 2 (AT_2) membrane-bound receptors on target cells and represents the "classical angiotensinogen

⬇ *Renin*

angiotensin I
Asp-Arg-Val-Tyr-Ile-His-Pro-Phe-*His-Leu*

⬇ *Angiotensin Converting Enzyme (ACE)*

angiotensin II   *ACE2*
Asp-Arg-Val-Tyr-Ile-His-Pro-*Phe* ➡   angiotensin(1-7)
                                    Asp-Arg-Val-Tyr-Ile-His-Pro

⬇ *Aminopeptidase A (APA)*

angiotensin III
Arg-Val-Tyr-Ile-His-Pro-Phe

⬇ *Aminopeptidases B/N*

angiotensin IV
Val-Tyr-Ile-His-Pro-Phe

Figure 1. The enzymes and the peptides of the "classical" and "non-classical" RAS

RAS", (Fig. 1) involved in the control of vascular tone and fluid homeostasis. Then several exopeptidases, which include aminopeptidases and/or carboxypeptidases, and endopeptidases further process the precursors and active peptides to intermediate peptides with various biological activities, which represents the "non-classical RAS" (Fig. 1).

The expression of selected RAS components is either induced or decreased in cancer, according to a cell-specific and cancer-specific pattern. RAS components have been associated with tumor vasculature defects and/or a more direct effect on tumor cells, supporting a favoring role for the RAS in human cancer progression. Inhibitors for the enzymes or antagonists for the receptors of the RAS (Fig. 2) have anti-tumor effects in human and in animal cancer models, which have been attributed to their effects on the tumor-associated vasculature and/or tumor cells.

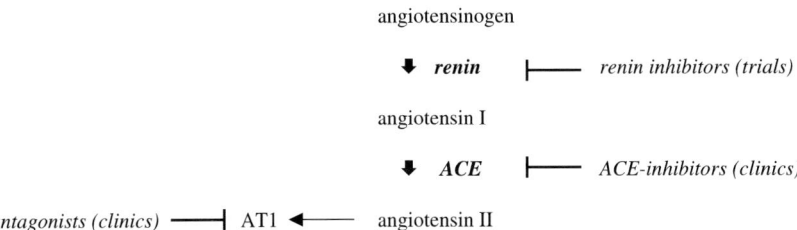

Figure 2. The inhibitors and antagonists of the "classical" RAS

Table 1. Chemical structures of representative drugs modifying the RAS which are in clinical use for cardiovascular diseases

Name	Structure	Target
Enalapril		angiotensin convertingenzyme (ACE) inhibitor
Valsartan		angiotensin receptor-1antagonist

Therefore the RAS protease inhibitors and receptor agonists/antagonists (Table 1) developed for treating cardiovascular disorders may have wider application in cancer than initially envisioned, which will be reviewed in this manuscript.

2.   THE RENIN-ANGIOTENSIN SYSYEM IN HUMAN CANCERS

The functions of the renin-angiotensin system (RAS) are well-characterized in vasoconstriction, the regulation of the hydric and electrolyte homeostasis, edema and the thickening of the vascular wall. The RAS also exerts a regulatory role in vascular cell migration, proliferation, death and/or survival functions. In cardiovascular diseases, clinical use of drugs targeting the RAS improves the conditions. These properties of the RAS make it a potential target to control the inappropriate functions of the tumor-associated vasculature which include defective perfusion, edema and high tumor interstitial pressure, and proliferation and recruitment of endothelial and mural cells of the tumor-associated angiogenic vessels. However, the involvement of other molecules, which are presently not completely defined, has also been postulated. The human RAS (Fig. 1) is composed of a precursor protein, angiotensinogen (AGT), from which the proteases renin (EC 3.4.23.15), angiotensin converting enzyme (ACE, EC 3.4.15.1), and several aminopeptidases (aminopeptidase A (APA) and aminopeptidases B/N), carboxypeptidases (prolyl-carboxypeptidase, and endopeptidases sequentally release families of peptides, the angiotensins (Ang) I, II, III, IV and (1-7), with subtle differences in biological functions, and acting on the 7-transmembrane G-protein coupled receptors (GPCR) angiotensin type 1 and type 2 receptors AT_1 et AT_2, and other receptors for the further-processed angiotensins. The RAS functions are endocrine in the blood via AT_1, and paracrine/autocrine in tissues other than the blood via AT_1, AT_2 and/or other Ang peptide receptors. The production and binding of angiotensin peptides locally formed depend on the relative expression of the proteases involved in their metabolism and on the relative expression of their cellular receptors. The RAS is expressed independently of the circulating RAS in non-vascular tissues (Hirasawa *et al* 2002; Humpel *et al* 1994; Inwang *et al* 1997; Juillerat-Jeanneret 1993; Juillerat-Jeanneret *et al* 1992, 2000, 2004; Kakinuma *et al* 1997, 1998; Milsted *et al* 1990; Suganuma *et al* 2004, 2005; Tahmasebi *et al* 1998, 2006).

In cancer, the role of the RAS has been mainly evaluated in the context of angiogenesis, however, some information exists suggesting a more direct role for the RAS in cancer progression. The secretion by tumor cells of factors involved in endothelial cell proliferation and permeability in response to the activation of the RAS, such as vascular endothelial growth factor/vascular permeability factor (VEGF/VPF), or involved in the proliferation and differentiation of perivascular cells and in the subsequent destabilization of the tumor vessels, such as the angiopoietins, transforming growth factor-β (TGF-β, epidermal growth factor (EGF) or platelet-derived growth factor (PDGF), has been suggested (Nadal *et al* 2002; Naito *et al* 1998; Otani *et al* 2000; Uemura *et al* 2003, 2005, 2006; Yamagishi *et al* 2003). The functions of the RAS are paracrine/autocrine in tissues other than the blood via the binding of angiotensin peptides locally formed to the AT_1 and/or AT_2 receptors (de Gasparo *et al* 2000; de Paepe *et al* 2002; Zhuo *et al* 1998), depending on the relative expression of the proteases involved in the metabolism of angiotensins and on the relative expression of their cellular receptors. These tissue functions include the control of cell proliferation and death (Achard *et al* 2001; Greco *et al* 2003; Kucerova *et al* 2003; Marshall *et al* 2000; Miyama *et al* 2002; Rivera *et al* 2001). Inhibitors of renin and ACE, and antagonists of the AT_1 receptor, modifying what can be named the "classical" RAS, have been developed and are in clinical use or under clinical evaluation in the context of cardiovascular disorders. However, a role in cancer of the "non-classical" RAS is emerging, whereas less studied, but possibly promising as target for therapy. The role and functions in cancer of *ACE inhibitors* and *antagonists to AT_1 receptors* of the "classical RAS" have been recently reviewed by many authrors (Molteni *et al* 2006; Deshayes and Nahmias 2005; Uemura *et al* 2006) and are starting to be well established thus only an overview will be provided here, whereas the potential roles and functions in cancer of *renin and its inhibitors*, or of the components of the "*non-classical RAS*" are just emerging. In order to question these issues, we will first compare the expression of the components of the RAS, either "classical" and "non-classical" in human tumors and adjacent tissue, then review what is known about their potential functions in cancer and the models that have been used to evaluate the functions and components of the RAS in cancer.

3.   THE "CLASSICAL" RAS IN CANCER

The concept of a localized tissue RAS has emerged, in addition to the circulating RAS and activation of the RAS has been demonstrated under neoplastic conditions. The local tumor RAS may i) enhance angiogenesis and microvessel density ii) promote tumor cell proliferation iii) participate in the remodeling of the tumor stroma. ACE inhibitors and antagonists to angiotensin receptors may delay tumor growth, in humans and experimental models of carcinomas, sarcomas, gliomas. Ang II is a potent mitogen, and Ang II/AT$_1$ can transactivate other receptors, such as EGFR, and induce the production of bioactive factors such as TGFβ or VEGF, as well as intracellular signaling pathways, such various tyrosine kinases, such as ERK (Molteni *et al* 2006; Deshayes and Nahmias 2005; Uemura *et al* 2006).

The RAS functions in cancer may also be mediated by interfering with the tumor stroma. Ang II is a fibrogenic factor, therefore Ang II effects in cancer may also be mediated by cancer-associated (myo)fibroblasts (Fujita *et al* 2005) or tumor-associated macrophages which express renin (Juillerat-Jeanneret *et al* 2000, 2004), AT$_1$ (Egami *et al* 2003) and ACE (Juillerat-Jeanneret *et al* 1997).

3.1.   Renin and Renin Inhibitors

In the context of the vascular system, renin (EC 3.4.23.15) is an aspartyl protease synthesized as a proenzyme and activated in the juxtaglomerular cells of the kidney, a modified myoepithelial cell of the wall of the afferent arteriole, and secreted into the blood where renin acts on its only known substrate, AGT, of which renin releases Ang I. Transcription of renin gene is regulated both in a tissue-specific and developmental manner. In this context AGT has no other function than being a precursor of Ang II. However, the kinetics characteristics of hydrolysis of AGT by renin are very unfavorable for an enzyme-catalyzed reaction. In the cklassical RAS, no function has been attributed to AGT and Ang I. In addition to the kidney, the renin gene and protein are expressed in other tissues than the kidney, and in particular in some cancers, and a intracellular receptor for renin has been described, suggesting other functions for this enzyme than the release of Ang I. In human cancers, the role of renin has been postulated to be the production of Ang I from AGT. Renin-secreting tumors of several non-renal origins have been described, and the expression of renin has been detected in different human cancers, including from the breast (Tahmasebi *et al* 1998, 2006), brain (Ariza *et al* 1998; Juillerat-Jeanneret *et al* 2004), prostate (Uemura *et al* 2006), pancreas (Leung 2004; Reddy *et al* 1995; Lam and Leung 2002). In breast cancer, ISH showed that the expression of renin mRNA was expressed by a band of myofibroblasts and myoepithelial cells surrounding the ductal epithelial cells expressing AT$_1$ in normal tissue and lobular in situ carcinoma (Inwang *et al* 1997; de Paepe *et al* 2002). In latter stage invasive cancer, this band was disrupted and attenuated. In the breast AGT and renin was expressed in normal, not in tumoral epithelial cells, in tumor associated fibroblasts and normal myoepithelial cells (Tahmasebi *et al*

1998, 2006). However, the effect of renin inhibition has been examined only in glioblastoma in our group (Juillerat-Jeanneret *et al* 2000, 2004) using piperidine renin inhibitors (Maerki *et al* 2004), to the best of my knowledge. In glioblastoma, no evidence for renin secretion by the tumor was found. Renin inhibition directly blocked glioblastoma cell proliferation, independently of extracellular production of angiotensin peptides which did not directly induce human glioblastoma cell proliferation, apoptosis and/or DNA synthesis (Juillerat-Jeanneret *et al* 2004), and evidence was strong for an intracellular effects of the renin inhibitors. Therefore the use of renin inhibitors developed to inhibit the circulating enzyme, and which are only poorly cell-permeable, must probably be reconsidered when addressing cancer (Juillerat-Jeanneret *et al* 2004). The anti-proliferative effects of renin in human glioblastoma cells was dependent on inhibition of serum-induced ERK phosphorylation (Juillerat-Jeanneret 2006). Therefore, a direct role of (intracellular) renin in the proliferation and/or survival of tumor cells may be postulated, not necessarily related to the extracellular production of angiotensin peptides.

3.2.   Angiotensin Converting Enzyme (ACE) and ACE-inhibitors

Angiotensin converting enzyme (ACE, EC 3.4.15.1) is an ectopeptidase expressed in most vascular beds, including cancer vasculature, and in the context of the cardio-vascular system, the role of ACE is to release Ang II from Ang I and to degrade bradykinin. However many peptidases other that renin and ACE have the potential to hydrolyse the various angiotensin peptides, which include exopeptidases and endopeptidases (Campbell *et al* 2003). ACE is a metalloprotease of wide specificity, which has many other bioactive peptide substrates than Ang I, therefore the effects of ACE-inhibitors, including in cancer, developed to treat cardiovascular diseases may be dependent on the inhibition of hydrolysis of substrates other than Ang I. Several controversial studies have been published, linking ACE expression and ACE inhibitors or ACE I/D polymorphism to cancer development and/or progression (Juillerat-Jeanneret *et al* 2000; Abali *et al* 2002; Frame *et al* 1996; Gonzalez-Zuloeta *et al* 2005; Lever *et al* 1998; Nakagawa *et al* 1995; Medeiros *et al* 2004; Small *et al* 1997, 1999; Yoshii *et al* 2002, 2005; Reddy *et al* 1995; Fujita *et al* 2005; Prontera *et al* 1999; Volpert *et al* 1996; Lindholm *et al* 2001; Friis *et al* 2001; Yasumatsu *et al* 2004; Noguchi *et al* 2003; Koh *et al* 2005; Haiman *et al* 2003; Freitas-Silva *et al* 2004; Röken *et al* 2006), and no clear picture can be obtained from these studies.

In breast cancer, ACE was expressed by normal and tumoral epithelial cells (Tahmasebi *et al* 2006). ACE inhibitors seem to have only a minor effect on cancer risk, incidence rate and tumor prevalence, but rather affect tumor progression and metastasis. ACE-inhibitors are not directly antiproliferative for cancer cells (Juillerat-Jeanneret *et al* 2000, 2004; Yasumatsu *et al* 2004), but can modify tumor apoptosis and are able to decrease angiogenesis, either alone (Small *et al* 1997, 1999; Yoshii *et al* 2002, 2005; Fujita *et al* 2005; Prontera *et al* 1999) or associated with interferon (IFN)-β (Noguchi *et al* 2003). ACE is highly expressed in the abnormal vessels of human glioblastoma, however, our own *in vitro* and *in vivo* studies did not convincingly demonstrate a clear advantage to ACE inhibition (lisinopril) in experimental glioblastoma in immunocompetent rats (Juillerat-Jeanneret *et al* 2000, 2004), whereas perindopril in nude mice reduced head and neck carcinoma growth and VEGF-dependent angiogenesis (Yasumatsu *et al* 2004). The thiol ACE-inhibitor captopril, but not the non-thiol ACE-inhibitor lisinopril, was able to inhibit the proliferation of ACE-negative breast carcinoma cells, to reduce their expression of estrogen-receptor, and to increase that of progesterone-receptor (Small *et al* 1997, 1999). ACE inhibitors may slow cancer progression (Lever *et al* 1998; Small *et al* 1997, 1999; Yoshii *et al* 2002; Yasumatsu *et al* 2004; Noguchi *et al* 2003; Hii *et al* 1998), mainly acting via their anti-angiogenic potential via AT_1, since Ang II may induce the release of VEGF expression by cancer cells (Suganuma *et al* 2004) and induce angiogenesis. ACE-inhibitors may also act as more general zinc metalloprotease inhibitors, acting as inhibitors of MMPs (Volpert *et al* 1996; Prontera *et al* 1999; Williams *et al* 2005), or via the release of the anti-angiogenic angiostatin (de Groot-Besseling *et al* 2004) independently of the RAS and of ACE inhibition (Gonzalez-Zuloeta *et al* 2005; Reddy *et al* 1995; Fujita *et al* 2005). Therefore, while the role of ACE inhibitors in cancer is not clear, it is related to tumor-associated angiogenesis and VEGF pathways, and not the survival of tumor cells themselves.

From genetic studies it was concluded that ACE polymorphism was involved in the lymph node metastic progression of gastric cancer (Ebert *et al* 2005; Röcken *et al* 2006), possibly associated with chymase polymorphisms (Sugimoto *et al* 2006). ACE polymorphism was not correlated to lung and renal cancer (Cheon *et al* 2000; Usmani *et al* 2000), but possibly involved in enhancing smoking-cancer association (Arima *et al* 2006). In prostate cancer and leukemia, ACE polymorphism was correlated to cancer progression (Medeiros *et al* 2004; Hajek *et al* 2003). ACE polymorphism may be associated with bladder and breast cancer risk and be an indicator of favourable outcome (Haiman *et al* 2003; Koh *et al* 2005; Kosugi *et al* 2006; Yaren *et al* 2006; Gonzalez-Zuloeta *et al* 2005), which may be dependent on the presence of anti-oxidants (Koh *et al* 2005; Yuan *et al* 2005).

3.3.   Angiotensin II (Ang II) and Angiotensin Receptors (AT_1 and AT_2)

In the classical RAS, all the functions of the RAS are considered mediated by Ang II and a G-protein-coupled receptor (GPCR), the Ang II type 1-receptor (AT_1) (de Gasparo *et al* 2000), with presently little known function for the AT_2 receptor (Nouet *et al* 2004) other than to antagonize AT_1-mediated effects, thus functioning as an AT_1 counter-receptor. Both AT_1 and AT_2 receptors are GPCR proteins of about 360 amino acids, sharing only 30% homology. Tissue-specific functions of AT_1 and/or AT_2 other than the regulation of the vascular tone include the regulation of cell growth and apoptosis, of production of reactive oxygen species, of hormone secretion and of inflammatory and fibrogenic reactions (Leung and Chappel 2003), all of each are mediated by Ang II and may be relevant for cancer. Ang II is a potent cell mitogen and migration-inducing factor, mediated either via autocrine or paracrine pathways. In cancer, AT_1 may exert growth stimulatory effects and AT_1 antagonists decrease tumor growth by inhibiting VEGF (Suganuma et al 2004). AT_1 antagonists have beneficial effects on tumor progression, vascularization and metastasis. AT_1 antagonism reduced the growth, progression and vascularization of several experimental cancers of different types (Fujita et al 2005; Egami et al 2003; Suganuma et al 2004; Uemura et al 2003, 2005, 2006; Miyama et al 2002; Arrieta et al), possibly mediated by AT_1 expressed on tumor vasculature (Fujita et al 2005; Miyama et al 2002). Long-term blockade of AT_1 leaves the AT_2 fully active. In the context of the vascular system and angiogenesis (Fujiyama et al 2001; Silvestre et al 2002), AT_2 antagonizes AT_1 effects, thus potentially having beneficial anti-cancer effects. However, AT_2 may also increase VEGF production (Walther et al 2003; Rizkalla et al 2003; Zhang et al 2004). Therefore the role of AT_2 and its antagonism in cancer is far from clear.

The expression, role and the AT_1- and AT_2-mediated signaling pathways in human cancers and cancer cells, including astrocytoma (Ariza et al 1988; Juillerat-Jeanneret et al 2004; Fogarty et al 2002), breast (de Paepe et al 2002; Muscella et al 2002; Greco et al 2003), ovarian (Suganuma et al 2004), skin (Takeda and Kondo 2001), cervix (Kikkawa et al 2004), prostate (Dinh et al 2001, 2002; Nassis et al 2001), pancreatic (Fujimoto et al 2001), gastric (Freitas-Silva et al 2004) has been recently reviewd (Deshayes and Nahmias 2005). Generally AT_1 expression was inhomogeneous but increased in cancers compared to non-tumoral tissue depending on the type and grade, and was correlated with tumor invasiveness.

AT_1 pro-angiogenic and growth-promoting vascular functions in cancer are mediated by Ang II. Consequently, AT_1 antagonists inhibit tumor growth, mediated by the blockade of Ang II-dependent tumor cells production of the pro-angiogenic peptide VEGF (Rivera et al 2001). AT_1 is expressed on tumor stromal smooth muscle cells and Ang II stimulates the migration of pericytes via TGF-β and PDGF receptors (Nadal et al 2002) and the expression of VEGF receptor by these cells (Otani et al 2000; Yamagishi et al 2003). Ang II can also stimulate the migration of stromal cells, including pericytes via TGF-β and PDGF receptors (Nadal et al 2002) and the expression of VEGF receptor by these cells (Otani et al 2000; Yamagishi et al 2003; Fujita et al 2005). Therefore, Ang II/AT_1 seems mainly involved in promoting angiogenesis and perivascular cell growth (Rivera et al, 2001; Miyama et al 2002) while AT_2 receptors may be growth inhibitory and pro-apoptotic (Berry et al 2000, 2001; Miura et al 2005), possibly involving Pax-2 (Zhang et al 2004). The proliferative effects of Ang II on tumor-associated human fibroblasts (Marshall et al 2000) involve AT_1 receptors.

AT_1 is expressed in *breast* cancer where it may exert growth stimulatory effects and regulate NO synthesis (Inwang et al 1997; de Paepe et al 2002; Greco et al 2003). Ang II increased the mitogenic signaling in human breast carcinoma cells, via the Ca^{2+}, PKC, EGF receptor and ERK pathways (de Paepe et al 2002; Greco et al 2003) and integrin β1 expression (Berry et al 2001, 2000). In breast cancer, ductal epithelial cells express AT_1 in normal tissue and in lobular *in situ* carcinoma

(Inwang *et al* 1997; de Paepe *et al* 2002). In latter stage invasive cancer, AT_1 and AT_2 mRNAs were detected (Tahmasebi *et al* 2006). Ang II/AT_1 reduces breast cancer cells adhesion and invasion, by reducing integrin $\alpha3$ and $\beta1$ expression via PKC signaling (Puddefoot *et al* 2006). In estrogen receptor-negative breast cancer cells, ER-independent oestrogen signaling may be mediated by AT_1, at least in part, to activate survival mechanisms (Lim *et al* 2006). In *pancreatic* cancer, the role of the Ang II/AT_1 has also been demonstrated in cancer cells growth and cancer progression (Hang *et al* 2004) mediated by the activation of the MAPK and NFkB pathways (Amaya *et al* 2004). In *colon* mucosa and cancer AT_1 is expressed and may exert growth stimulatory effects and regulate NO synthesis (Inwang *et al* 1997; de Paepe *et al* 2002; Hirasawa *et al* 2002; Kucerova *et al* 2003). In *prostate* cancer (Uemura *et al* 2005, 2006; Dinh *et al* 2001, 2002; Nassis *et al* 2001; Fabiani *et al* 2001), the RAS is over expressed, cancer cells secrete Ang II, Ang II is mitogenic and AT_1 antagonists inhibit the growth of prostate cancer cells and tumors, possibly mediated by cross-talk with the stroma. In *ovarian* cancers, Ang II stimulates *in vitro* tumor cell proliferation, invasion, VEGF secretion (Kikkawa *et al* 2004; Suganuma *et al* 2004, 2005; Watanabe *et al* 2005; Ino *et al* 2006) and these effects were inhibited by AT_1 antagonists (Suganuma *et al* 2005). In human ovarian cancer patients, AT_1 expression was restricted to tumor cells, membrane and cytoplasm, but not stromal or non-tumoral epithelial cells, correlated with a poor patient outcome and to VEGF expression and microvessel density, but not with tumor grade and stage or tumor proliferation index (Ino *et al* 2006). In human *glioblastoma*, we have shown the selective expression of AT_1 and AT_2 in human glioblastoma (Juillerat-Jeanneret *et al* 2004), however AT_1 blockade had no effect on glioblastoma cell growth, while AT_2 blockade decreased growth. Ang peptides did not play any direct role in glioblastoma cell growth, apoptosis and/or DNA synthesis (Juillerat-Jeanneret *et al* 2003). In a C6-cells glioblastoma rat model, losartan, an AT_1 antagonist, reduced tumor growth, vascular density, cell proliferation and mitotic index (Rivera *et al* 2001).

Therefore, AT_1 favors cancer development by increasing tumor angiogenesis, while the function of AT_2 in is not known with certainty. AT_2 receptor is mainly expressed in development and repair, and in cancer it may be important in cell proliferation and angiogenesis. AT_2 blockade may inhibit tumor growth (Uemura *et al* 2006). In tumor angiogenesis, AT_1 induces the VEGF and angiopoietin/Tie-2 receptor tyrosine kinases (Otani *et al* 2000; Imanishi *et al* 2004; Fujiyama *et al* 2001). AT_2 deficiency in mice attenuates susceptibility to lung cancer, possibly meidiated by lung stromal fibroblasts and TGFβ (Kanehira *et al* 2005). AT_1 can transactivate and AT_2 trans-inactivate (Uemura *et al* 2003; Greco *et al* 2003; Elbaz *et al* 2000) the EGF receptor in prostate and breast cancer cells activating the ERK, STAT3, PKC or SHP-1 pathways. AT_2 activates unconventional signaling pathways not involving classical GPCR-mediated pathways. AT_2 can activate cellular protein tyrosine and serine/threonine phosphatases (Stoll *et al* 2001; Lehtonen *et al* 2004; Moore *et al* 2004), blocking AT_1-mediated ERK activation. AT_2 trans-inactivates EGF-, FGF- and IGF-receptors (Stoll *et al* 2001). Feedback activation of AT_2 by

AT_1 blockade is anti-fibrotic (Okada *et al* 2004). However, off-target effects may exist. AT_2 antagonists may also recognize non-Ang II binding sites different form AT_2/Ang II sites, mainly on activated cells of the macrophage lineage (Egidy *et al* 1997). In addition, inhibition of Ang II effects potentiates the effects of anti-tumoral molecules (Yasumaru *et al* 2003).

In conclusion several studies have shown a direct effect of the RAS on tumor cells, but the effects of the components of the RAS may also be indirect, mediated by the tumor stroma: pro-angiogenic effect on vascular cells, profibrotic effects on tumor-associated (myo)fibroblasts and presently poorly defined on tumor-associated macrophages.

In summary, the RAS may exert its effects in cancer at two levels:
1) by directly controlling tumor cell proliferation, resistance to cell death and/or survival. These effects seem to involve the enzyme renin and the AT_2 receptor. However the cellular signaling pathways and mechanisms involved are not known.
2) by controlling the proliferation and functions of the tumor-associated vascular system. These effects seem mediated by Ang II and AT_1 receptor, and to involve the interactions between endothelial cells and pericytes, mediated by TGF-β, VEGF and PDGF, and their associated receptors. However, the mechanisms involved are not yet clearly established.

Therefore it can be expected that within the next years the interest of the RAS in cancer may be shifted toward the cancer stroma. Published information demonstrates that the RAS is involved in the survival of normal and tumor cells, as a regulator of the functions of tumor vasculature and stroma. Ang II binding to AT_1 receptors on tumor cells will result in the production of angiogenic factors, which will induce the proliferation/death, migration of vascular cells, vascular permeability defects and increased intratumoral hydrostatic pressure which are associated with human tumors. These defects in the differentiation of tumor-associated vascular cells result in a poor intratumoral distribution of anti-cancer drugs and are associated with resistance to treatment.

ACE inhibitors and AT_1 antagonists, blocking Ang II production and action, have beneficial effects on cancer at the steps of tumor progression, vascularization and metastasis. AT_1 is over-expressed by tumor and stromal (endothelial cells, fibroblasts and macrophages) cells. A direct role for renin and AT_2 is less clear in the context of cancer.

4.   THE "NON-CLASSICAL" RAS IN CANCER

The human "non-classical RAS" is composed of a precursor protein, angiotensinogen (AGT), expressed in human cancer (Juillerat-Jeanneret *et al* 2004; Milsted *et al* 1990) and having functions other than being a precursor of Ang II, from which several aminopeptidases (aminopeptidase A (APA, EC 3.4.11.7) (Fournié-Zaluski *et al* 2004; Juillerat-Jeanneret *et al* 2000, 2003, 2004) and aminopeptidases B/N (Juillerat-Jeanneret *et al* 2003, 2004), and carboxypeptidase (prolyl-carboxypeptidase (EC 3.4.21.26) (Santos *et al* 2000) and ACE2 sequentally release families of peptides, the angiotensins (Ang) III, IV (von Bohlen and Halbach 2003) and (1-7) (Santos *et al* 2000), with subtle differences in biological functions, and acting on the 7-transmembrane G-protein coupled receptors (GPCR) AT_1 et AT_2 and on other receptors.

4.1.   Angiotensinogen (AGT)

AGT belongs to the superfamily of the non-inhibitory serpins (serine protease inhibitors), which have the potential to decrease angiogenesis in several cancer models. In human cancer AGT inhibits VEGF-induced or FGF-induced angiogenesis (Célérier *et al* 2002). In glioblastoma AGT is involved in the maintenance of the normal functions of the cerebral vasculature (Kakinuma *et al* 1998) and in AGT-ko mice some angiotensin peptides have the potential to restore these functions (Kakinuma *et al* 1998). We have demonstrated that human glioblastoma cell lines express AGT mRNA, that AGT is released by tumor cells in vivo in humans, but AGT did not modify glioblastoma cell proliferation (Juillerat-Jeanneret *et al* 2004). Thus AGT is expressed and secreted by glioblastoma and is involved in vascular functions of brain tumors.

4.2.   (Pro)Renin and (Pro)Renin-Receptors

In humans, most of the renin exitst in its enzymatically inactive form, prorenin. Many tissues can synthesize prorenin, but the juxtaglomerular cells are the exclusive site for processing of prorenin to active renin. Thus intracellular functions of (pro)rennin can be postulated. We have shown that the mRNAs for renin and renin-receptor are co-expressed in human glioblastoma and glioblastoma cells (Juillerat-Jeanneret *et al* 2004), as well as other cancers (Juillerat-Jeanneret et al, unpublished results), and that renin inhibitors (Table 2) with the potential to enter cells and inhibit human glioblastoma cell growth (Juillerat-Jeanneret *et al* 2004), can inhibit serum-induced ERK phosphorylation (Juillerat-Jeanneret 2006).

   The mannose-6-phosphate may be a receptor for cellular uptake of (pro)rennin (van Kesteren *et al* 1997). Another cellular receptor for (pro)renin has been described (Nguyen *et al* 2002), identical to CAPER (Schefe *et al* 2006) and whose C-terminal is similar to V-ATPase. Prorenin/renin binding to this receptor in cells is linked to intracellular signaling pathways, such as extracellular-regulated kinase (ERK) phosphorylation, or TGF-β secretion and these effects may be angiotensin-independent (Huang *et al* 2006). The primary location of the (pro)renin receptors is perinuclear in human cells which allow direct interaction with a transcription factor and gene regulation (Schefe *et al* 2006).

   Therefore an intracellular renin-angiotensin system may be responsible for the pathological role of the RAS. However, no information has been published formally establishing a role for renin-receptors in cancer.

Table 2. Chemical structures of the renin inhibitors evaluated in human glioblastoma cells

RO0663525

pepstatin

remikiren

4.3.   Aminopeptidases A (APA), Ang III and Ang III AT₃ Receptor(s)

Aminopeptidases A (APA, Glu-aminopeptidase EC 3.4.11.7, and Asp-aminopeptidase EC 3.4.11.21) release Ang III (des-Asp1-Ang II) from Ang I/II, with subtle differences in biological functions compared to Ang II, but still able to bind on the 7-transmembrane G-protein coupled receptors (GPCR) AT_1 and AT_2. In cancer, APA can control angiogenesis and tumor growth in mice (Marchio *et al* 2004; Suganuma *et al* 2004, 2005). In human glioblastoma, we have shown that APA activity is upregulated in the abnormal tumor vasculature and that Ang III is the main angiotensin peptide produced in these tumors, depending on the secretion by tumor cells of not yet identified soluble factors which are not dependent on tumor cell hypoxia (Juillerat-Jeanneret *et al* 2003). APA increase in activated brain-derived endothelial cells is inhibited by glucocorticoid or TGF-β exposure (Juillerat-Jeanneret *et al* 2000) with a concomitant induction of ACE

(Juillerat-Jeanneret *et al* 2000). Thus, glioblastoma-derived factors increase APA expression in glioblastoma vascular cells, and TGF-β decreases this expression. We have shown that APA is not involved in the proliferation of brain-derived endothelial cells and have postulated that it is related to increased vascular permeability and tumor edema (Juillerat-Jeanneret *et al* 2000). A central role for Ang III for permeability defects of tumor vasculature is in accordance with the obseravtion that in AGT-ko mice, blood-brain barrier (BBB) function is lost and can be restored by Ang II or Ang IV, but not Ang III (Kakinuma *et al* 1997, 1998). Increased APA expression was also shown in cervical (Suganuma *et al* 2004; Fujimura *et al* 2000), prostate (Bogenrieder *et al* 1997) and kidney (Nanus *et al* 1998) cancers and in the blood of experimental breast cancer in rat (Carrera *et al* 2006). In endometrial and uterine cancers it has been involved in tumor growth, angiogenesis and VEGF production (Ino *et al* 2004). The effect of APA inhibitors has been evaluated only for kinase regulation in thyroid cancer (Ochedalska *et al* 2002), and APA inhibitors antagonize Ang II effects in prostate cancer cells (Lawnicka *et al* 2004).

Ang III may act on AT_1 and AT_2, with slightly different affinity than Ang II, mimicking some of the functions of Ang II, but also displaying Ang III-selective functions, such as chemokine production and cell-growth regulation (Ruiz-Ortega et al 2000) or may act on a poorly-defined AT_3 receptor (Chaki and Inagami 1992). The role of the AT_3 receptor of Ang III is not known. Therefore in cancer, APA is most probably related to dysfunctions of cancer-associated vasculature, resulting from defects of the TGFβ pathways.

4.4.   Aminopeptides B, Ang IV (Ang3-8) and AT_4 Receptor(s); ACE2, Ang(1-7) and Ang(1-7) Receptor(s)

Several peptidases, including aminopeptidases B/N (EC 3.4.11.6)/EC 3.4.11.14) activities, prolyl-carboxypeptidase (EC 3.4.21.26) and ACE2 (Warner *et al* 2004) further process angiotensin peptides to Ang IV (von Bohlen und Halbach 2003) or Ang (1-7) (Gallagher and Tallant 2000; Santos *et al* 2004), respectively. Vascular surface markers in brain cancers include aminopeptidases and we and others have shown that these enzymes are increased in neoplasms of the central nervous system, i.e. aminopeptidase A (Juillerat-Jeanneret *et al* 2000, 2003) and insulin-regulated aminopeptidase (IRAP) (Fernando *et al* 2005). IRAP and aminopeptidase B activities are increased in the serum of rats with experimental breast cancer (Carrera *et al* 2006). However, the expression and/or activity of these aminopeptidases has been evaluated only in few studies in a limited number of cancers.

Ang IV or Ang (1-7) peptides are no longer able to use the cognate AT_1 and AT_2 receptors, but other specific receptors. Ang IV acts on the AT_4 receptor, which has been identified as the transmembrane aminopeptidase, insulin-regulated membrane aminopeptidase IRAP. IRAP is associated with the GLUT4 vesicular glucose transporter (Chai *et al* 2004), which may be of interest in cancer. The expression of the AT_4 receptor has been demonstrated in the glandular epithelium of normal prostate and was decreased in cancer, similar to AT_2 (Dinh *et al* 2001). A high affinity binding site for Ang(1-7) has been reported (Tallant *et al* 1997; Tom *et al* 2003), which may be anti-proliferative, anti-apoptotic, NO-generating. Ang(1-7) has been involved in inhibiting lung cancer cell proliferation (Gallagher and Tallant 2004) but inducing cell proliferation in astrocytoma (Fogarty *et al* 2002). APA and IRAP bind the peptide Ang IV (Albiston *et al* 2001, 2003; Chai *et al* 2004; Demaeght *et al* 2006) which then acts as an inhibitor of their enzymatic activities (Goto *et al* 2006; Lew *et al* 2003; Lee *et al* 2003). Therefore ligands for such aminopeptidases may have a potential interest in cancer therapy. We have shown decreased Aminopeptidase B/Aminopeptidase N activities in brain tumor vasculature in human glioblastoma (Juillerat-Jeanneret *et al* 2000), suggesting blockade of further processing of Ang III to Ang IV in these tumors. Therefore these enzymes and peptides may be potentially important in cancer, however their functions are not presently clearly established in tumor progression and the development of selective inhibitors or receptor antagonists is just starting.

In summary, published information demonstrates that the "non-classical RAS" is involved in cancer by mechanisms not necessarily involving the binding of angiotensin peptides to their $AT_{1/2}$ receptors. The "non-classical RAS" is a regulator of angiogenesis mediated by AGT and of the functions of tumor vasculature mediated by the overproduction of Ang III, resulting in vascular permeability defects. Interestingly, the end-peptide of the cascade, Ang IV, may be important in regulating these defects, being able to regulate its own production. These effects are either causative, or more probably reactive, responses to secretion of tumor-derived factors. The functions of the (pro)renin-receptor in cancer have not yet been investigated, however from the presently existing information it can be inferred that it will be involved in the regulation of the functions of cancer cells.

5.   DISCUSSION

In the last years, the selective expression of the components of the RAS in human cancers has been demonstrated, and some information has suggested that specific components, and the associated inhibitors, agonists and antagonists, of this system, i.e renin, angiotensinogen, ACE, Ang II, AT_1 and AT_2, aminopeptidases A/B/N may be important for cancer progression and for the development of disorders of cancer-associated vasculature. The expression of selected RAS components is either induced or decreased in cancer, according to a cell-specific and cancer-specific pattern. RAS components have been associated with tumor vasculature defects supporting a favoring role for the RAS in human cancer progression. The components of the "classical RAS", in particular the axis ACE-Ang II-AT_1 have been involved in favoring tumor-associated angiogenesis (Fig. 3). Therefore ACE inhibitors associated with AT_1 antagonists may likely prove useful in cancer treatment in combination with other chemotherapeutics.

The treatment of human cancers is limited by the systemic toxicity of chemostatic or chemotoxic anti-cancer agents and by the existence of drug resistance mechanisms. The use in this context of molecules which have shown efficiency

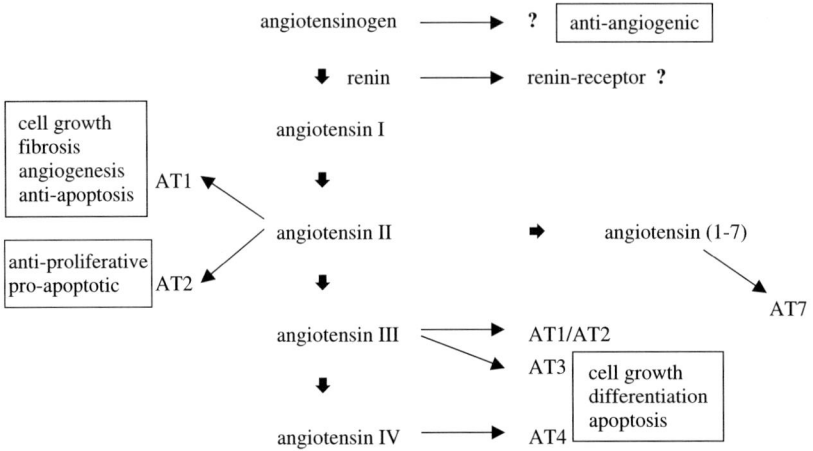

Figure 3. The potential functions of the receptors of the RAS in cancer

in cancer-unrelated human disorders, and which have also shown an unexpected efficiency in cancer cells and cancer-associated stromal cells, may be a way to improve cancer treatment and overcome resistance mechanisms. The therapeutic agents developed in the context of cardiovascular disorders and which target the renin-angiotensin system (RAS) have shown such a potential and deserve evaluation in the field of cancer. This approach offers the advantages of getting immediate access to drugs already tested in humans, without long chemical and biological development. However, before designing means to treat cancer by targeting the RAS, it is necessary to better define the characteristics of the cell populations expressing it and with the potential to respond to RAS inhibitors and antagonists, and to understand the exact molecules of the RAS and the biological mechanisms behind these effects. In particular the intracellular expression of these enzymes and receptors and the intracellular distribution which may be necessary to achieve for their associated inhibitors and antagonists, is important to consider.

The published information also suggests the involvement of other molecules of the RAS, which are presently not defined, but may be represented by components of the "non-classical RAS". However, only partial information presently exists and it will be necessary to investigate in more details these possibilities.

REFERENCES

Abali H, Gullu IH, Engin H, Haznedaroglu IC, Erman M, Tekuzman G, 2002, Old antihypertensives as novel antineoplastics: angiotensin I-converting enzyme inhibitors and angiotensin II type 1 receptor antagonists. *Med Hyp*. **59**: 344–348.

Achard JM, Fournier A, Mazouz H, Caride VJ, Penar PL, Fernandez LA, 2001, Protection against ischemia: a physiological function of the renin-angiotensin system. *Biochem Pharm*. **62**: 261–271.

Albiston AL, Mustafa T, McDowall SG, Mendelsohn FA, Lee J, Chai SY, 2003, AT4 receptor is insulin-regulated membrane aminopeptidase: potential mechanisms of memory enhancement. *Trends Endocrin Metab.* **14**: 72–77.

Albiston AL, McDowall SG, Matsacos D, Sim P, Clune E, Mustafa T, Lee J, Mendelsohn FA, Simpson RJ, Connolly LM, Chai SY, 2001, Evidence that the angiotensin IV (AT(4)) receptor is the enzyme insulin-regulated aminopeptidase. *J Biol Chem.* **276**: 48623–48626.

Amaya K, Ohta T, Kitagawa H, Kayahara M, Takamura H, Fujimura T, Nishimura GI, Shimizu K, Miwa K, 2004, Angiotensin II activates MAP kinase and NF-κB through angiotensin II type 1 receptor in human pancreatic cancer cells. *Int J Oncol.* **25**: 849–856.

Arrieta O, Guevara P, Escobar E, Garcia.Navarette R, Pineda B, Sotelo J, 2005, Blockage of angiotensin II type 1 receptor decreases the synthesis of growth factors and induces apoptosis in C6 cultured cells and C6 rat glioma. *Br J Cancer.* **92**: 1247–1252.

Arima H, Kiyohara Y, Tanizaki Y, Nakabeppu Y, Kubo M, Kato I, Suishi K, Tsuneyoshi M, Fujishima M, Ida M, 2006, Angiotensin-I-converting enzyme gene polymorphism modifies the smoking-cancer association: the Hisayama Study. *Eur J Cancer Prev.* **15**: 196–201.

Ariza A, Fernandez LA, Inagami T, Kim JH, Manuelidis EE, 1988, Renin in glioblastoma multiform and its role in neovascularization. *Am J Clin Pathol.* **90**: 437–441.

Berry MG, Goode AW, Puddefoot JR, Vinson GP, Carpenter R, 2000, Integrin beta1 upregulation in MCF-7 breast cancer cells by angiotensin II. *Eur J Surg Oncol.* **26**: 25–29.

Berry C, Touyz R, Dominiczak AF, Webb RC, Johns DG, 2001, Angiotensin receptors: signaling, vascular pathophysiology, and interactions with ceramide. *Am J Physiol.* **281**: H2337–H2365.

Bogenrieder T, Finstad CL, Freeman RH, Papandreou CN, Scher HI, Albino AP, Reuter VE, Nanus DM, 1997, Expression and localization of aminopeptidase A, aminopeptidase N, and dipeptidyl peptidase IV in benign and malignant human prostate tissue. Prostate. **33** : 225–232.

Campbell DJ, 2003, The renin-angiotensin and the kallikrein-kinin systems. *Int J Biochem Cell Biol.* **35**: 784–791.

Carrera MP, Ramirez-Exposito MJ, Duenas B, Dolores Mayas M, Jesus Garcia M, de la Chica S, Cortes P, Ruiz-Sanjuan M, Martinez-Martos JM, 2006, Insulin-regulated aminopeptidase/placental leucil Aminopeptidase (IRAP/P-lAP) and angiotensin IV-forming activities are modified in serum of rats with breast cancer induced by N-methyl-nitrosourea. *Anticancer Res.* **26**: 1011–1014.

Célérier J, Cruz A, Lamandé N, Gasc JM, Corvol P, 2002, Angiotensinogen and its cleaved derivatives inhibit angiogenesis. *Hypertension* **39**: 224–228.

Chai SY, Fernando R, Peck G, Ye SY, Mendelsohn FA, Jenkins TA, Albiston AL, 2004, The angiotensin IV/AT4 receptor. *Cell Mol Life Sci.* **61**: 2728–2737.

Chaki S, Inagami T, 1992, A newly found angiotensin II receptor subtype mediates cyclic-GMP formation in differentiated Neuro-2A cells. *Eur J Pharmol.* **225**: 355–356.

Cheon KT, Choi KH, Lee HB, Park SK, Rhee YK, Lee YC, 2000, Gene polymorphisms of endothelial nitric oxide synthase and angiotensin-converting enzyme in patients with lung cancer. *Lung.* **178**: 351–360.

De Gasparo M, Catt KJ, Inagami T, Wright JW, Unger T, 2000, International union of pharmacology. XXIII. The angiotensin II receptors. *Pharm Rev.* **52**: 415–472.

De Groot-Besseling RR, Ruers TJ, van Kraats AA, Poelen GJ, Ruiter DJ, de Waal RM, Westphal JR, 2004, Anti-tumor activity of a combination of plasminogen activator and captopril in a human melanoma xenograft. *Int J Cancer.* **112**: 329–334.

Demaegdt H, Lenaerts PJ, Swales J, De Backer JP, Laeremans H, Le MT, Kersemans K, Vogel LK, Michotte Y, Vanderheyden P, 2006, Vauquelin G. Angiotensin AT(4) receptor ligand interaction with cystinyl aminopeptidase and aminopeptidase N: [(125)I]Angiotensin IV only binds to the cystinyl aminopeptidase apo-enzyme. *Eur J Pharm.* **546**: 19–27.

De Paepe B, Verstraeten VLMR, De Potter CR, Vakaet LA, Bullock GR7, 2001, Growth-stimulatory angiotensin II type 1 receptor is upregulated in breast hyperplasis and *in situ* carcinoma but not in invasive carcinoma. *Histochem Cell Biol.* **116**: 247–254.

De Paepe B, Verstraeten VLMR, De Potter CR, Bullock GR, 2002, Increased angiotensin II type-1 receptor density in hyperplasi, DCIS and invasive carcinoma of the breast is paralleled with increased NO expression. *Histochem Cell Biol.* **117**: 13–19.

Deshayes F, Nahmias C, 2005, Angiotensin receptors: a new role in cancer ?. *Trends Endocrinol Metab.* **16**: 293–299.

Dinh DT, Frauman AG, Sourial M, Casley DJ, Johnston CI, Fabiani ME, 2001, Identification, distribution and expression of angiotensin II receptors in the normal human pprostate and benign prostatic hyperplasia. *Endocrinology.* **142**: 1349–1356.

Dinh DT, Frauman AG, Somers GR, Ohishi M, Zhou J, Casley DJ, Johnston CI, Fabiani ME, 2002, Evidence for activation of the rennin-angiotensin system in the human prostate: increased angiotensin II and reduced AT(1) receptor expression in benign prostatic hyperplasis. *J Pathol.* **196**: 213–219.

Ebert MPA, Landeckel U, Westphal S, Dierkes J, Glas J, Folwaczny C, Roessner A, Stolte M, Malfertheiner P, Röcken C, 2005, The nagiotensin I-converting enzyme gene insertion/deletion polymorphism is linked to early gastric cancer. *Cancer Epidemiol Biomarkers Prev.* **14**: 2987–28989.

Egami K, Murohara T, Shimada T, Sasaki K, Shintani S, Sugaya T, Ishii M, Akagi T, Ikeda H, Matsuishi T, Imaizumi T, 2003, Role of host angiotensin II type 1 receptor in tumor angiogenesis and growth. *J Clin Invest.* **112**: 67–75.

Egidy G, Friedman J, Viswanathan M, Wahl LM, Saavedra JM, 1997, CGP-42112 partially activates human monocytes and reduces their stimulation by lipopolysaccharides. Am J Physiol. **273**: C826–C833.

Elbaz N, Bedecs K, Masson M, Sutren M, Strosberg AD, Nahmias C, 2000, Functional trans-activation of insulin receptor kinase by growth-inhibitory angiotensin II AT$_2$ receptor. *Mol Endocrinol.* **14**: 795–804.

Fabiani ME, Hawkes DJ, Frauman AG, Tikellis C, Johnston CI, Wilkinson-Berka JL, 2003, Regulation of angiotensin II receptors in the prostate of the transgenic (mren-2)27 rats: effects of angiotensin-converting enzyme inhibition. *Int J Biochem Cell Biol.* **35**: 973–983.

Fernando RN, Larm J, Albiston AL, Chai SY, 2005, Distribution and cellular localization of insulin-regulated aminopeptidase in the rat central nervous system. *J Comp Neurol.* **487**: 372-390.

Fogarty DJ, Sanchez-Gomez MV, Matute C, 2002, Multiple angiotensin receptor subtypes in normal and tumor astrocytes in *vitro*. *Glia.* **39**: 304–313.

Fournie-Zaluski MC, Fassot C, Valentin B, Djordjijevic D, Reaux-Le Goazigo A, Corvol P, Roques BP, Llorens-Cortes C, 2004, Brain renin-angiotensin system blockade by systemically active aminopeptidase A inhibitors: a potential treatment of salt-dependent hypertension. Proc Nat Acad Sci USA *101*: 7775–7780.

Frame KL, Patton K, Reed MJ, Ghilchik MW, Parish DC, 1996, Angiotensin converting enzyme and enkephalinase in human breast cyst fluid. *Br J Cancer.* **74**: 807–813.

Freitas-Silva M, Pereira D, Coelho C, Bicho M, Lopes C, Medeiros R, 2004, Angiotensin I-converting enzyme gene insertion/deletion polymorphism and endometrial human cancer in normotensive and hypertensive women. *Cancer Genet Cytogenet.* **155**: 42–46.

Friis S, Sorensen HT, Mellemkjaer L, McLaughlin JK, Nielsen GL, Blot WJ, Olsen JH, 2001, Angiotensin-converting enzyme inhibitors and the risk of cancer: a population-based cohort study in Denmark. *Cancer.* **92**: 2462–2470.

Fujimura H, Ino K, Nagasaka T, Nakashima N, Nakazato H, Kikkawa F, Mizutani S, 2000, Aminopeptidase A expression in cervical neoplasia and its relationship to neoplastic transformation and progression. *Oncology.* **58**: 342–352.

Fujita M, ayashi I, Yamashina S, Fukamizu A, Itoman M, Majima M, 2005, Angiotensin type 1a receptor signaling-dependent induction of vascular endothelial graowth factor in stroma is relevant to tumor-associated angiogenesis and tumor growth. Carcinogenesis. **26**: 271–279.

Fujiyama S, Matsubara H, Nozawa Y, Maruyama K, Mori Y, Tsutsumi Y, Masaki H, Uchiyama Y, Koyama Y, Nose A, Iba O, Tateishi E, Ogata N, Jyo N, Higashiyama S, Iwasaka T, 2001, Angiotensin AT(1) and AT(2) receptors differentially regulate angiopoietin-2 and vascular endothelial growth factor expression and angiogenesis by modulating heparin binding-epidermal growth factor (EGF)-mediated EGF receptor transactivation. *Circ Res.* **88**: 22–29.

Fijimoto Y, Sasaki T, Tsuchida A, Chayama K, 2001, Angiotensin II type 1 receptor expression in human pancreatic cancer and growth inhibition by angiotensin II type 1 receptor antagonist. *FEBS Lett.* **495**: 197–200.

Gallagher PE, Tallant EA, 2004, Inhibition of human lung cancer cell growth by angiotensin-(1-7). *Carcinogenesis*. **25**: 2045–2052.

Gonzalez-Zuloeta Ladd AM, Vasquez AA, Sayed-Tabatabarei FA, Coebergh JW, Hofman A, Niajou O, Stricker B, van Duijn C, 2005, Angiotensin-converting enzyme gene insertion/deletion polymorphism and breast cancer risk. *Cancer Epidemiol Biomarkers Prevent*. **14**: 2143–2146.

Goto Y, Hattori A, Ishii Y, Mizutani S, Tsujimoto M, 2006, Enzymatic properties of human aminopeptidase A. Regulation of its enzymatic activity by calcium and angiotensin IV. *J Biol Chem*. **281**: 3503–3513.

Greco S, Muscella A, Elisalvatore P, Storelli C, Mazzotta A, Manca C, Marsigliante S, 2003, Angiotensin II activates extracellular signal regulated kinases via protein kinase C and epidermal growth factor receptor in breast cancer cells. *J Cell Physiol*. **196**: 370–377.

Haiman C,Henderson SO, Bretsky P, Kolonel LN, Henderson BE, 2003, Genetic variation in angiotensin I-converting enzyme (ACE) and breast cancer risk: the multiethnic cohort. *Cancer Res*. **63**: 6984–6987.

Hajek D, Tomiska M, Krahulcova E, Druckmuller M, Florianova M, Izakovicova-Holla L, Vacha J, 2003, I/D ACE gene polymorphism in survival of leukemia patients – hypothesis and pilot study. *Medical Hypotheses*. **61**: 80–85.

Hang H, Li SZ, Xu GM, Tu ZX, Gong YF, 2004, Angiotensin II type 1 receptor mRNA and its protein expression in human pancreatic cancer cell lines. *Chinese J Dig Dis*. **5**: 68–71.

Hii SI, Nicol DL, Gotley DC, Thompson LC, Green MK, Jonsson JR, 1998, Captopril inhibits tumour growth in a xenograft model of human renal cell carcinoma. *Br J Cancer*. **77**: 880–883.

Hirasawa K, Sato Y, Hosoda Y, Yamamoto T, Hanai H, 2002, Immunohistological localization of angiotensin II receptor and local renin-angiotensin system in human colonic mucosa. *J Histochem Cytochem*. **50**: 275–282.

Huang Y, Wongamorntham S, Kasting J, McQuillan D, Owens RT, Yu L, Noble NA, Border W, 2006, Renin increases mesangial cell transforming growth factor b1 and matrix proteins through receptor-mediated, angiotnsin II-independent mechanisms. *Kidney Int*. **69**: 105–113.

Humpel C, Lippoldt A, Strömberg I, Bygdeman M, Wagner J, Hilgenfeldt U, Ganten D, Fuxe K, Olson L, 1994, Human angiotensinogen is highly expressed in human cortical grafts. *Glia*. **10**: 186–192.

Imanishi T, Hano T, Nishio I, 2004, Angiotensin II potentiates vascular endothelial growth factor-induced proliferation and network formation of endothelial progenitor cells. *Hypertens Res*. **27**: 101–108.

Ino K, Shibata K, Kajiyama H, Yamamoto E, Nagasaka T, Nawa A, Nomura S, Kikkawa F, 2006, Angiotensin II type 1 receptor expression in ovarian cancer and its correlation with tumor angiogenesis and patient survival. *Br J Cancer*. **94**: 552–560.

Inwang ER, Puddefoot JR, Brown CL, Goode AW. Marsigliante S, Ho MM, Payne JG, Vinson GP, 1997, Angiotensin II type 1 receptor expression in human breast tissue. *Br J Cancer*. **75**: 1279–1283.

Juillerat-Jeanneret L, Aguzzi A, Wiestler OD, Darekar P, Janzer RC, 1992, Dexamethasone regulates the activity of enzymatic markers of cerebral endothelial cell lines. *In Vitro Cell. Dev Biol*. **28A**: 537–543.

Juillerat-Jeanneret L. 1993, Modulation of proteolytic activity in tissues following chronic inhibition of angiotensin converting enzyme. *Biochem Pharm*. **45**: 1447–1454.

Juillerat-Jeanneret L, Aubert JD, Leuenberger P, 1997, Peptidases in human bronchoalveolar lining fluid, macrophages and epithelial cells: dipeptidylaminopeptidase IV/CD26, aminopeptidase N/CD13 and dipeptidyl carboxypeptidase / angiotensin converting enzyme. *J Lab Clin Med*. **130**: 603–614.

Juillerat-Jeanneret L, Lohm S, Hamou MF, Pinet F, 2000, Regulation of aminopeptidase A in human brain tumor vasculature : evidence for a role of TGF-¯β *Lab Invest*. **80**: 973–980.

Juillerat-Jeanneret L, Monnet-Tschudi F, Zürich MG, Lohm S, Duijvestijn AM, Honegger P, 2003, Regulation of peptidase activity in a three-dimensional aggregate model of brain tumor vasculature. *Cell Tissue Res*. **311**: 53–59.

Juillerat-Jeanneret L, Célérier J, Chapuis Bernasconi C, Nguyen G, Wostl W, Maerki HP, Janzer RC, Corvol P, Gasc JM, 2004, Renin and angiotensinogen expression and function in growth and apoptosis of human glioblastoma. *Br J Cancer*. **90**: 1059–1068.

Juillerat-Jeanneret L, 2006, Targeting the renin-angiotensin system and the endothelin axis in human brain cancer. In *Progress in brain cancer research*. Frank Columbus, ed. *in press*.

Juillerat-Jeanneret L, 2006, Inhibiting the enzymes of the endothelin and renin-angiotensin systems in cancer. *Curr Enzyme Inhibit.* **2**: 353–362.

Kakinuma Y, Hama H, Sugiyama F, Goto K, Murakami K, Fukamizu A, 1997, Anti-apoptotic action of angiotensin fragments to neuronal cells from angiotensinogen knock-out mice. *Neurosc Lett.* **232**: 167–170.

Kakinuma Y, Hama H, Sugiyama F, Yagami K, Goto K, Murakami K, Fukamizu A, 1998, Impaired blood-brain barrier function in angiotensinogen-deficient mice. *Nature Medicine.* **4**: 1078–1080.

Kanehira T, Tani T, Takagi T, Nakano Y, Howard EF, Tamura M, 2005, Angiotensin II type 2 receptor gene deficiency attenuates susceptibility to tobacco-specific nitrosamine-induced lung tumorigeneisi: involvement of transforming growth factor-β-dependent cell growth attenuation. *Cancer Res.* **65**: 7660–7665.

Kikkawa F, Mizuno M, Shibata K, Kajiyama H, Morita T, Ino K, Nomura S, Mizutani S, 2004, Activation of invasiveness of cervical carcinoma cells by angiotensin II. *Am J Obstet Gynecol.* **190**: 1258–1263.

Koh WP, Yuan JM, van den Berg D, Lee HP, Yu MC, 2005, Polymorphism in angiotensin II type 1 receptor and angiotensin I-converting enzyme genes and breast cancer risk among Chinese women in Singapore. *Carcinogenesis.* **26**: 459–464.

Kosugi M, Miyajima A, Kikuchi E, Honguchi Y, Murai M, 2006, Angiotensin II type 1 receptor antagonist candesartan as an angiogenic inhibitor in a xenpgraft model of bladder cancer. *Clin Cancer Res.* **12**: 2888–2893.

Kucerova D, Zelezna B, Sloncova E, Sovova VV, 2003, Angiotensin II receptors on colorectal carcinoma cells. *Int J Mol Med.* **2**: 593–595.

Lam KY, Leung PS, 2002, Regulation and expression of renin-angiotensin system in human pancreas and pancreatic endocrine tumours. *Eur J Endocrinol.* **146**: 567–572.

Lamszus K, Brockmann MA, Eckerich C, Bohlen P, May C, Mangold U, Fillbrandt R, Westphal M, 2005, Inhibition of glioblastoma angiogenesis and invasion by combined treatments directed against vascular endothelial growth factor receptor-2, epidermal growth factor receptor, and vascular endothelial-cadherin. *Clin. Cancer Res.* **11**: 4934–4940.

Lawnicka H, Potocka AM, Juzala A, Fournié-Zaluski MC, Pawlikovski M, 2004, Angiotensin II and its fragments (angiotensin III anf IV) decrease the growth of DU-145 prostate cancer *in vitro*. *Med Sci Monit.* **10**: BR410–413.

Lever AF, Hole DJ, Gillis CR, McCallum IR, MacKinnon PL, Meredith PL, Murray LS, Reid JL, Robertson JW, 1998, Do inhibitors of angiotensin-I-converting enzyme protects against risk of cancer ? *Lancet* **352**: 179–184.

Lee J, Mustafa T, McDowall SG, Mendelsohn FA, Brennan M, Lew RA, Albiston AL, Chai SY, 2003, Structure-activity study of LVV-hemorphin-7: angiotensin AT4 receptor ligand and inhibitor of insulin-regulated aminopeptidase. *J Pharm Exp Ther.* **305**: 205–211.

Lehtonen JY, Daviel L, Nahmias C, Horiuchi M, Dzau VJ, 2004, Analysis of functional domains of angiotensin II type 1 receptor involved in apoptosis. *Mol Endicrinol.* **13**: 1051–1060.

Leung PS, 2004, The peptide hormone angiotensin II: its new functions in tissues and organs. *Curr protein Pept Sci.* **5**: 267–273.

Leung PS, Chappel MC, 2003, A local pancreatic renin-angiotensin system: endocrine and exocrine roles. *Int J Biochem Cell Biol.* **35**: 838–846.

Lew RA, Mustafa T, Ye S, McDowall SG, Chai SY, Albiston AL, 2003, Angiotensin AT4 ligands are potent, competitive inhibitors of insulin regulated aminopeptidase (IRAP). *J Neurochem.* **86**: 344–350.

Lim KT, Cosgrave N, Hill AD, Young LS, 2006, Nongenomic oestrogen signaling in oestrogen receptor negative breast cancer cells: a role for the angiotensin II receptor AT1. *Breast Cancer Res.*

Lindholm LH, Anderson H, Ekbom T, Hansson L, Lanke J, Dahlof B, de Faire U, Forsen K, Hedner T, Linjer E, Schersten B, Wester P, Moller T, 2001, Relation between drug treatment and cancer in hypertensives in the Swedish Trial of Old Patients with Hypertension 2: a 5-year, prospective, randomized, controlled trial. *Lancet.* **358**: 539–544.

Maerki HP, Binggeli A, Bittner B, Bohner-Lang V, Breu V, Bur D, Coassolo PH, Clozel JP, D'Arcy A, Doebeli H, Fischli W, Funk CH, Foricher J, Giller T, Gruninger F, Guenzi A, Guller R, Hartung T, Hirth G, Jenny CH, Kansy M, Klinkhammer U, Lave T, Lohri B, Luft FC, Mervaala EM, Muller DN,

Muller M, Montavon F, Oefner CH, Qiu C, Reichel A, Sanwald-Ducray P, Scalone M, Schleimer M, Schmid R, Stadler H., Treiber A, Valdenaire O, Vieira E, Waldmeier P, Wiegand-Chou R, Wilhelm M, Wostl W, Zell M, Zell R, 2001, Piperidine renin inhibitors: from leads to drug candidates. *Il Farmaco.* **56**: 21–27.

Marchio S, Lahdenranta J, Schlingenmann RO, Valdembri D, Wesseling P, Arap MA, Hajitou A, Ozawa MG, Trepel M, Giordano RJ, Nanus DM, Dijkman HBPM, Oosterwijk E, Sidman RL, Cooper MD, Bussolino F, Pasqualini R, Arap W, 2004, Aminopeptidase A is a functional target in angiogenic blood vessels. *Cancer Cell.* **5**: 151–162.

Marshall RP, McAnulty RJ, Laurent GJ, 2000, Angiotensin II is mitogenic for human lung fibroblasts via activation of the type 1 receptor. *Am J Resp Crit Care Med.* **161**: 1999–2004.

Medeiros R, Vasconcelos A, Costa S, Pinto D, Lobo F, Morais A, Oliveira J, Lopes C, 2004, Linkage of angiotensin I-converting enzyme gene insertion/deletion polymorphism to the progression of human prostate cancer. *J Pathol.* **202**: .330–335.

Milsted A, Barna BP, Ransohoff RM, Brosnihan KB, Ferrario CM, 1990, Astrocyte cultures derived from human brain tissue express angiotensinogen mRNA. *Proc Nat Acad Sci USA.* **87**: 5720–5723.

Miura S, Karnik SS, Saku K, 2005, Constitutively active homo-oligomeric angiotensin II type 2 receptor induces cell signaling independent of receptor conformation and ligand stimulation. *J Biol Chem.* **280**: 18237–18244.

Miyama A, Kosaka T, Asano T, Seta K, Kawai T, Hayakawa M, 2002, Angiotensin II type 1 antagonist prevents pulmonary metastasis of murine renal cancer by inhibiting tumor angiogenesis. *Cancer Res.* **62**: 4176–4179.

Molteni A, Heffelfinger S, Moulder JE, Uhal B, Castellani WJ, 2006, Potential deployment of angiotensin I converting enzyme inhibitors and of angiotensin II type 1 and type 2 receptor blockers in cancer chemotherapy. *Anti-cancer Agents Med Chem.* **6**: 451–460.

Moore SA, Huang N, Hinthrong O, Andres RD, Grammatopoulos TN, Weyhenmeyer JA, 2004, Human angiotensin II type 2 receptor inhibition of insulin mediated ERK2 activity via a a G-protein signaling pathway. *Mol Brain Res.* **124**: .62–69.

Muscella A, Greco S, Elia MG, Storelli C, Marsigliante S, 2002, Angiotensin II stimulation of Na+/K+ ATPase activity and cell growth by calcium-independent pathways in MCF-7 breast cancer cells. *J Endocrinol.* **173**: 315–323.

Nadal JA, Scicli GM, Carbini LA, Scicli AG, 2002, Angiotensin II stimulates migration of retinal miscrovascular pericytes : involvement of TGF-beta and PDGF-BB. Am J Physiol. **282**: H739–H748.

Naito S, Shimizu S, Maeda S, Wang J, Paul R, Fagin JA, 1998, Ets-1 is an early response gene activated by ET-1 and PDGF-BB in vascular smooth muscle cells. Am J Physiol. **274**: C472–C480.

Nakagawa T, Kubota T, Kabuto M, Kodera T, 1995, Captopril inhibits glioma cell invasion in vitro: involvement of matrix metalloproteinases. *Anticancer Res.* **15**: 1985–1989.

Nanus DM, Bogenrieder T, Papandreou CN, Finstad CL, Lee A, Vlamis V, Motzer RJ, Bander NH, Albino AP, Reuter VE, 1998, Aminopeptidase A expression and enzymatic activity in primary human renal cancers. Int J Oncol. **13**: 261–267.

Nassis L, Frauman AG, Ohishi M, Zhuo J, Casley DJ, Johnston CI, Fabiani ME, 2001, Localization of angiotensin-converting enzyme in the human prostate: pathological expression of begnign prostatic hyperplasia. J Pathol.*195*: 571–579.

Nouet S, Amzallag N, Li JM, Louis S, Seitz I, Cui TX, Alleaume AM, Di Benedetto M, Boden C, Masson M, Strosberg AD, Horiuchi M, Couraud PO, Nahmias C, 2004, Trans-inactivation of receptor tyrosine kinases by novel angiotensin II AT$_2$ receptor-interacting protein, ATIP. J Biol Chem. *279*: 28989–28997.

Nguyen G, Delarue F, Burcklé C, Bouzhir L, Giller T, Sraer JD, 2002, Pivotal role of the renin/prorenin receptor in angiotensin II production and cellular response to renin. *J Clin Invest.* **109**: 1417–1427.

Noguchi R, Yoshii H, Kuriyama S, Yoshii J, Ikenaka Y, Yanase K, Namisaki T, Kitade M, Yamasaki M, Mitoro A, Tsujinoue H, Imazu H, Masaki T, Fukui H, 2003, Combination of interferon-β and the angiotensin-converting enzyme inhibitor, perindopril, attenuates murine hepatocellular carcinoma development and angiogenesis. Clin Cancer Res. **9**: 6038–6045.

Ochedalska AL, Rebas E, Kunert-Radek J, Fournié-Zaluski MC, Pawlikowski M, 2002, Angiotensin II and IV stimulate the activity of tyrosine kinases in estrogen-induced rat pituitary tumors. Biochem Biophys Res Com. **297**: 931–933.

Okada H, Watanabe Y. Inoue T, Kobayashi T, Kikula T, Kanno Y, Ban S, Suzuki H, 2004, Angiotensin II type 1 receptor blockade attenuates renal fibrogenis in a immune-mediated nephritic kidney through counter-activation of angiotensin II type 2 receptor. *Biochem Biophys Res Comm*. **314**: 403–408.

Otani A, Takagi H, Oh H, Suzuma K, Matsumura M, Ikeda E, Honda Y, 2000, Angiotensin II-stimulated vascular endothelial growth factor expression in bovine retinal pericytes. *Invest Ophthal Vis Sci*. **41**: 1192–1199.

Prontera C, Mariani B, Rossi C, Poggi A, Rotilio D, 1999, Inhibition of gelatinase A (MMP-2) by Batimastat and captopril reduces tumor growth and lung metastases in mice bearing Lewis lung carcinoma. Int J Cancer. **81**: 761–766.

Puddefoot JR, Udeozo UKI, Barker S, Vinson GP, 2006, The role of angiotensin II in the regulation of breast cancer cells adhesion and invasion. Endocrine-Related Cancer. **13**: 895–903.

Reddy MK, Baskaran K, Molteni A, 1995, Inhibitors of angiotensin-converting enzyme modulate mitosis and gene expression in pancreatic cancer cells. *Proc Nat Acad Sc USA*. **210**: 221–226.

Rivera E, Arrieta O, Guevara P, Duarte-Rojo A, Sotelo J, 2001, AT1 receptor is present in glioma cells, its blockage reduces the growth of rat glioma. *Br J Cancer*. **85**: 1396–1399.

Rizkalla B, Forbes JM, Cooper ME, Cao Z, 2003, Increased renal vascular endothelial growth factor and angiopoietins ba angiotensin II infusion is mediated by both AT1 and AT_2 receptors. *J Am Soc Nephrol*. **14**: 3061–3071.

Röcken C, Lendeckel U, Dierkes J, Westphal S, Carl-McGrath S, Peters B, Krüger S, Malfertheiner P, Roessner A, Ebert MPA, 2006, The number of lymph node metastases in gastric cancer correlates with angiotensin I-converting enzyme gene insertion/deletion polymorphism. *Clin Cancer Res*. **11**: 2526–2529.

Ruiz-Ortega M, Lorenzo O, Egido J, 2000, Angiotensin III increases MCP-1 and activates NF-kappa B and AP-1 in cultured mesangial and mononuclear cells. Kid Int. **57**: 2285–2298.

Sansom CE, Hoang MV, Turner AJ, 1998, Molecular modeling and site-directed mutagenesis of the active site of endothelin converting enzyme. Prot Engin. **11**: 1235–1241.

Santos RA, Campagnole-Santos MJ, Andrade ESP, 2000, Angiotensin-(1-7): an update. *Reg Peptides*. **91**: 45–62.

Schefe JH, Menk M, Reinemund J, Effertz K, Hobbs RM, Pandolfi PP, Ruiz P, Unger T, Funke-Kaiser H, 2006, A novel signal transduction cascade involving direct physical interaction of the rennin/prorenin receptor with the transcription factor promyelocytic zing finger protein. *Circ Res*. **99**: 1355–1366.

Silvestre JS, Tamarat R, Senbonmatsu T, Icchiki T, Ebrahimian T, Iglarz M, Besnard S, Duriez M, Inagami T, Levy BI, 2002, Antiangiogenic effect of angiotensin II type 2 receptor in ischemia-induced angiogenesis in mice hindlimb. *Circ Res*. **90**: 1072–1079.

Small W, Molteni A, Kim, YT, Taylor JM, Chen Z, Ward WF, 1997, Captopril modulates hormone receptor concentration and inhibits proliferation of human mammary ductal carcinoma cells in culture. Breast Cancer Res Treatment. **44**: 217–224.

Small W, Molteni A, Kim, YT, Taylor JM, Ts'ao CH, Ward WF, 1999, Mechanism of captopril toxicity to a human mammary ductal carcinoma cell line in the presence of copper. Breast Cancer Res Treatment. **55**: 223–229.

Stoll M, Unger T, 2001, Angiotensin and its AT_2 receptor: new insight into an old system. Regul Pept. **99**: 175–182.

Suganuma T, Ino K, Shibata K, Nomura S, Kajiyama H, Kikkawa F, Tsuruoka N, Mizutani S, 2004, Regulation of aminopeptidase A expression in cervical carcinoma: role of tumor-stromal interaction and vascular endothelial growth factor. *Lab Invest*. **84**: 639–648.

Suganuma T, Ino K, Shibata K, Kajiyama H, Nagasaka T, Mizutani S, Kikkawa F, 2005, Functional expression of the angiotensin II type 1 receptor in human ovarian carcinoma cells and its blockade therapy resulting in suppression of tumor invasion, angiogenesis, and peritoneal dissemination. *Clin Cancer Res*. **11**: 2686–2694

Sugimoto M, Furuta T, Shirai N, Ikuma M, Sugimura H, Hishida A, 2006, Influence of chymase and angiotensin I-converting enzyme gene polymorphism on gastric cancer risk in Japan. *Cancer epidemiol Biomarkers Prev.* **15**: 1929–1934.

Tahmasebi M, Puddefoot JR, Inwang ER, Goode AW, Carpenter R, Vinson GP, 1998, Transcription of the prorenin gene in normal and diseased breast. *Eur J Cancer.* **34**: 1777–1782.

Tahmasebi M, Barker S, Puddefoot JR, Vinson GP, 2006, Localization of renin-angiotensin system (RAS) components in breast. *Br J Cancer.* **95**: 67–74.

Takeda H, Kondo S, 2001, Differences between squamous cell carcinoma and keratoacanthoma in angiotensin type-1 receptor expression. *Am J Pathol.* **158**: 1633–1637,

Tallant EA, Lu X, Weiss RB, Chappell MC, Ferrario CM, 1997, Bovine aortic endothelial cells contain an angiotensin(1-7) receptor. *Hypertension.* **29**: 388–393.

Tom B, Dendorfer A, Danser AHJ, 2003, Bradykinin, angiotensin-(1-7), and ACE inhibitors: how they interact. *Int J Biochem Cell Biol.* **35**: 792–801.

Uemura H, Ishiguro H, Nakaigawa N, Nagashima Y, Miyoshi Y, Fujinami K, Sakaguchi A, Kubota Y, 2003, Angiotensin II receptor blocker shows antiproliferative activity in prostate cancer cells: a possibility of tyrosine kinase inhibitor of growth factor. Mol Cancer Ther. **2** yy: 1139–1147.

Uemura H, Hasumi H, Kawahara T, Sugiura S, Miyoshi Y, Nakaigawa N, Teranichi J, Fujinami K, Noguchi K, Ishiguro H, Kubota Y, 2005, Pilot study of angiotensin II receptor blocker in advanced hormone refractory prostate cancer. *Int J Clin Oncol.* **10**: 405–410.

Uemura H, Hasumi H, Ishiguro H, Teranichi J, Miyoshi Y, Kubota Y, 2006, Renin-angiotensin system is an important factor in hormone refractory prostate cancer. *Prostate.* **66**: 822–830.

Uemura H, Ishiguro H, Kubota Y, 2006, Angiotensin II receptor blocker: possibility of antitumor agent for prostate cancer. *Mini-Rev Med Chem.* **6**: 835–844.

Usmani BA, Janeczko M, Shen R, Mazumdar M, Papandreou CN, Nanus DM, 2000, Analysis of the insertion/deletion polymorphism of the human angiotensin converting enzyme (ACE) gene in patients with renal cancer. *Br J Cancer.* **82***: 550–552.*

Van Kesteren CAM, Danser AHJ, Derkx FHM, Dekkers DHW, Lamers JMJ, Saxena PR, Schalekamp MA, 1997, Mannose-6-phosphate receptor-mediated internalization and activation of prorenin by cardiac cells. *Hypertension.* **30**: 1389–1396.

Volpert OV, Ward WF, Lingen MW, Chesler L, Solt DB, Johnson MD, Molteni A, Polverini PJ, Bouck NP, 1996, Captopril inhibits angiogenesis and slows the growth of experimental tumors in rats. J Clin Invest. **98**: 671–679.

Von Bohlen und Halbach O, 2003, Angiotensin IV in the central nervous system. *Cell Tissue Res.* **311**: 1–9.

Walther T, Menrad A, Orzechowski HD, Siemeister G, Paul M, Schirner M, 2003, Differential regulation of *in vivo* angiogenesis by angiotensin II receptors. *FASEB J.* **17**: 2061–2067.

Warner FJ, Smith AI, Hooper NM, Turner AJ, 2004, Angiotensin-converting enzyme-2: a molecular and cellular perspective. *Cell Mol Life Sci,* **61:** 2704.

Watanabe T, Barker TA, Berk BC, 2005, Angiotensin II and the endothelium: diverse signals and effects. *Hypertension.* **45**: 163–169.

Williams RN, Parson SL, Morris TM, Rowlands BJ, Watson SA, 2005, Inhibition of matrix metalloproteinase activity and growth of gastric adenocarcinoma cells by an angiotensin converting enzyme inhibitor in in vitro and murine models. *EJSO.* **31**: 1042–1050.

Yamagishi S, Amano S, Inagaki Y, Okamoto T, Inoue H, Takeuchi M, Choei H, Sasaki N, Kikuchi S, 2003, Angiotensin II-type 1 receptor interaction upregulates vascular endothelial growth factor messenger RNA levels in retinal pericytes. *Drugs Exp Clin Res.* **29**: 75–80.

Yaren A, Turgut S, Kursunluoglu R, Oztop I, Ketten C, Erdem E, 2006, Association between the polymorphism of the angiotensin converting enzyme gene and tumor size of breast cancer in premenopausal patients. *Tohoku J Exp Med.* **210**: 109–116.

Yasumaru M, Tsuji S, Tsujii M, Irie T, Komori M, Kimura A, Nishida T, Kakiuchi Y,Kawai N, Murata H, Horimoto M, Sasaki Y, Hayashi N, Kawano S, Hori M, 2003, Inhibition of angiotensin II activity enhanced the antitumor effect of cyclooxygenase-2 inhibitors via insulin-loke growth factor 1 receptor pathways. *Cancer Res.* **63**: 6726–6734.

Yasumatsu R, Nakashima T, Masuda M, Ito A, Kuratomi Y, Nagakawa T, Komune S, 2004, Effects of the angiotensin-1 converting enzyme inhibitor perindopril on tumor growth and angiogenesis in head and neck squamous cell carcinoma cells. *J Cancer Res Clin Oncol.* **130**: 567–573.

Yoshiji H, Kuriyama S, Fukui H, 2002, Perindopril: possible use in cancer therapy. *Anti-cancer Drugs.* **13**: 221–228.

Yoshii H, Kuriyama S, Fukui H, 2002, Angiotensin-converting enzyme inhibitors may be an alternative anti-angiogenic strategy in the treatment of liver fibrosis and hepatocellular carcinoma. Possible role of vascular endothelilal growth factor. Tumour Biol. **23**: 348–356.

Yoshii H, Yoshii J, Ikenaka Y, Noguchi R, Tsujinoue H, Nakatani T, Imazu H, Yanase K, Kuriyama S, Fukui H, 2002, Inhibition of the renin-angiotensin system attenuates liver-enzyme-altered preneoplastic lesions and fibrosis development in rats. J Hepatol. **37**: 22–30.

Yoshii H, Yoshii J, Ikenaka Y, Noguchi R, Yanase K, Tsujinoue H, Imazu H, Fukui H, 2002, Suppression of the renin-angiotensin system attenuates vascular endothelial growth factor-mediated tumor development and angiogenesis in murine hepatocellular carcinoma cells. Int J Oncol. **20**: 1227–1231.

Yoshii H, Noguchi R, Kuriyama S, Yoshii J, Ikenaka Y, 2005, Combination of interferon and angiotensin-converting enzyme inhibitor, perindopril, suppresses liver carcinogenesis and angiogenesis in mice. Oncology Reports. **13**: 491–495.

Yoshiji H, Kuriyama S, Fukui H, 2002, Perindopril: possible use in cancer therapy. Anti-cancer. *Drugs.* **13**: 221–228.

Yuan JM, Koh WP, Sun CL, Lee HP, Yu MC, 2005, Green tea intake, ACE gene polymorphism and breast cancer risk among Chinese women in Singapore. Carcinogenesis. **26**: 1389–1394.

Zhang X, Lassila M, Cooper ME, Cao Z, 2004, Retinal expression of vascular endothelial growth factor is mediated by angiotensin type 1 and type 2 receptors. Hypertension. **43**: 276–281.

Zhuo J, Moeller I, Jenkins T, Chais Y, Allen AM, Ohishi M, Mendelsohn FA, 1998, Mapping tissue angiotensin-converting enzyme and angiotensin AT1, AT_2, and AT4 receptors. *J Hyp.* **16**: 2027–2037.

CHAPTER 11

THE SKELETAL MUSCLE RAS IN HEALTH AND DISEASE

DAVID R. WOODS

Department of Medicine, Royal Victoria Infirmary, Queen Victoria Road, Newcastle, NE1 4LP, U.K.

1. INTRODUCTION

A local renin-angiotensin system (RAS) may be suggested by evidence of gene expression of RAS components within the tissue as well as physiological responsiveness of this gene expression. This chapter will focus on the evidence supporting the existence of the constituent elements of a physiologically functional paracrine muscle RAS. Further, this chapter will consider the effect of local skeletal muscle RAS in health on human exercise performance and in disease in relation to heart failure, insulin resistance, sarcopenia and osteoporosis.

1.1. The Circulating Renin-Angiotensin System

Renin cleaves angiotensinogen to generate the non-pressor decapeptide angiotensin I. The octapeptide angiotensin II is then derived primarily by the action of angiotensin-converting enzyme (ACE) which may either be circulating (after release by a carboxypeptidase) or an integral membrane protein (Beldent *et al* 1993; Zisman 1998). ACE also catalyses inactivation of bradykinin and thus ACE simultaneously generates a potent vasoconstrictor (angiotensin II) and inactivates a potent vasodilator (bradykinin).

The original concept of a circulating RAS producing angiotensin II has evolved with our understanding about the function, receptors and existence of other effector peptides, for example angiotensin-(1-7), angiotensin III and angiotensin IV. In addition, the existence of a local RAS has been established in several tissues and our understanding as to their role continues to develop. Recent data implicate a skeletal muscle RAS with local de novo angiotensin II production and intrinsic ACE activity that is physiologically responsive. Moreover, pharmacological manipulation

Po Sing Leung (ed.), Frontiers in Research of the Renin-Angiotensin System on Human Disease, 221–245.
© 2007 *Springer.*

of specific aspects of the RAS in addition to genetic studies suggest that a muscle RAS may have significant functional implications in both health and disease.

1.2.   Local Renin-Angiotensin Systems

A local RAS may be suggested by evidence of gene expression of RAS components within the tissue as well as physiological responsiveness of this gene expression. Local generation of angiotensin II and the demonstration of physiologically active angiotensin II receptors within the tissue are also key features. Local RAS have been described in the pancreas (Leung *et al* 2000; Sernia 2001), heart (Danser *et al* 1999 and reviewed in De Mello and Danser 2000), lung (Pieruzzi *et al* 1995) brain (reviewed in Allen *et al* 1999) and in adipose tissue (Jonsson *et al* 1994).

As has been suggested (Danser *et al* 1999) local angiotensin II production may depend either on in-situ synthesis of all RAS components or uptake of various constituents from the circulation. Or, as in the case of the skeletal muscle RAS, a combination of in-situ synthesis and uptake.

2.   SKELETAL MUSCLE RENIN-ANGIOTENSIN SYSTEM

2.1.   Skeletal Muscle ACE

The first suggestion of a relatively independent human skeletal muscle ACE arose from vastus lateralis muscle biopsy specimens that demonstrated muscle ACE activity did not correlate with serum ACE (Reneland *et al* 1994). Hind-limb skeletal muscles from rats, dogs and guinea pigs have demonstrated not only the presence of ACE in skeletal muscle membranes but intact paracrine kininase-II activity (Dragovic *et al* 1996). Muscle tissue was differentially centrifuged to obtain the skeletal muscle membrane fraction, incubated with bradykinin in the presence or absence of an ACE inhibitor, and the ability to hydrolyze bradykinin assessed. Approximately 50% of kininase activity in rat and dog skeletal muscle membrane was found to be due to ACE (Dragovic *et al* 1996). Cultured skeletal muscle myoblast cells also demonstrate ACE activity confirming that the ACE in the membrane fraction was from muscle and not derived from homogenized blood vessels and nerves (Dragovic *et al* 1996). Other workers have also demonstrated an effect of ACE on bradykinin degradation in rabbit skeletal muscle membranes (Ward *et al* 1995). Significantly, Ward et al also demonstrated functionality of skeletal muscle ACE in the conversion of angiotensin I to angiotensin II.

More recently immunohistochemistry of human muscle biopsies has localized ACE to the endothelial cells of capillaries in skeletal muscle (Schaufelberger *et al* 1998). ACE gene expression was found to be variable and, quantified by the number of ACE-mRNA transcripts, was related to muscle fibre area with an inverse relationship to capillary density (Schaufelberger *et al* 1998).

Local ACE is an important determinate of muscle function since isolated rat muscle perfused with a solution excluding ACE, renin, and angiotensinogen, still demonstrate marked vasoconstriction to topical Ang I that is prevented by ACE inhibition (Vicaut and Hou 1993). Any local variation in ACE expression might therefore influence angiotensin II generation and bradykinin degradation.

Indeed, there is evidence that muscle ACE gene expression can be functionally upregulated. Following two-kidney, one clip (2K1C) hypertension for 4 weeks, incremental doses of infused angiotensin I in isolated rat hindlimbs produces a dose-dependent increase in venous angiotensin II that is greater in 2K1C rats than controls (Muller et al 1997). An infusion of renin also increases angiotensin II to a greater extent in 2K1C rats compared to control. It would therefore appear that the skeletal muscle vascular bed can upregulate ACE with a functional increase in the conversion of exogenous and locally generated angiotensin I to angiotensin II.

2.2.   Skeletal Muscle Angiotensin II Receptors

There are two angiotensin II receptors: type 1 (AT_1) and type 2 (AT_2). Most of the known effects of angiotensin II, including vasoconstriction, hypertrophy, cellular growth, catecholamine release, and aldosterone secretion, are mediated by AT_1 (Matsubara 1998; Timmermans *et al* 1993; Munzenmaier and Green, 1996). The AT_2 receptor appears to attenuate the effects of angiotensin II at the AT_1 receptor (Nouet and Nahmias 2000). AT_1 receptor stimulation causes myocyte hypertrophy whereas AT_2 inhibits proliferative processes (Matsubara 1998). The AT_2 receptor also mediates vasodilation (Munzenmaier and Green, 1996) via the paracrine effects of bradykinin activating the endothelial bradykinin type 2 receptor–mediated nitric oxide system (Tsutsumi et al 1999). Similarly, the AT_1 receptor stimulates catecholamine synthesis in the adrenal while AT_2 reduces it (Takekoshi et al. 2002).

Since angiotensin II binds to AT_1 and AT_2 with a similar affinity the cellular response may depend on the relative expression, or responsiveness, of these receptors within individual tissues. The AT_2 receptor subtype is highly expressed in foetal tissue but dramatically decreases after birth (Viswanathan *et al* 1991), being restricted to a few tissues such as brain, adrenal, uterus heart, lung, myometrium and ovary (Timmermans *et al* 1993, Horiuchi *et al* 1999, Matsubara 1998, Allen *et al* 2000). Although AT_2 receptors exist in human right atrial appendages (Goette *et al* 2000), the tubules and glomeruli of human kidneys (Mifune *et al*, 2001) and the colon (Hirasawa 2002) the AT_1 receptor predominates.

Both AT_1 and AT_2 receptors exist throughout the rat skeletal muscle microcirculation (Nora *et al* 1998) and in the skeletal muscle fibres (Linderman and Greene 2001). However, in human skeletal muscle published evidence only confirms the presence of the AT_1 receptor although both receptors may exist in foetal-stage skeletal muscle (Malendowicz *et al* 2000). Administration of a specific AT_2 antagonist in humans does not affect basal forearm blood flow (Phoon and Howes 2001) but conversely the rat demonstrates a greater blood pressure rise with angiotensin II infusion during coexistent AT_2 antagonism compared to angiotensin II alone (Munzenmaier and Green, 1996).

2.3.   Skeletal Muscle Angiotensin II

The peripheral vasculature is an important site of angiotensin I conversion in humans (Admiraal *et al* 1993; Gasic *et al* 1990). Angiotensin II (in addition to renin and angiotensinogen) mRNA and protein have recently been demonstrated by reverse transcriptase polymerase chain reaction and immunohistochemistry within the skeletal muscle microvessels of the rat (Agoudemos and Greene 2005). The vascular endothelium accounts for much of the angiotensin II production (Ohishi *et al* 1997; Phillips *et al* 1993) and it is conceptually reasonable to consider skeletal muscle angiotensin II a product of the skeletal muscle vascular bed. However, it is interesting to note that the concentration of angiotensin II in the skeletal muscle microvessels exceeds that of plasma (Agoudemos and Greene 2005). Intracellular accumulation of angiotensin II following endocytosis of AT_1 receptors with angiotensin II from the circulation (Thomas 1999) could facilitate a cellular mechanism whereby stored angiotensin II may be subsequently used locally.

Further, half the angiotensin II in the venous drainage of skeletal muscle may be secondary to local de novo angiotensin II synthesis from the conversion of both locally produced and circulating angiotensin I (Danser *et al* 1992). Following constant infusion of 125I-Ang I into the left ventricle of pigs 67% of venous angiotensin I and 59% of venous angiotensin II across the skeletal muscle vascular bed was found to be derived from de novo production. Angiotensin I production in skeletal muscle may therefore contribute to the circulating pool and a proportion of circulating angiotensin II may be derived from local sources (Danser *et al* 1992a).

In healthy humans incremental doses of infused angiotensin I and angiotensin II exert the same maximal effect in decreasing forearm blood flow (FBF), with similar potencies (Saris *et al* 2000). Forearm fractional angiotensin I-to-II conversion is only 36%, ACE inhibition reduces this to 1% and abolishes the effects of angiotensin I, suggesting that locally generated angiotensin II is functionally important (Saris *et al* 2000). Since the extraction rates for angiotensin I across vascular beds are high, it is likely that local vascular ACE has a significant contribution to angiotensin II reaching the peripheral arterioles (Campbell 1985; Hilgers *et al* 1989; Admiraal *et al* 1990; Admiraal *et al* 1993). Indeed further evidence for the role of local muscle angiotensin II comes from the observation that although angiotensin II is a strong vasoconstrictor when applied to the intravascular space when it is applied to the interstitial space using microdialysis techniques it has minimal effect on the perfusion of skeletal muscle (Boschmann *et al* 2003a). This suggests that interstitial angiotensin II is less important for blood flow regulation than intravascular angiotensin II (Boschmann *et al* 2003a). Angiotensin II has also been shown to have a tissue-specific effect, again suggestive of the importance of local RAS and local regulation. Interstitial angiotensin II stimulates lipolysis in adipose tissue while inhibiting lipolysis and glucose uptake in muscle (Boschmann *et al* 2003a), effects that were not apparently mediated by changes in regional blood flow.

3.   SKELETAL MUSCLE RAS IN HEALTH AND PERFORMANCE

AT_1 mediated angiotensin II is crucial for optimal overload-induced skeletal muscle hypertrophy (Gordon *et al* 2001). In surgically-induced plantaris and/or soleus muscle overload inhibiting endogenous angiotensin II production by ACE inhibition markedly attenuates muscle hypertrophy which is restored by local angiotensin II perfusion. AT_1 receptor antagonism also attenuates hypertrophy but is not rescued by angiotensin II perfusion. It is locally elevated angiotensin II that is vital since the contralateral soleus does not recover the hypertrophic response despite angiotensin II entering the systemic circulation, inducing cardiac hypertrophy similar to the perfused soleus. (Gordon *et al* 2001). Further support for functional skeletal muscle AT_1 receptors being required for training-related increases in both muscle mass and contractile force was reported recently. Daily AT_1 blockade in rats undergoing eccentric contraction training (24 contractions twice a week for 4 weeks) prevented a training-induced increase in muscle mass and muscle contractile force compared to controls (McBride 2006).

Angiotensin II may also be important in the redirection of blood flow from type I muscle fibres to the type II fibres (Rattigan *et al* 1996) that are favoured in power performance (a sprinter may have 80% fast twitch fibres, an endurance athlete 20%). Nitric oxide (NO) opposes angiotensin II-induced increases in arterial pressure and in skeletal muscle resistance during dynamic exercise (Symons *et al* 1999). Acute exercise stimulates NO release and may have a synergistic role with prostaglandin in mediating vasodilatation and hyperaemia during muscular contraction since their inhibition during acute exercise reduces microvascular flow in human quadriceps (Boushel *et al* 2002). Recently, microdialysis in human calf muscle has confirmed an elevation of tissue bradykinin with exercise (Langberg *et al* 2002) perhaps supporting a role for bradykinin-NO induced hyperaemia. Interestingly, the oxidative capacity of muscle (greatest in the type 1 fibres that correlate with efficiency in cyclists) (Coyle *et al* 1992) is in direct correlation and may be interdependent with muscle kallikrein (Shinojo *et al* 1987). Genetic studies support these findings as the DD genotype of the ACE gene, associated with increased bradykinin degradation, has also been associated with significant blunting of NO vasodilatory responses in forearm vessels (Butler *et al* 1999).

Angiotensin II infused into rat hindlimbs increases the contraction-induced oxygen uptake and the tension during tetanic stimulation (Rattigan *et al* 1996). Greater local angiotensin II production may therefore facilitate muscle contraction for maximal power, possibly at the cost of muscle efficiency. Indeed, following angiotensin II administration in rats (Brink *et al* 1996) there is a reduction in metabolic efficiency with skeletal muscle wasting secondary to enhanced protein degradation (Brink *et al* 2001) caused predominantly by an anorexigenic response (Brink *et al* 1996).

Other actions of angiotensin II that might influence performance in health include the facilitation of sympathetic transmission by enhancing noradrenaline release from peripheral sympathetic nerve terminals and the CNS (Saxena 1992, Story and Ziogas 1987). Other potential mechanisms include angiotensin II as a direct stimulator of cellular growth (both hypertrophic and hyperplastic) (Campbell-Boswell and Robertson 1989, Daemen *et al* 1991), and the induction of various endogenous growth factors; fibroblast growth factor, transforming growth factor-ß$_1$, platelet derived growth factor (Dzau 1994, Huckle and Earp 1994, Rosendorff, 1996).

A series of gene-environment interaction studies focussing on the human ACE gene have revealed further insight into the effect of skeletal muscle RAS in health and performance. The ACE gene contains a polymorphism consisting of the presence (insertion, I) or absence (deletion, D) of a 287 base pair sequence in intron 16 (Rigat *et al* 1990). Hence, three genotypes exist: II, ID and DD, the distributions of which within a Caucasian population are roughly 25, 50 and 25% respectively. Although this polymorphism occurs in an intron it is an exceptionally strong and consistent marker for ACE activity in many different Caucasian populations (Cambien *et al* 1994, Busjahn *et al* 1997, Danser *et al* 1998, Agerholm-Larsen *et al* 1999, Kohno *et al* 1999, Rossi *et al* 1999, Martinez *et al* 2000) and accounts for up to 47% of the variance in plasma ACE (Rigat *et al* 1990). ACE is consistently highest in the DD subjects, intermediate in the ID and lowest in the II subjects. The ACE polymorphism also appears to be a determinant of ACE at a cellular level (Costerousse *et al* 1993; Danser *et al* 1995; Davis *et al* 2000; Mizuiri *et al* 2001) and thus may influence angiotensin II production.

The contractile responses of internal mammary arteries to angiotensin I and II and the maximal angiotensin II-induced response suggest that angiotensin I conversion is greatest in the presence of the D allele (Buikema *et al* 1996). This may be secondary to increased tissue conversion of angiotensin I since DD subjects have a significantly enhanced forearm vasoconstrictor response to angiotensin I infusion that is not accompanied by differences in serum angiotensin II levels (van Dijk *et al* 2000). This may therefore reflect a difference in local angiotensin II production within the peripheral muscular bed alone although other workers have found greater plasma angiotensin II concentrations following angiotensin I infusion in DD subjects (Brown *et al* 1998; Ueda *et al* 1995).

The ACE polymorphism also affects bradykinin degradation, this being least in II subjects with low tissue and circulating ACE (Brown *et al* 1998). Reduced bradykinin degradation may favourably alter substrate metabolism in II subjects with improvements in the efficiency and contractile function of skeletal muscle, beneficial effects in endurance exercise.

In addition, a reduction in ACE activity leads not only to an attenuation of angiotensin II production and a decrease in bradykinin degradation but also to an increase in Ang-(1–7) (as it is not converted to Ang-(1-5) by ACE) (Ferrario and Iyer 1998). This may further favour vasodilation and potential substrate delivery. Ang-(1-7) can be generated by several enzymes including neutral endopeptidase 24.11 (NEP), from angiotensin I, bypassing the prerequisite formation of angiotensin II. NEP is expressed in cultured human skeletal muscle adult myoblasts and myotubes (Vaghy *et al* 1995). The actions of Ang-(1-7) are most often opposite those of angiotensin II and include an anti-proliferative effect on VSMC and a vasodilator effect not mediated by AT$_1$ or AT$_2$ but via the synthesis and release of

vasodilator prostaglandins and NO (Stroth and Unger 1997). Conversely, geneti-
cally determined high ACE expression in rats is associated with low circulating and
tissue NEP activity (Oliveri *et al* 2001) suggesting the existence of a modulating
effect of ACE expression on NEP activity. This could determine lower ang-(1-7)
tissue levels in addition to higher angiotensin II.

It could be expected that a reduction in ACE with a favourable effect on
angiotensin II, bradykinin and Ang-(1-7) metabolism may translate into a potential
advantage in human performance. This indeed would appear to be the case with an
excess of II subjects in elite runners with a significant linear trend of increasing I
allele frequency with distance run (Myerson *et al* 1999). Similarly, elite Australian
rowers exhibit an excess of the I allele and the II genotype (Gayagay *et al* 1998).
In addition the I allele has also been found in significantly higher frequency in the
fastest 100 South African-born finishers in the South African Ironman Triathlon
(Collins *et al* 2004) and in elite very-long-distance (25 km) swimmers (Tsianos
et al 2004). Interestingly rowers exhibit a preponderance of type 1 muscle fibres
similar to endurance runners. As discussed in section 4 it is a reduction in type 1
fibres that is blamed for some of the reduction in muscle efficiency in CHF that
is reversed by reducing ACE activity (akin to the effect of the I allele). Recently,
in 41 untrained healthy young volunteer subjects skeletal muscle biopsies from the
vastus lateralis demonstrated that II subjects had higher percentages of slow-twitch
type I fibres and a lower percentages of fast-twitch type IIb fibres than DD subjects
with a linear trend for decreases in type I fibres and increases in type IIb fibres
from the II through the ID to the DD genotypes (Zhang *et al* 2003).

Conversely the D allele has been associated with power-oriented performance,
being found in excess in short-distance swimmers (Woods *et al* 2001) and other
power-oriented athletes (Nazarov *et al* 2001). Although not all reports support these
findings the common denominator among negative studies has been the selection of
athletes from mixed sporting disciplines, cohorts that are unlikely to yield reliable
information in a population association study (Taylor *et al* 1999; Karjilainen *et al*
1999; Rankinen *et al* 2000).

In prospective training studies the I allele has also been associated with greater
improvement in endurance performance (Montgomery *et al* 1998) and the D allele
with greater strength gains in the quadriceps muscle (Folland *et al* 2000).

In the search for a physiological link between the ACE genotype and elite human
performance the study of central cardio-respiratory factors such as $\dot{V}O_{2max}$ has
revealed no consistent effect (Hagberg *et al* 1998; Rankinen *et al* 2000; Woods
et al 2002; Sonna *et al* 2002). This is corroborated by a genome-wide scan for
markers linked with $\dot{V}O_{2max}$ that found none on chromosome 17, the location of the
ACE gene (Bouchard *et al* 2000).

Greater endurance of a fairly small muscle group, the upper arm, for II subjects after
training (Montgomery *et al* 1998), and an increased arterio-venous oxygen difference
during maximal exercise in II postmenopausal women (Hagberg *et al* 1998) suggests
that the influence of ACE may instead be due to local muscle effects. Further, examination of delta efficiency (DE, the ratio of the change in work performed min^{-1} to

Key points: Performance and the muscle RAS

1. Locally elevated angiotensin II mediated by skeletal muscle AT_1 receptors are crucial in overload-induced skeletal muscle hypertrophy (Gordon *et al* 2001) and the muscle mass and contractile force response to eccentric contraction training is mediated by AT_1 receptors (McBride 2006).
2. Angiotensin II increases the contraction-induced oxygen uptake and the tension during tetanic stimulation (Rattigan *et al* 1996).
3. A series of gene-environment interaction studies regarding the ACE gene have suggested that the DD genotype, associated with greater ACE activity, is associated with increased angiotensin II (Brown *et al* 1998; Ueda *et al* 1995) and enhanced performance in power-orientated events (Woods *et al* 2001; Nazarov *et al* 2001) and with greater strength gains in the quadriceps muscle in response to training (Folland *et al* 2000).
4. Conversely, the I allele, associated with reduced ACE has been associatedwith enhanced endurance performance (Myerson *et al* 1999; Gayagay *et al* 1998; Collins *et al* 2004; Tsianos *et al* 2004).
5. The endurance enhancement associated with the I allele is not thought to be due to central cardio-respiratory factors (Woods *et al* 2002) but to local muscle effects mediated by the RAS such as an improvement in muscle efficiency (Williams *et al* 2000) and a higher percentage of slow-twitch type I fibres and a lower percentages of fast-twitch type IIb fibres (Zhang *et al* 2003).

Figure 1. Performance and the muscle RAS

the change in energy expended min^{-1}), the most valid measure of the efficiency of muscular contraction (Gaesser and Brooks 1975) reveals that DE rises significantly with training only in those of II genotype (Williams *et al* 2000). This is supported by the greater peripheral tissue oxygenation and lesser rise in lactate, reflecting greater muscle efficiency, that occurs in II compared to DD subjects during exercise in patients with chronic airways disease (Kanazawa *et al* 2002).

Taken together the data would suggest that the D allele is associated with power-oriented athletic performance. This may be secondary to the effect of a greater ACE level on local angiotensin II production via the skeletal muscle RAS and its subsequent hypertrophic effect on muscle growth and subsequently strength. Conversely, it may be that a reduction in ACE has local muscle effects via the skeletal muscle RAS that increase muscle efficiency and contribute to the enhanced endurance associated with the I allele (Fig. 1).

4.   SKELETAL MUSCLE RAS AND HEART FAILURE

Congestive heart failure (CHF) is a condition associated not just with altered cardiac function and metabolism but also a generalised skeletal muscle myopathy. Increased RAS activity with elevated plasma and tissue angiotensin II is an important contributor to cardiac and vascular remodelling in patients with CHF (Unger *et al*

2002). This has a detrimental effect on skeletal muscle perfusion and fibre type ratio with a subsequent reduction in peak aerobic capacity (LeJemtel et al 1986; Minotti et al 1991; Harridge et al 1996; Coats 1996). Exercise capacity does not correlate with the degree of left ventricular (LV) dysfunction (Sullivan & Hawthorne, 1995) but peak oxygen consumption does correlate closely with ultra-structural changes in skeletal muscle (Munzel et al 1993). A reduction in ACE may mediate peripheral muscle effects that contribute to the efficacy of ACE inhibition. Recently ACE inhibition in rats post-myocardial infarction (MI) was found to prevent MI-induced alterations in skeletal (gastrocnemius) muscle mitochondrial function and to preserve the mRNAs concentration of mitochondrial transcriptional factors. (Zoll et al 2006). Defects in sarcoplasmic reticulum calcium-transport in the hind-leg skeletal muscle of rats following myocardial infarction can also be attenuated by ACE inhibition or angiotensin receptor blocker (ARB) therapy (Shah et al 2004).

ACE inhibition also enhances peak aerobic capacity and induces improvement in skeletal muscle perfusion in patients with CHF (Mancini et al 1987; Drexler et al 1989) though not necessarily in healthy subjects (Predel et al 1994). Chronic therapy with ACE inhibitors in CHF improves endothelial function, peripheral oxygen extraction and exercise performance greater than acute improvements in cardiac output (Drexler et al 1991).

CHF is associated with elevated circulating levels of angiotensin II and muscle wasting, an important predictor of poor outcome (Coats 1996). Angiotensin II induced muscle loss is associated with reduced skeletal muscle IGF-1 expression (Brink et al 1997) while circulating levels may be normal (Hambrecht et al 2002). Using skeletal muscle–specific IGF-1–transgenic mice it has recently been demonstrated that these changes are prevented by over expression of muscle-specific IGF-1 (Song et al 2005). Aldosterone too, has recently been demonstrated in rats to be capable of directly inducing myocyte apoptosis in skeletal muscle, an effect that can be reduced by pre-treatment with the aldosterone antagonist spironolactone (Burniston et al 2005).

Maximum oxidative capacity and effective muscle mass measured by 31P magnetic resonance spectroscopy during aerobic exercise decrease by 30% and 65% respectively in CHF (Kemp et al 1996). This is corroborated by muscle biopsies demonstrating reduced muscle oxidative capacity (Mettauer et al 2001; Drexler et al 1992) and a reduction in mitochondrial density that correlates with peak VO2 (Drexler et al 1992). In addition, rat models of CHF demonstrate alterations in skeletal muscle fibre ratio with an increased proportion of fatigue-sensitive fast type-II fibres and a decreased proportion of slow-twitch, fatigue-resistant type 1 fibres (De Sousa et al 2000). The proportion of slow-twitch type 1 fibres also falls in humans with CHF (Sullivan, 1990, Drexler et al 1992), perhaps contributing to the reduced metabolic efficiency seen (Kemp et al 1996), an effect that is preserved by ACE inhibition (Sabbah et al 1996).

Slow twitch fibres have a high oxidative capacity but the muscle of CHF patients reveal a decrease in citrate synthase activity and a concomitant reduction in oxidative capacity (De Sousa et al 2000). ACE inhibitors improve peak $\dot{V}O_2$ in CHF specifically by reducing the limitation due to peripheral muscle factors (Jondeau et al

---

Key points: Heart failure and the muscle RAS

1. CHF is associated with an up-regulated RAS and elevated circulating levels of angiotensin II. Muscle wasting is an important predictor of poor outcome in CHF (Coats 1996) and aldosterone can directly induce myocyte apoptosis in skeletal muscle (Burniston et al 2005).
2. A reduction in ACE in rats post-MI prevents MI-induced alterations in skeletal muscle mitochondrial function and preserves the mRNAs concentration of mitochondrial transcriptional factors (Zoll et al 2006).
3. Defects in sarcoplasmic reticulum calcium-transport in the hind-leg skeletal muscle of rats following MI can be attenuated by ACE inhibition or ARB therapy (Shah et al 2004).
4. ACE inhibitors improve peak $\dot{V}O_2$ in CHF specifically by reducing the limitation due to peripheral muscle factors (Jondeau et al 1997).
5. ACE is up-regulated in CHF. ACE gene expression in muscle biopsies from patients with CHF relates to muscle fibre area with an inverse relationship to capillary density (Schaufelberger et al 1998). A decreased capillary-to-fibre ratio occurs in CHF (De Sousa et al 2000, Drexler 1992) but ACE inhibitors improve peripheral oxygen extraction and exercise performance greater than acute improvements in cardiac output (Drexler et al 1991).
6. Maximum oxidative capacity of muscle is reduced in CHF (Kemp et al 1996, Mettauer et al 2001; Drexler et al 1992) and there is a decreased proportion of slow-twitch, fatigue-resistant, high oxidative capacity type 1 fibres (De Sousa et al 2000), an effect that ACE inhibition may preserve (Sabbah et al 1996).

Figure 2. Heart failure and the muscle RAS

1997). Moreover, these effects are partly mediated via antagonism of angiotensin II since AT_1 receptor blockade activates the perfusion of exercising muscle (raised delta $\dot{V}O_2$/delta work rate, a measure of aerobic work efficiency) (Guazzi et al 1999). A decreased capillary-to-fibre ratio also occurs in CHF (De Sousa et al 2000, Drexler 1992) which may negatively impact on substrate delivery and hence muscle efficiency and therefore performance. ACE, up-regulated in CHF, may be key to this effect since ACE expression has an inverse relationship to capillary density (Schaufelberger et al 1998).

It becomes apparent that part of both the clinical state of CHF, with an upregulated RAS, and part of the mechanism of response to treatment is mediated by effects localized to skeletal muscle with the skeletal muscle RAS as a central focus (Fig. 2).

5.   SKELETAL MUSCLE RAS AND INSULIN RESISTANCE

In a retrospective sub-study of the SOLVD trial (Vermes et al 2003) of 291 non-diabetic patients (of which 153 were on enalapril and 138 on placebo) 40 patients developed diabetes during follow-up. There was a highly significant difference between the groups: 9 (5.9%) of the new diabetics were in the enalapril group and

31 (22.4%) in the placebo group. Multivariate analysis revealed ACE inhibition as the most powerful predictor for risk reduction of developing diabetes especially in patients with impaired fasting plasma glucose. CHF is an insulin-resistant state and it is possible that an improvement in CHF with ACE inhibition may simply be the mechanism.

However, a similar effect of ACE inhibition on reducing the development of diabetes has been found in patients despite the absence of LV dysfunction.

In the HOPE trial (which demonstrated reduced mortality in patients at high risk of ischaemic heart disease even in the absence of LV dysfunction) over a treatment period of 4.5 years, a reduction in ACE with Ramipril reduced the incidence of developing diabetes (relative risk reduction) by 34% (Yusuf et al 2000). This effect persisted 2 and a half years after the trial had ended (Bosch et al 2005). ACE inhibition in hypertensives using lisinopril in the ALLHAT study also reduced the rates of new DM compared with amlodipine (relative risk reduction of 30%) (ALLHAT investigators 2002). A 22% relative risk reduction in new onset diabetes was also found with ARB therapy in CHF in the CHARM trial (Yusuf et al 2005) and a 23% relative risk reduction in new diabetes with another ARB, valsartan, compared to amlodipine in hypertensives (Julius et al 2004). In a similar vein the recent DREAM trial in patients without cardiovascular disease but with impaired glucose tolerance or impaired fasting glucose found that while ACE inhibition did not reduce progression to diabetes it did increase regression to normoglycaemia (Bosch et al 2006).

Overall the effect of RAS blockade improving insulin resistance and reducing new onset of type 2 diabetes is mounting. A recent meta-analysis of 10 randomised controlled trials with almost 70,000 hypertensives and 5727 patients with CHF demonstrated a 22% relative risk reduction in new type 2 diabetes with ACE inhibition or ARB treatment compared to placebo or other drugs (some admittedly diabetogenic such as atenolol, some metabolically neutral such as amlodipine) (Scheen 2004). The fascination now lies with the underlying mechanism (Fig. 3).

CHF is an insulin-resistant state with neurohormonal activation both increasing peripheral insulin resistance and decreasing insulin secretion (Paolisso et al 1991). While an improvement in CHF status with ACE inhibition may simply be the mechanism it is also possible that an effect on skeletal muscle RAS plays a part since a reduction in ACE enhances muscle perfusion and insulin-mediated glucose disposal (Donnelly 1992; Kudoh et al 2000) and interstitial angiotensin II is known to impair muscle glucose uptake (Boschmann et al 2003a).

Selective skeletal muscle ACE inhibition in humans by local retrodialysis increases interstitial glucose and decreases the serum interstitial gradient for glucose by facilitating transcapillary glucose transport (Muller et al 1997; Frossard et al 2000). Similarly, acute ACE inhibition enhances insulin-stimulated glucose transport activity in rat skeletal muscle. Chronic ACE inhibition with enalapril also improves insulin resistance in humans (Morel et al 1995).

The male heterozygous TG(mREN2)27 rat has elevated local tissue angiotensin II and demonstrates insulin resistance. Using this model the chronic administration

---

Key points: Insulin resistance and the muscle RAS

1. Interstitial angiotensin II impairs muscle glucose uptake (Boschmann *et al* 2003a).
2. Selective skeletal muscle ACE inhibition facilitates transcapillary glucose transport (Muller *et al* 1997; Frossard *et al* 2000).
3. In the insulin resistant TG(mREN2)27 rat ARB treatment increases insulin-mediated glucose transport in type IIb epitrochlearis and type I soleus muscles (Sloniger *et al* 2005).
4. Angiotensin II-induced NADPH oxidase activation impairs insulin signalling in skeletal muscle cells (Wei *et al* 2006).
5. Several studies (SOLVD, HOPE, the ALLHAT study, CHARM, DREAM etc) have demonstrated a reduction in onset of diabetes or improvement in glycaemia with ACE inhibition or an ARB (Vermes *et al* 2003; Yusuf *et al* 2000; The ALLHAT investigators 2002; Yusuf *et al* 2005; Julius *et al* 2004; Bosch *et al* 2006).
6. The interaction between ACE, bradykinin degradation and muscle GLUT4 translocation (Shiuchi *et al* 2002; Henriksen and Jacob 2003; Wong *et al* 2006).

Figure 3. Insulin resistance and muscle RAS

of the ARB irbesartan increases whole-body insulin sensitivity and insulin-mediated glucose transport in both type IIb epitrochlearis and type I soleus muscles compared with vehicle-treated rats with an increase in glycogen synthase activation due to insulin in the soleus muscle (Sloniger *et al* 2005).

Very recently it has been found that angiotensin II markedly enhances NADPH oxidase activity and consequent reactive oxygen species (ROS) generation in L6 myotubes (Wei *et al* 2006). Angiotensin II-induced generation of ROS (which inactivate nitric oxide) contribute to the development of insulin resistance in skeletal muscle. The effects of angiotensin II on NADPH oxidase activity and ROS generation are blocked by the ARB losartan (Wei *et al* 2006). Further, angiotensin II prevents insulin-induced tyrosine phosphorylation of the insulin receptor substrate 1 (IRS1) and prevents glucose transporter-4 (GLUT4) translocation to the plasma membrane in L6 myotubes. These effects were reversed by pre-treating myotubes with the ARB losartan. These are potential mechanisms by which ARB and ACE inhibition, working via a reduction in skeletal muscle angiotensin II activity, reduce the onset of new diabetes in patients with an otherwise upregulated RAS in CHF. Similarly, it could also explain the increased regression to normoglycaemia seen with these agents in patients with impaired glucose tolerance and impaired fasting glycaemia.

Other workers (Zhao *et al* 2006) have found that increasing angiotensin II in the rat either by infusion or by inducing unilateral renal artery stenosis (2K1C) also increases muscle ROS and upregulates NADPH oxidase which then disrupts the normal nitric-oxide-dependent attenuation of sympathetic vasoconstriction in exercising muscle. Using a ROS scavenger this effect of angiotensin II in exercising muscle was prevented. These are potentially very important effects on sympathetic vasoregulation in exercising skeletal muscle, especially when the RAS is upregulated in CHF.

Bradykinin administration also enhances muscle glucose uptake, an effect which can be completely abolished by pre-treatment with either a B2 bradykinin receptor antagonist or a nitric oxide synthase inhibitor (Henriksen et al 1999), suggesting that a B2 bradykinin receptor mediated increase in nitric oxide production in skeletal muscle facilitates glucose uptake (Henriksen et al 1999, Shiuchi et al 2001). This may at least in part be due to a B2 bradykinin-NO mediated increase in GLUT4 translocation (Shiuchi et al 2002, Henriksen and Jacob 2003). Bradykinin also acts as a potent vasodilator via the release of nitric oxide (Rett et al 1989). Muscle work increases muscle blood flow and glucose uptake in humans, an effect reproduced by bradykinin infusion in the human forearm (Dietze et al 1996). Indeed, a concomitant increase in bradykinin in the venous effluent from working muscle occurs. However, if the bradykinin -generating protease in muscle tissue (kallikrein) is inhibited with aprotinin these responses are significantly diminished (Dietze et al 1996). Agents which inhibit both ACE and neutral endopeptidase, such as the vasopeptidase inhibitor omapatrilat, have been found to raise tissue bradykinin levels and enhance muscle glucose uptake in animal models via the bradykinin-nitric oxide pathway, although the exact mechanism of increased muscle glucose uptake is not certain (Wong et al 2006).

These are important mechanisms by which ACE inhibition, working via a reduction in skeletal muscle bradykinin degradation, could improve insulin resistance and reduce the onset of new diabetes in patients with an otherwise upregulated RAS in CHF.

Microdialysis techniques have demonstrated that angiotensin II decreases local blood flow in a dose-dependent manner and inhibits lipolysis in human gastrocnemius muscle (Goossens et al 2004). They also demonstrated that local angiotensin II stimulation appeared to cause a dose-dependent biphasic response, with an antilipolytic effect at physiological concentrations but either no effect or a lipolytic effect at higher concentrations. The authors comment on the fact that the effect of angiotensin II may be dose and tissue-specific: angiotensin II has been shown to exert a lipolytic effect in adipose tissue and an antilipolytic effect in skeletal muscle tissue (Boschmann et al 2003b) with subtle effects of interstitial angiotensin II on skeletal muscle perfusion and metabolism (Boschmann et al 2006). This further supports the importance of local RAS. Although there have been apparent inconsistencies in the literature regarding the apparent variable effects of angiotensin II in different tissues this may just reflect physiological fine tuning of local tissue RAS. In support of this, for example, is the simple observation that under hyperinsulinaemic euglycaemic conditions, infusion of angiotensin II has divergent effects on regional arterial blood flow with a reduction in renal blood flow but an increase in skeletal muscle blood flow (Fliser et al 2000).

Considering one of the potential mechanisms involving the skeletal muscle RAS associated with a reduction in ACE seen with the I allele on human performance and the effect of a reduction in ACE pharmacologically in CHF, namely a change in muscle fibre type, it is interesting to note the effect this may have on insulin resistance. Animal studies have suggested that fibre composition of skeletal muscle may be linked to insulin resistance. In fructose-fed insulin-resistant rats the ratio of type 1 fibres in the soleus muscle decreases compared to controls but ACE inhibition results in a recovery of type 1 fibres and a normalisation of the ratio similar to controls (Ura *et al* 1999). As type 1 fibres are those which have the greatest oxidative metabolism, such an effect of ACE inhibition on muscular fibre composition may contribute to improve glucose uptake by the skeletal muscles and thus increase insulin sensitivity. Certainly in the study by Ura et al (Ura *et al* 1999) the ACE inhibitor effect on fibre type was associated with an improvement in insulin resistance (Ura et al 1999).

6.   SKELETAL MUSCLE RAS, SARCOPENIA AND OSTEOPOROSIS

As outlined in section 4 skeletal muscle RAS appears to have a role in CHF and may be central to the effects of some therapies. Similarly, the skeletal muscle RAS may have a role in sarcopenia and possibly osteoporosis.

A study of 641 women with hypertension (but without CHF) (Onder *et al* 2002) has found that those who had taken ACE inhibitors continuously had a significantly lower average 3-year decline in knee extensor muscle strength compared with continuous or intermittent users of other anti-hypertensive drugs and those who had never used anti-hypertensives. Further, average 3-year decline in walking speed in continuous ACE inhibitor users was significantly less than in intermittent users of ACE inhibitors and continuous or intermittent users of other anti-hypertensive drugs and those who had never used anti-hypertensive drugs. Similarly, in 2431 elderly patients with hypertension but without CHF treatment with an ACE inhibitor was associated with a larger lower extremity muscle mass as assessed by DEXA scan than with other classes of anti-hypertensives (Di Bari *et al* 2004).

In addition ACE inhibition may help preserve bone mineral density (BMD). Improving strength has a positive effect on BMD (Rhodes *et al* 2000) and grip strength is an independent predictor of BMD (Kroger *et al* 1994). An open, prospective study of 134 patients with low-to-moderate hypertension and stable BMD were randomized to various anti-hypertensives. ACE inhibitors had a beneficial effect on BMD and calcium metabolism in these subjects. When analysed by ACE I/D polymorphism DD subjects demonstrated the greatest improvement in BMD, perhaps reflecting a greater effect on their higher baseline ACE levels (Perez-Castrillon *et al* 2003a). In an earlier study (Perez-Castrillon *et al* 2003b) the same authors had found hypertensive postmenopausal women with the II genotype to have a greater spinal BMD than the ID or DD subjects.

In postmenopausal women ACE levels appear to affect the muscle and bone response to HRT. Improvement in maximal voluntary force of the abductor pollicis brevis muscle in those taking HRT has been found to be strongly ACE genotype-dependent with those with the I allele associated with lower ACE levels having the greatest response. A similar effect was found in the BMD response to HRT in Ward's triangle and the spine (Woods *et al* 2001).

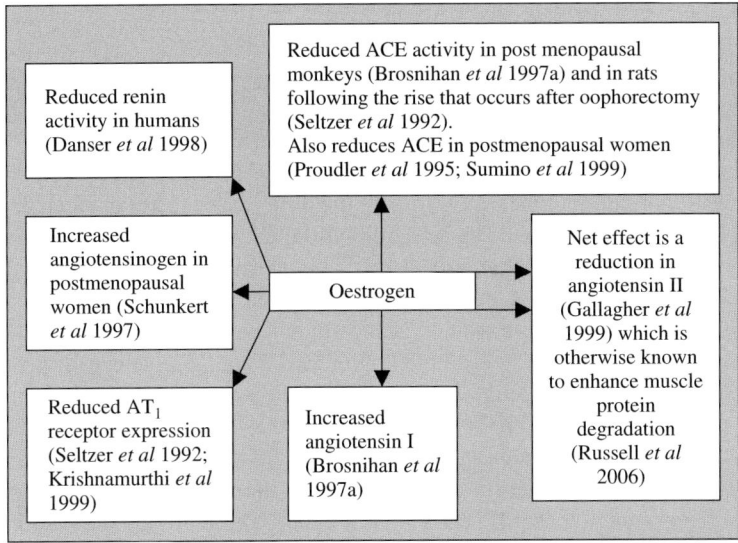

Figure 4. Important interactions exist between oestrogen and the RAS. These interactions may mediate the apparent benefits a reduction in ACE has on muscle strength and bone mineral density

Important interactions between oestrogen and the RAS exist (Fig. 4). Oophorectomy produces significant increases in ACE activity and angiotensin II binding in the rat anterior pituitary, both of which return to normal after oestrogen replacement including a decrease in anterior pituitary AT_1 receptor numbers (Seltzer et al., 1992). ACE activity is also reduced in postmenopausal monkeys treated with HRT (Brosnihan et al., 1997a). This reduction in ACE activity after oestrogen treatment is associated with a significant increase in plasma Ang I and renin and a reduced formation of angiotensin II. Furthermore, oestradiol replacement therapy decreases not only serum ACE activity in rats following oophorectomy but also reduces ACE activity in kidney and aorta tissue extracts (Brosnihan et al., 1997b).

HRT also stimulates the synthesis of angiotensinogen (Schunkert et al., 1997) but reduces renin (Danser et al., 1998) and serum ACE activity (Proudler et al., 1995; Sumino et al., 1999). The overall effect in the rat, where oestrogen treatment reduces tissue ACE mRNA, is a reduction in angiotensin II (Gallagher et al., 1999) which is a potent stimulator of osteoclastic bone resorption (Hatton et al., 1997). In addition oestrogen replacement in rats reduces AT_1 receptor expression (Krishnamurthi et al., 1999).

In summary oestrogen augments both tissue and circulating levels of angiotensinogen and angiotensin I but does not increase angiotensin II secondary to the overriding reduction in ACE activity (Brosnihan et al., 1997a). Further, the angiotensin II/angiotensin I ratio, an in vivo index of ACE activity, is significantly reduced by oestrogen treatment. In rats treated with oestrogen following oophorectomy the reduced tissue ACE and circulating angiotensin II is also associated with elevated circulating levels of Ang-(1-7), a vasodilator, and puts the net balance of oestrogen on the RAS in favour of vasodilation (Brosnihan *et al.*, 1997b). HRT also increases plasma levels of bradykinin in hypertensive postmenopausal women (Sumino *et al.*, 1999) which, considering the bradykinin release from working skeletal muscle (Rett *et al.*, 1990) may have an effect on both substrate delivery and local vasoregulation.

More recently, angiotensin I has been found to induce protein degradation in skeletal muscle in murine myotubes with a parabolic dose-response curve (Sanders *et al.*, 2005). This effect was inhibited by ACE inhibition, suggesting it was mediated by angiotensin II formation. In the same study angiotensin II induced skeletal muscle degradation with a similar dose-response curve. In both cases this effect was thought to be mediated via upregulation of the ubiquitin-proteasome proteolytic pathway. Again using murine myotubes both angiotensin I and angiotensin II were found to enhance protein degradation with a similar dose-response curve in the activation of protein kinase C (PKC) (Russell *et al* 2006). Both PKC and NF-kappaB activation appear to be required for the induction of proteasome expression and protein degradation by angiotensin II since their inhibition by specific inhibitors attenuates the effect of angiotensin II (Russell *et al* 2006). Therefore the interaction between oestrogen and the skeletal muscle RAS could potentially explain some of the effects seen with variations in ACE on muscle strength and hence bone density.

7.   CONCLUSIONS

A physiologically functional skeletal muscle RAS exists. It is capable of de novo angiotensin II production and interaction with the kallikrein-kinin system. A pharma-cological or genetically-mediated reduction in ACE activity appears to have significant effects via skeletal muscle RAS in reversing the decline in physical performance due to peripheral muscle factors in those with CHF. Similar pivotal roles for skeletal muscle RAS have been identified in relation to human performance in health, insulin resistance and effects that may halt or slow the decline in muscle strength in ageing. A greater understanding of the skeletal muscle RAS has implications not just for elite human performance but also for the treatment of many disease states including CHF, insulin resistance, diabetes and the effects of aging.

REFERENCES

Admiraal P, Danser AHL, Jong MS, Pieterman H, Derkx FHM, Schalekamp MADH. 1993 Regional angiotensin II production in essential hypertension and renal artery stenosis. *Hypertension.* **21**: 173–184.

Admiraal PJJ, Derkx FHM, Danser AHJ, Pieterman H & Schalekamp MADH. 1990 Metabolism and production of angiotensin I in different vascular beds in subjects with hypertension. *Hypertension.* **15**: 44–55.

Agerholm-Larsen B, Tybjserg-Hansen A, Schnohn P, Nordestgaard BG. 1999 ACE gene polymorphism explains 30–40% of variability in serum ACE activity in both women and men in the population at large: the Copenhagen City Heart study. *Atherosclerosis.* **147**: 425–7.

Agoudemos MM, Greene AS. 2005 Localization of the renin-angiotensin system components to the skeletal muscle microcirculation. *Microcirculation.* **12**: 627–36.

Allen AM, MacGregor DP, McKinley MJ, Mendelsohn FAO. 1999 Angiotensin II receptors in the human brain. *Reg Pep.* **79**: 1–7.

Allen AM, Zhuo J, Mendelsohn FA. 2000 Localization and function of angiotensin AT1 receptors. *Am J Hypertens* **13**: 31S–38S

ALLHAT Officers and Coordinators for the ALLHAT Collaborative Research Group. 2002 Major outcomes in high-risk hypertensive patients randomized to angiotensin-converting enzyme inhibitor or calcium channel blocker vs diuretic: the Antihypertensive and Lipid-Lowering Treatment to Prevent Heart Attack Trial (ALLHAT). *JAMA.* **288**: 2981–2997.

Beldent V, Michaud A, Wei L, Chauvet M.-T. & Corvol P. 1993 Proteolytic release of human angiotensin-converting enzyme. Localisation of the cleavage site. *J Biol Chem.* **268**: 26428–26434.

Bosch J, Lonn E, Pogue J, Arnold JM, Dagenais GR, Yusuf S; HOPE/HOPE-TOO Study Investigators. 2005 Long-term effects of ramipril on cardiovascular events and on diabetes: results of the HOPE study extension. *Circulation.* **112**: 1339–46.

Bosch J, Yusuf S, Gerstein HC, Pogue J,Sheridan P, Dagenais G, Diaz R, Avezum A, Lanas F, Probstfield J, Fodor G, Holman RR. 2006 Effect of ramipril on the incidence of diabetes. *N Engl J Med.* **355**: 1551–62.

Boschmann M, Adams F, Klaus S, Sharma AM, Luft FC, Jordan J. 2003b Differential response to interstitial angiotensin II in normal weight and obese men. *Int J Obes Relat Metab Disord* **27**: S52.

Boschmann M, Adams F, Schaller K, Franke G, Sharma AM, Klaus S, Luft FC, Jordan J. (2006) Hemodynamic and metabolic responses to interstitial angiotensin II in normal weight and obese men. *J Hypertens.* **24**: 1165–71

Boschmann M, Jordan J, Adams F, Christensen NJ, Tank J, Franke G, Stoffels M, Sharma AM, Luft FC, Klaus S 2003a Tissue-specific response to interstitial angiotensin II in humans. *Hypertension* 41: 37–41.

Bouchard C, Rankinen T, Chagnon YC, Rice T, Perusse L, Gagnon J, Borecki I, An P, Leon AS, Skinner JS, Wilmore JH, Province M, Rao DC. 2000 Genomic scan for maximal oxygen uptake and its response to training in the HERITAGE Family Study. *J Appl Physiol.* **88**: 551–559.

Boushel R, Langberg H, Gemmer C, Olesen J, Crameri R, Scheede C, Sander M, Kjaer M. 2002 Combined inhibition of nitric oxide and prostaglandins reduces human skeletal muscle blood flow during exercise. *J Physiol* **543**: 691–8.

Brink, M., Wellen, J., and Delafontaine, P. 1996. Angiotensin II causes weight loss and decreases circulating insulin-like growth factor I in rats through a pressor-independent mechanism. *J. Clin. Invest.* **97**: 2509–2516.

Brink M, Price SR, Chrast J, Bailey JL, Anwar A, Mitch WE, Delafontaine P. 2001 Angiotensin II induces skeletal muscle wasting through enhanced protein degradation and down-regulates autocrine insulin-like growth factor I. *Endocrinology.* **142**: 1489–96.

Brosnihan KB, Weddle D, Anthony MS, Heise C, Li P, and Ferrario CM. 1997a Effects of chronic hormone replacement on the renin-angiotensin system in cynomolgus monkeys. *J. Hypertens.* **15**, 719–726.

Brosnihan KB, Li P, Ganten D, Ferrario CM. 1997b Estrogen protects transgenic hypertensive rats by shifting the vasoconstrictor-vasodilator balance of RAS. *Am. J. Physiol.* **273** (*Regulatory Integrative Com. Physiol.*), R1908–R1915.

Brown NJ, Blais C, Gandhi SK and Adam A. 1998 ACE Insertion/Deletion Genotype Affects Bradykinin Metabolism. *J Cardiovasc Pharmacol.* **32**: 373–377.

Buikema H, Pinto YM, Rooks G, Grandjean JG, Schunkert H, van Gilst WH. 1996 The deletion polymorphism of the angiotensin-converting enzyme gene is related to phenotypic differences in human arteries. *Eur Heart J.* **17**: 787–94.

Burniston JG, Saini A, Tan LB, Goldspink DF. 2005 Aldosterone induces myocyte apoptosis in the heart and skeletal muscles of rats in vivo. *J Mol Cell Cardiol.* **39**: 95–399.

Busjahn A, Knoblauch H, Knoblauch M, Bohlender J, Menz M, Faulhaber HD, Becker A, Schuster H, Luft FC. 1997 Angiotensin-converting enzyme and angiotensinogen gene polymorphisms, plasma levels, cardiac dimensions: a twin study. *Hypertension.* **29**: 165–70.

Butler R, Morris AD, Burchell B, Struthers AD. 1999 *DD* Angiotensin-Converting Enzyme Gene Polymorphism Is Associated With Endothelial Dysfunction in Normal Humans. *Hypertension.* **33**: 1164–1168.

Cambien F, Costerousse O, Tiret L, Poirier O, Lecerf L, Gonzales MF, Evans A, Arveiler D, Cambou JP & Luc G. 1994 Plasma level and gene polymorphism of angiotensin-converting enzyme in relation to myocardial infarction, *Circulation.* **90**: 669–676.

Campbell D J. 1985 The site of angiotensin production. *J Hypertens.* **3**: 199–207.

Campbell-Boswell M & Robertson ALJ. 1989 Effects of angiotensin II and vasopressin on human smooth muscle cells in vitro. *Exp Mol Pathol.* **35**: 265–276.

Coats AJ. 1996 The "muscle hypothesis" of chronic heart failure. *J Mol Cell Cardiol* **28**: 2255–2262.

Collins M, Xenophontos SL, Cariolou MA, Mokone GG, Hudson DE, Anastasiades L, Noakes TD. 2004 The ACE gene and endurance performance during the South African Ironman Triathlons. *Med Sci Sports Exerc.* **36**: 1314–20.

Costerousse O, Allegrini J, Lopez M & Alhenc-Gelas F. 1993 Angiotensin-I converting enzyme in human circulating mononuclear cells: genetic polymorphism of expression in T-lymphocytes. *Biochem J.* **290**: 33–40.

Coyle EF, Sidossis LS, Horowitz JF & Beltz JD. 1992 Cycling efficiency is related to the percentage of Type I muscle fibers. *Med Sci Sports Exerc.* **24**: 782–788.

Daemen MJAP, Lombardi DM, Bosman FT & Schwartz SM. 1991 Angiotensin II induces smooth muscle cell proliferation in the normal and injured rat arterial wall. *Circ Res.* **68**: 450–456.

Danser AH, Derkx FH, Hense HW, Jeunemaitre X, Riegger GA, Schunkert H. 1998 Angiotensinogen (M235T) and angiotensin-converting enzyme (I/D) polymorphisms in association with plasma renin and prorenin levels. *J Hypertens.* **16**: 1879–1883.

Danser AH, Derkx FH, Schalekamp MA, Hense HW, Riegger GA, and Schunkert H. 1998 Determinants of interindividual variation of renin and prorenin concentrations: evidence for a sexual dimorphism of (pro)renin levels in humans. *J. Hypertens.* **16**, 853–862.

Danser AH, Koning MM, Admiraal PJ, Sassen LM, Derkx FH, Verdouw PD & Schalekamp MA. 1992 Production of angiotensins I and II at tissue sites in intact pigs, *Am J Physiol.* **263**: H429–437.

Danser A, Saris JJ, Schuijt MP, van Kats JP. 1999 Is there a local renin-angiotensin system in the heart. *Cardiovasc res.* **44**: 252–265.

Danser AH, Schalekamp MA, Bax WA, van-den-Brink AM, Saxena PR, Riegger GA & Schunkert H. 1995 Angiotensin converting enzyme in the human heart. Effect of the deletion/insertion polymorphism. *Circulation.* **92**: 1387–1388.

Davis GK, Millner RW, Roberts DH. 2000 Angiotensin converting enzyme (ACE) gene expression in the human left ventricle: effect of ACE gene insertion/deletion polymorphism and left ventricular function. *Eur J Heart Fail* 2: 253–6.

De Mello WC, Danser AH. 2000 Angiotensin II and the heart: on the intracrine renin-angiotensin system. *Hypertension.* **35**: 1183–1188.

De Sousa E, Veksler V, Bigard X, Mateo P, Ventura-Clapier R. 2000 Heart failure affects mitochondrial but not myofibrillar intrinsic properties of skeletal muscle. *Circulation* **102**: 1847–53.

Di Bari M, van de Poll-Franse LV, Onder G, Kritchevsky SB, Newman A, Harris TB, Williamson JD, Marchionni N, Pahor M. 2004 Antihypertensive medications and differences in muscle mass in older persons: the Health, Aging and Body Composition Study. *J Am Geriatr Soc.* **52**: 961–6.

Dietze GJ, Wicklmayr M, Rett K, Jacob S, Henriksen EJ. 1996 Potential role of bradykinin in forearm muscle metabolism in humans. *Diabetes* **45**: S110–S114.

Donnely R. 1992 Angiotensin-converting enzyme inhibitors and insulin sensitivity: metabolic effects in hypertension, diabetes, and heart failure. *J Cardiovasc Pharmacol* **20**: S38–45.

Dragovic T, Minhall R, Jackman HL, Wang L-X & Erdos EG. 1996 Kininase II-type enzymes. Their putative role in muscle energy metabolism, *Diabetes. Suppl 1*, S34–37.

Drexler H, Munzel T, Riede U, Just H. 1991 Adaptive changes in the periphery and their therapeutic consequences. *Am J Cardiol* **67**: 29C–34C.

Drexler H, Riede U, Munzel T, Konig H, Funke E & Just H. 1992 Alterations of skeletal muscle in chronic heart failure. *Circulation* **85**: 1751–1759.

Drexler H, Banhardt U, Meinertz T, Wollschlager H, Lehmann M, Just H. 1989 Contrasting peripheral short-term and long-term effects of converting enzyme inhibition in patients with congestive heart failure: a double-blind, placebo-controlled trial., *Circulation* **79**: 491–502.

Dzau VJ. 1994 Cell biology and genetics of angiotensin in cardiovascular disease. *J Hypertens.* **12**: S3–10.

Ferrario CM and Iyer SN. 1998 Angiotensin-(1-7): a bioactive fragment of the renin-angiotensin system. *Reg. Pep.* **78**: 13–18.

Fliser D, Dikow R, Demukaj S, Ritz E. 2000 Opposing effects of angiotensin II on muscle and renal blood flow under euglycemic conditions. *J Am Soc Nephrol* **11**: 2001–6.

Folland J, Leach B, Little T, Hawker K, Myerson S, Montgomery H, and Jones D. Angiotensin-converting enzyme genotype affects the response of human skeletal muscle to functional overload. *Exp Physiol* **85**: 575–9, 2000.

Frossard M, Joukhadar C, Steffen G, Schmid R, Eichler HG, Muller M. 2000 Paracrine effects of angiotensin-converting-enzyme- and angiotensin-II-receptor- inhibition on transcapillary glucose transport in humans. *Life Sci.* **66**: PL147–54.

Gaesser GA, & Brooks GA. 1975 Muscular efficiency during steady-state exercise: effects of speed and work rate. *J Appl Physiol* **38**: 1132–1139.

Gallagher PE, Li P, Lenhart JR, Chappell MC, and Brosnihan KB. 1999 Estrogen regulation of angiotensin-converting enzyme mRNA. *Hypertension.* **33**, 323–328.

Gasic S, Heinz G, Kleinbloesm C. 1990 Quantitative evidence of peripheral conversion of angiotensin within the human leg: effects of local angiotensin I administration and angiotensin converting enzyme inhibition on regional blood flow and angiotensin II balance across the leg. *Naunyn Schmiedebergs Arch Pharmacol.* **342**: 436–440.

Gayagay G, Yu B, Hambly B, Boston T, Hahn A, Celermajer DS, and Trent RJ. 1998 Elite endurance athletes and the ACE I allele-the role of genes in athletic performance. *Hum Genet.* **103**: 48–50.

Goette A, Arndt M, Röcken C, Spiess A, Staack T, Geller JC, Huth C, Ansorge S, Klein HU, Lendeckel U. 2000 Regulation of Angiotensin II Receptor Subtypes During Atrial Fibrillation in Humans. *Circulation.* **101**: 2678–81.

Goossens GH, Blaak EE, Saris WHM and van Baak MA. 2004 Angiotensin II-Induced Effects on Adipose and Skeletal Muscle Tissue Blood Flow and Lipolysis in Normal-Weight and Obese Subjects *The J of Clin Endocrin & Metab* **89**: 2690–2696.

Gordon S, Davis BS, Carlson CJ, Booth FW. 2001 Angiotensin II is required for optimal overload-induced skeletal muscle hypertrophy. *Am J Physiol Endocrinol Metab.* **280**: E150–9.

Guazzi M, Palermo P, Pontone G, Susini F, Agostoni P. 1999 Synergistic efficacy of enalapril and losartan on exercise performance and oxygen consumption at peak exercise in congestive heart failure. *Am J Cardiol* **84**: 1038–43.

Hagberg J, Ferrell M, McCole RE, Wilund SD, and Moore, G.E. 1998 VO2 max is associated with ACE genotype in postmenopausal women. *J Appl Physiol* **85**: 1842–6.

Hambrecht, R. Schulze PC, Gielen S, Linke A, Mobius-Winkler S, Yu J, Kratzsch J J, Baldauf G, Busse MW, Schubert A, Adams V, Schuler G. 2002. Reduction of insulin-like growth factor-I expression in the skeletal muscle of noncachectic patients with chronic heart failure. *J. Am. Coll. Cardiol.* **39**: 1175–1181.

Harridge SD, Magnusson G, & Gordon A. 1996 Skeletal muscle contractile characteristics and fatigue resistance in patients with chronic heart failure. *Eur Heart J.* **17**: 896–901.

Hatton R, Stimpel M, and Chambers TJ. 1997 Angiotensin II is generated from angiotensin I by bone cells and stimulates osteoclastic bone resorption in vitro. *J. Endocrinol.* **152**, 5–10.

Henriksen EJ, Jacob S. (2003) Modulation of metabolic control by angiotensin converting enzyme (ACE) inhibition. *J Cell Physiol* **196**: 171–9.

Henriksen EJ, Jacob S, Kinnick TR, Youngblood EB, Schmit MB, Dietze GJ. 1999 ACE inhibition and glucose transport in insulinresistant muscle: roles of bradykinin and nitric oxide. *Am J Physiol* **277**: R332–6.

Hilgers K, Kuczera M, Wilhelm MJ, Wiecek A, Ritz E, Ganten D, Mann JFE. 1989 Angiotensin formation in the isolated rat hindlimb. *J Hypertens.* **7**: 789–798.

Huckle WR & Earp HS. 1994 Regulation of cell proliferation and growth by angiotensin II. *Prog Growth Factor Res.* **5**: 177–194.

Hirasawa K, Sato Y, Hosoda Y, Yamamoto T, Hanai H. 2002 Immunohistochemical localization of angiotensin II receptor and local renin-angiotensin system in human colonic mucosa. *J Histochem Cytochem* 50: 275–82.

Horiuchi M, Akishita M, Dzau VJ. 1999 Recent progress in angiotensin II type 2 receptor research in the cardiovascular system. *Hypertension.* **33**: 613–621.

Jondeau G, Dib JC, Dubourg O & Bourdarias JP. 1997 Relation of functional improvement in congestive heart failure after quinapril therapy to peripheral limitation, *Am J Cardiol.* *79*, 635–638.

Jonsson JR, Game PA, Head RJ & Frewin DB. 1994 The expression and localisation of the angiotensin-converting enzyme mRNA in human adipose tissue, *Blood Pressure.* *3*, 72–75.

Julius S, Kjeldsen SE, Weber M, Brunner HR, Ekman S, Hansson L, Hua T, Laragh J, McInnes GT, Mitchell L, Plat F, Schork A, Smith B, Zanchetti A; VALUE trial group. 2004 Outcomes in hypertensive patients at high cardiovascular risk treated with regimens based on valsartan or amlodipine: the VALUE randomised trial. *Lancet.* **363**: 2022–2031.

Kanazawa H, Otsuka T, Hirata K, Yoshikawa J. 2002 Association between the angiotensin-converting enzyme gene polymorphisms and tissue oxygenation during exercise in patients with COPD, *Chest* **121**: 697–701.

Karjalainen J, Kujala UM, Stolt A, Mantysaari M, Viitasalo M, Kainulainen K, and Kontula K. 1999 Angiotensinogen Gene M235T polymorphism predicts left ventricular hypertrophy in endurance athletes. *J Am Coll Cardiol* **34**: 494–9.

Kemp GJ, Thompson CH, Stratton JR, Brunotte F, Conway M, Adamopoulos S, Arnolda L, Radda GK & Rajagopalan B. 1996 Abnormalities in exercising skeletal muscle in congestive heart failure can be explained in terms of decreased mitochondrial ATP synthesis, reduced metabolic efficiency, and increased glycogenolysis. *Heart* **76**: 35–41.

Kohno M, Yokokawa K, Minami, M, Kano H, Yasunari K, Hanehira T, Yoshikawa J 1999 Association between angiotensin-converting enzyme gene polymorphisms and regression of left ventricular hypertrophy in patients treated with angiotensin-converting enzyme inhibitors. *Am J Med.* **106**: 544–9.

Krishnamurthi K, Verbalis JG, Zheng W, Wu Z, Clerch LB and Sandberg K. 1999 Estrogen regulates Anmgiotensin AT1 receptor expression via cytosolic proteins that bind to the 5' leader sequence of the receptor mRNA. *Endocrinology* **140**, 5435–5438.

Kroger H, Tuppurainen M, Honkanen R, Alhava E, and Saarikoski S. 1994 Bone mineral density and risk factors for osteoporosis—a population-based study of 1600 perimenopausal women. *Calcif. Tissue Int.* **55**, 1–7.

Kudoh A, Matsuki A. 2000 Effects of angiotensin-converting enzyme inhibitors on glucose uptake. *Hypertension* **36**: 239–44.

Langberg H, Bjorn C, Boushel R, Hellsten Y, Kjaer M. 2002 Exercise-induced increase in interstitial bradykinin and adenosine concentrations in skeletal muscle and peritendinous tissue in humans. *J Physiol* **542**: 977–83.

LeJemtel T, Maskin CS, Lucido D, Chadwick BJ. 1986 Failure to augment maximal limb blood flow in response to one-leg versus two-leg exercise in patients with severe heart failure. *Circulation* **74**: 245–251.

Leung PS, Carlsson PO. 2001 Tissue renin-angiotensin system: its expression, localization, regulation and potential role in the pancreas. *J Mol Endocrinol* , **26**: 155–164.

Linderman J, Greene AS. 2001 Distribution of angiotensin II receptor expression in the microcirculation of striated muscle. *Microcirculation.* **8**: 275–81.

Malendowicz SL, Ennezat PV, Testa M, Murray L, Sonnenblick EH, Evans T, LeJemtel TH. 2000 Angiotensin II Receptor Subtypes in the Skeletal Muscle Vasculature of Patients With Severe Congestive Heart Failure. *Circulation.* **102**: 2210.

Mancini D, Davis L, Wexler JP Chadwick B, Le Jemtel TH. 1987 Dependence of enhanced maximal exercise performance on increased peak skeletal muscle perfusion during long-term captopril therapy in heart failure. *J Am Coll Cardiol* **10** 845–850.

Martinez EPA, Escribano J, Sanchis C, Carrion L, Artigao M, Divison JA, Masso J, Vidal A, Fernandez JA. 2000 Angiotensin-converting enzyme (ACE) gene polymorphisms, serum ACE activity and blood pressure in a Spanish-Mediterranean population. J Hum Hypertens 14, 131–5.

Matsubara H. 1998 Pathophysiological role of angiotensin II type 2 receptor in cardiovascular and renal diseases. *Circ Res.* **83**: 1182–1191.

McBride TA. 2006 AT1 receptors are necessary for eccentric training-induced hypertrophy and strength gains in rat skeletal muscle. *Exp Physiol.* **91**: 413–21.

Mettauer B, Zoll J, Sanchez H, Lampert E, Ribera F, Veksler V, Bigard X, Mateo P, Epailly E, Lonsdorfer J, Ventura-Clapier R. 2001 Oxidative capacity of skeletal muscle in heart failure patients versus sedentary or active control subjects. *J Am Coll Cardiol* **8**: 947–54.

Minotti JR, Christoph I, Oka R, Weiner MW, Wells L & Massie BM. 1991 Impaired skeletal muscle function in patients with congestive heart failure. Relationship to systemic exercise performance. *J Clin Invest* **88**: 2077–2082.

Mizuiri S, Hemmi H, Kumanomidou H, Iwamoto M, Miyagi M, Sakai K, Aikawa A, Ohara T, Yamada K, Shimatake H, Hasegawa A. Angiotensin-converting enzyme (ACE) I/D genotype and renal ACE gene expression. Kidney Int. 2001 Sep;60(3): 1124–30.

Montgomery HE, Marshall RM, Hemingway H, Myerson S, Clarkson P, Dollery C, Hayward M, Holliman DE, Jubb M, World M, Thomas EL, Brynes AE, Saeed N, Barnard M, Bell JD, Prasad K, Rayson M, Talmud PJ, & Humphries SE. 1998 Human gene for physical performance. *Nature* **393**: 221–222.

Morel Y, Gadient A, Keller U, Vadas L, Golay A. 1995 Insulin sensitivity in obese hypertensive dyslipidemic patients treated with enalapril or atenolol. *J Cardiovasc Pharmacol.* **26**: 306–311.

Mifune M, Sasamura H, Nakazato Y, Yamaji Y, Oshima N, Saruta T. 2001 Examination of angiotensin II type 1 and type 2 receptor expression in human kidneys by immunohistochemistry. *Clin Exp Hypertens* **23**: 257–66.

Muller M, Fasching P, Schmid R, Burgdorff T, Waldhausl W, Eichler HG. 1997 Inhibition of paracrine angiotensin-converting enzyme in vivo: effects on interstitial glucose and lactate concentrations in human skeletal muscle. *Eur J Clin Invest.* **27**: 825–30.

Munzel T, Kurz S & Drexler H. 1993 Are alterations of skeletal muscle ultrastructure in patients with heart failure reversible under treatment with ACE-inhibitors? *Herz* **18**: 400–405.

Munzenmaier D, Greene AS. 1996 Opposing actions of angiotensin II on microvascular growth and arterial blood pressure. *Hypertension.* **27**: 760–5.

Myerson S, Hemingway H, Budget R, Martin J, Humphries S, & Montgomery H. 1999 Human angiotensin I-converting enzyme gene and endurance performance. *J Appl Physiol.* **87**: 1313–1316.

Nazarov IB, Woods DR, Montgomery HE, Shneider OV, Kazakov VI, Tomilin NV, and Rogozkin VA. 2001 The Angiotensin Converting Enzyme I/D polymorphism in Russian athletes., *Eur. J. Hum. Genet.* **9**: 797–801.

Nouet, S and Nahmias C. Signal transduction from the Angiotensin II AT$_2$ receptor. 2000 *Trends in Endocrin and Metab* **11**: 1–6.

Nora E, Munzenmaier DH, Hansen-Smith FM, Lombard JH, Greene AS. 1998 Localization of the angiotensin II type 2 receptor in the microcirculation of skeletal muscle. *Am J Physiol.* **275**: H1395–H1403.

Ohishi M, Ueda M, Rakugi H, Okamura A, Naruko T, Becker A, Hiwada K, Kamitani A, Kamide K, Higaki J, and Ogihara T. 1997 Upregulation of angiotensin-converting enzyme during the healing process after injury at the site of percutaneous transluminal coronary angioplasty in humans. *Circulation.* **96**: 3328–3337.

Oliveri C, Ocaranza MP, Campos X, Lavandero S, Jalil JE. 2001 Angiotensin I-Converting Enzyme Modulates Neutral Endopeptidase Activity in the Rat. *Hypertension.* **38**: 650.

Onder G, Penninx BW, Balkrishnan R, Fried LP, Chaves PH, Williamson J, Carter C, Di Bari M, Guralnik JM, Pahor M. 2002 Relation between use of angiotensin-converting enzyme inhibitors and muscle strength and physical function in older women: an observational study. *Lancet.* **359**: 926–30.

Paolisso G, De Riu S, Marrazzo G, Verza M, Varrichio M, D'Onofrio F. Insulin resistance and hyper-insulinemia in patients with chronic congestive heart failure. *Metabolism.* 1991; 40: 972–977.

Perez-Castrillon JL, Silva J, Justo I, Sanz A, Martin-Luquero M, Igea R, Escudero P, Pueyo C, Diaz C, Hernandez G, and Duenas A. 2003a Effect of quinapril, quinapril-hydrochlorothiazide, and enalapril on the bone mass of hypertensive subjects: relationship with angiotensin converting enzyme polymorphisms. *Am J Hypertens* **16**: 453–9.

Perez-Castrillon JL, Justo I, Silva J, Sanz A, Martin-Escudero JC, Igea R, Escudero P, Pueyo C, Diaz C, Hernandez G, and Duenas A. 2003b Relationship between bone mineral density and angiotensin converting enzyme polymorphism in hypertensive postmenopausal women. *Am J Hypertens* **16**: 233–5.

Phillips SK, Rook, KM, Siddle NC, Bruce SA & Woledge, R. C. (1993) Muscle weakness in women occurs at an earlier age than in men, but strength is preserved by hormone replacement therapy. *Clin Sci.* **84**: 95–98.

Phoon S, Howes LG. 2001 Role of angiotensin type 2 receptors in human forearm vascular responses of normal volunteers. *Clin Exp Pharmacol Physiol* **28**: 734–6.

Pieruzzi F, Abassi ZA, Keiser HR. 1995 Expression of renin-angiotensin system components in the heart, kidneys, and lungs of rats with experimental heart failure., *Circulation.* **92**: 3105–12.

Predel HG, Rohden C, Heine O, Prinz U and Rost RE. 1994 ACE inhibition and physical exercise: studies on physical work capacity, energy metabolism, and maximal oxygen uptake in well-trained, healthy subjects. *J Cardiovasc Pharmacol.* **23**: Suppl 1, S25–28.

Proudler AJ, Hasib Ahmed AI, Crook D, Fogelman I, Rymer JM and Stevenson JC. 1995 Hormone replacement therapy and serum angiotensin-converting-enzyme activity in postmenopausal women. *Lancet* **346**, 89–90.

Rankinen T, Wolfarth B, Simoneau J, Maier-Lenz D, Rauramaa R, Rivera MA, Boulay MR, Chagnon YC, Perusse L, Keul J, and Bouchard C. 2000 No association between the angiotensin-converting enzyme ID polymorphism and elite endurance athlete status. *J Appl Physiol* **88**: 1571–1575.

Rattigan S, Dora KA, Tong AC & Clark MG. 1996 Perfused skeletal muscle contraction and metabolism improved by angiotensin II-mediated vasoconstriction. *Am J Physiol.* **271**: E96–103.

Reneland R & Lithell H. 1994 Angiotensin-converting enzyme in human skeletal muscle. A simple in vitro assay of activity in needle biopsy specimens. *Scand J Clin Lab Invest.* **54**: 105–111.

Rett K, Wicklmayr M, Fink E, Maerker E, Dietze G, and Mehnert H. 1989 Local generation of kinins in working skeletal muscle tissue in man. *Biol. Chem. Hoppe. Seyler* **370**, 445–9.

Rett K, Wicklmayr M, and Dietze GJ. 1990 Metabolic effects of kinins: Historical and recent developments. *J Cardiovasc Pharmacol* **15**: S57–59.

Rhodes EC, Martin AD, Taunton JE, Donnelly M, Warren J and Elliot J. 2000 Effects of one year of resistance training on the relation between muscular strength and bone density in elderly women. *Br. J. Sports Med.* **34**, 18–22.

Rigat B, Hubert C, Alhenc-Gelas F, Cambien F, Corvol P & Soubrier F. 1990 An insertion/deletion polymorphism in the angiotensin-1-converting enzyme gene accounting for half the variance of serum enzyme levels. *J Clin Invest.* **86**: 1343–1346.

Rosendorff C. 1996 The renin-angiotensin system and vascular hypertrophy. *J Am Coll Cardiol.* **28**: 803–812.

Rossi GP, Narkiewicz K, Cesari M, Winnicki M, Bigda J, Chrostowska M, Szczech R, Pawlowski R, Pessina AC. 1999 Genetic determinants of plasma ACE and renin activity in young normotensive twins. *J Hyperten.* **17**: 647–55.

Russell ST, Wyke SM, Tisdale MJ. 2006 Mechanism of induction of muscle protein degradation by angiotensin II. Cell Signal. **18**: 1087–96.

Sabbah HN, Shimoyama H, Sharov VG, Kono T, Gupta RC, Lesch M, Levine TB & Goldstein S. 1996 Effects of ACE inhibition and beta-blockade on skeletal muscle fibre types in dogs with moderate heart failure. *Am J Physiol* **270**: H115–H120.

Sanders PM, Russell ST, Tisdale MJ. 2005 Angiotensin II directly induces muscle protein catabolism through the ubiquitin-proteasome proteolytic pathway and may play a role in cancer cachexia. *Br J Cancer.* **93**: 425–34.

Saris J, van Dijk MA, Kroon I, Schalekamp MA, Danser AH. 2000 Functional importance of angiotensin-converting enzyme-dependent in situ angiotensin II generation in the human forearm. *Hypertension.* **35**: 764–8.

Saxena PR. 1992 Interaction between the renin-angiotensin-aldosterone and sympathetic nervous systems. *J Cardiovasc Pharmacol.* **19**: S80–88.

Schaufelberger M, Drexler H, Schieffer E & Swedberg K. 1998 Angiotensin-converting enzyme gene expression in skeletal muscle in patients with chronic heart failure. *J Card Fail.* **4**: 185–191.

Scheen AJ. 2004 Renin-angiotensin system inhibition prevents type 2 diabetes mellitus. Part 1. Meta-analysis of randomised clinical trials. *Diab Metab.* 30: 487–96.

Schunkert H, Danser AHJ, Hense HW, Derkx FH, Kurzinger S, and Riegger GA. 1997 Effects of estrogen replacement therapy on the renin-angiotensin system in postmenopausal women. *Circulation.* **95**, 39–45.

Seltzer A, Pinto JE, Viglione PN, Correa FM, Libertun C, Tsutsumi K, Steele MK, and Saavedra JM. 1992 Estrogens regulate angiotensin-converting enzyme and angiotensin receptors in female rat anterior pituitary. *Neuroendocrinology* **55**, 460–7.

Sernia C. (2001) A critical appraisal of the intrinsic Pancreatic Angiotensin-generating system., *J Pancreas.* 2, 50–55.

Shah KR, Ganguly PK, Netticadan T, Arneja AS, Dhalla NS. 2004 Changes in skeletal muscle SR Ca2+ pump in congestive heart failure due to myocardial infarction are prevented by angiotensin II blockade. *Can J Physiol Pharmacol.* **82**: 438–47.

Shimojo N, Chao J, Chao L, Margolius HS, Mayfield RK. 1987 Identification and characterization of a tissue kallikrein in rat skeletal muscles. *Biochem J.* **243**: 773–8.

Shiuchi T, Nakagami H, Iwai M, Takeda Y, Cui T, Chen R, Minokoshi Y, Horiuchi M. 2001 Involvement of bradykinin and nitric oxide in leptin-mediated glucose uptake in skeletal muscle. *Endocrinology* **142**: 608–12. (2001)

Shiuchi T, Cui TX, Wu L, Nakagami H, Takeda-Matsubara Y, Iwai M, Horiuchi M. 2002 ACE inhibitor improves insulin resistance in diabetic mouse via bradykinin and NO. *Hypertension* **40**: 329–34

Song Y-H, Li Y, Du J, Mitch WE, Rosenthal N and Delafontaine P. 2005 Muscle-specific expression of IGF-1 blocks angiotensin II–induced skeletal muscle wasting. *J. Clin. Invest.* **115**: 451–458.

Sonna LA, Sharp MA, Knapik JJ, Cullivan M, Angel KC, Patton JF, and Lilly CM. 2001 Angiotensin-converting enzyme genotype and physical performance during US Army basic training. *J Appl Physiol* **91**: 1355–1363.

Sloniger JA, Saengsirisuwan V, Diehl CJ, Kim JS, Henriksen EJ. 2005 Selective angiotensin II receptor antagonism enhances whole-body insulin sensitivity and muscle glucose transport in hypertensive TG(mREN2)27 rats. *Metabolism.* **54**: 1659–68.

Story DF, Ziogas J. 1987 Interaction of angiotensin II with noradrenergic transmission. *Trends Pharmacol Sci.* **8**: 269–71.

Strassburg S, Springer J, Anker SD. 2005 Muscle wasting in cardiac cachexia. *Int J Biochem Cell Biol.* **37**: 1938-47.

Stroth U, Unger T. 1999 The renin-angiotensin system and its receptors. *J Cardiovasc Pharmacol.* **33** (Suppl. 1): S21–8.

Sullivan M, Green H & Cobb F. 1990 Skeletal muscle biochemistry and histology in ambulatory patients with long-term heart failure. *Circulation* **81**: 518–527.

Sumino H, Ichikawa S, Kanda T, Sakamaki T, Nakamura T, Sato K, Kobayashi I, and Nagai R. 1999 Hormone replacement therapy in postmenopausal women with essential hypertension increases circulating plasma levels of bradykinin. *Am. J.Hypertens.* **12**, 1044–7.

Sullivan MJ, & Hawthorne MH. 1995 Exercise intolerance in patients with chronic heart failure. *Prog Cardiovasc Dis.* **38:** 1–22.

Symons JD, Stebbins CL, Musch TI. 1999 Interactions between angiotensin II and nitric oxide during exercise in normal and heart failure rats. *J Appl Physiol.* **87**: 574–81.

Thomas W. 1999 Regulation of angiotensin II type 1 (AT1) receptor function. *Regul Pept.* **79**: 9-23.

Timmermans PB, MW, M., P. C. Wong, A. T. Chiu, W. F. Herblin, P. Benfield, D. J. Carini, R. J. Lee, R. R. Wexler, J. M. Saye, and R. D. Smith. (1993) Angiotensin II receptors and angiotensin II receptor antagonists. *Pharmacol. Rev.* **45**, 205–25

Tsianos G, Sanders J, Dhamrait S, Humphries S, Grant S, Montgomery H. 2004 The ACE gene insertion/deletion polymorphism and elite endurance swimming. *Eur J Appl Physiol.* **92**: 360–2.

Takekoshi K, Ishii K, Shibuya S, Kawakami Y, Isobe K, Nakai T. 2002 Angiotensin II type 2 receptor counter-regulates type 1 receptor in catecholamine synthesis in cultured porcine adrenal medullary chromaffin cells. *Hypertension* **39**: 142–8.

Taylor RR, Mamotte CDS, Fallon K, and Bockxmeer FM. 1999 Elite athletes and the gene for angiotensin-converting enzyme. *J. Appl. Physiol.* **87**: 1035–37.

Tsutsumi Y, Matsubara H, Masaki H, Kurihara H, Murasawa S, Takai S, Miyazaki M, Nozawa Y, Ozono R, Nakagawa K, Miwa T, Kawada N, Mori Y, Shibasaki Y, Tanaka Y, Fujiyama S, Koyama Y, Fujiyama A, Takahashi H, Iwasaka T. 1999 Angiotensin II type 2 receptor overexpression activates the vascular kinin system and causes vasodilation. J Clin Invest **104**: 925–35.

Ueda S, Elliott HL, Morton JJ, Connell JMC. 1995 Enhanced Pressor Response to Angiotensin I in Normotensive Men With the Deletion Genotype (DD) for Angiotensin-Converting Enzyme. *Hypertension.* **25**: 1266–69.

Unger T. 2002 The role of the renin-angiotensin system in the development of cardiovascular disease. *Am J Cardiol* **89**(2A): 3A–9A.

Vaghy PL, Russell JS, Lantry LE, Stephens RE, Ward PE. 1995 Angiotensin and bradykinin metabolism by peptidases identified in cultured human skeletal muscle myocytes and fibroblasts. *Peptides.* **16**: 1367–73.

van Dijk MA, Kroon I, Kamper AM, Boomsma F, Danser AH, Chang PC. 2000 The angiotensin-converting enzyme gene polymorphism and responses to angiotensins and bradykinin in the human forearm. *J Cardiovasc Pharmacol.* **35**: 484–90.

Vermes E, Ducharme A, Bourassa MG, Lessard M, White M, Tardif J-C. 2003 Enalapril Reduces the Incidence of Diabetes in Patients With Chronic Heart Failure Insight From the Studies Of Left Ventricular Dysfunction (SOLVD) *Circulation.* **107**: 1291

Vicaut E, Hou. X. 1993 Arteriolar constriction and local renin-angiotensin system in rat microcirculation. *Hypertension.* **21**: 491–7.

Viswanathan M, Tsutsumi K, Correa FMA, and Saavedra JM. 1991 Changes in the expression of angiotensin receptor subtypes in the rat aorta during development. *Biochem. Biophys. Res. Commun.* **179**: 1361–1367.

Ward PE, Russell JS & Vaghy PL. 1995 Angiotensin and bradykinin metabolism by peptidases identified in skeletal muscle. *Peptides.* **16**: 1073–1078.

Wei Y, Sowers JR, Nistala R, Gong H, Uptergrove GM, Clark SE, Morris EM, Szary N, Manrique C, Stump CS. 2006 Angiotensin II-induced NADPH oxidase activation impairs insulin signaling in skeletal muscle cells. *J Biol Chem.* **281**: 35137–46

Williams AG, Rayson MP, Jubb M, World M, Woods DR, Hayward M, Martin J, Humphries SE & Montgomery HE. 2000 The ACE gene and muscle performance, *Nature* **403**: 614.

Wong V, Szeto L, Uffelman K, Fantus IG, Lewis GF. 2006 Enhancement of muscle glucose uptake by the vasopeptidase inhibitor, omapatrilat, is independent of insulin signaling and the AMP kinase pathway. *J Endocrinol.* **190**: 441–50.

Woods D, Onambele G, Woledge R, Skelton D, Bruce S, Humphries S and Montgomery H. 2001 Angiotensin-I converting enzyme genotype-dependent benefit from hormone replacement therapy in isometric muscle strength and bone mineral density. *J Clin Endocrinol Metab.* **86**: 2200–4.

Woods DR, World M, Rayson MP, Williams AG, Jubb M, Jamshidi Y, Hayward M, Mary DASG, Humphries SE, Montgomery HE. 2002 Endurance enhancement related to the human angiotensin I-converting enzyme I-D polymorphism is not due to differences in the cardiorespiratory response to training. *Eur J Appl Physiol* **86**: 240–244.

Woods DR, Hickmann M, Jamshidi Y, Brull D, Vassiliou V, Jones A, Humphries S, Montgomery H. 2001 Elite swimmers and the D allele of the ACE I/D polymorphism. *Hum. Genet.* **108**: 230–2.

Yusuf S, Ostergren JB, Gerstein HC, Pfeffer MA, Swedberg K, Granger CB, Olofsson B, Probstfield J, McMurray JV; Candesartan in Heart Failure-Assessment of Reduction in Mortality and Morbidity Program Investigators. 2005 Effects of candesartan on the development of a new diagnosis of diabetes mellitus in patients with heart failure. *Circulation.* **112**: 48–53.

Yusuf S, Sleight P, Pogue J, Bosch J, Davies R & Dagenais G. 2000 Effects of an angiotensin-converting-enzyme inhibitor, ramipril, on cardiovascular events in high-risk patients. The Heart Outcomes Prevention Evaluation Study Investigators. *N Engl J Med* **342:** 145–53.

Zhang B, Tanaka H, Shono N, Miura S, Kiyonaga A, Shindo M, Saku K. 2003 The I allele of the angiotensin-converting enzyme gene is associated with an increased percentage of slow-twitch type I fibers in human skeletal muscle. *Clin Genet.* **63**: 139–44.

Zhao W, Swanson SA, Ye J, Li X, Shelton JM, Zhang W, Thomas GD. 2006 Reactive oxygen species impair sympathetic vasoregulation in skeletal muscle in angiotensin II-dependent hypertension. *Hypertension.* **48**: 637–43.

Zisman, L. S. 1998 Inhibiting tissue Angiotensin-converting enzyme. A pound of flesh without the blood? *Circulation.* **98**: 2788–2790.

Zoll J, Monassier L, Garnier A, N'Guessan B, Mettauer B, Veksler V, Piquard F, Ventura-Clapier R, Geny B. 2006 ACE inhibition prevents myocardial infarction-induced skeletal muscle mitochondrial dysfunction. *J Appl Physiol.* **101**: 385–91.

CHAPTER 12

LOCAL ANGIOTENSIN GENERATION AND AT₂ RECEPTOR ACTIVATION

JOEP H.M. VAN ESCH AND A.H. JAN DANSER

Department of Pharmacology, Erasmus MC, Rotterdam, The Netherlands

1. INTRODUCTION

The renin-angiotensin system (RAS) plays an important role in the regulation of blood pressure and body fluid homeostasis. Traditionally, the RAS has been viewed as a circulating system ("circulating" RAS). However, it is now well-established that angiotensin (Ang) generation also occurs at tissue sites ("tissue" RAS). The complexity of the system has increased even further now that we know that Ang II activates more than one receptor, that Ang II has metabolites which activate their own receptors, and that there may even be receptors for renin and prorenin. This review summarizes the latest insights on tissue angiotensin generation and focuses in particular on the activation of the Ang II type 2 (AT_2) receptor by locally generated Ang II.

2. THE RENIN-ANGIOTENSIN SYSTEM

2.1. Renin, Prorenin and (Pro)Renin Receptors

Renin belongs to the family of aspartyl proteases and has only one known substrate, angiotensinogen, the precursor of all angiotensin peptides. Structure analysis revealed that renin consists of 2 homologous lobes which form a cleft containing the active site. Renin has an inactive precursor, prorenin, in which the active site is covered by the prosegment.

The renin gene was cloned in the 1980s in human, rat and mouse. Most species have one renin gene (*ren-1ᶜ*), although some mouse strains have two renin genes, *ren-1ᵈ* and a submandibular variant, designated as *ren-2*. The *ren-2* gene is encoding for a nonglycosylated prorenin, as opposed to the *ren-1* gene which can be glycosylated at three asparagine residues. The renin gene is located on chromosome 1 in human and mouse, whereas it is localized on chromosome 13 in rat.

Po Sing Leung (ed.), Frontiers in Research of the Renin-Angiotensin System on Human Disease, 247–272.
© 2007 *Springer.*

The renin gene encodes for pre-prorenin consisting of a presegment of 23 amino acids, a prosegment of 43 amino acids and the actual renin protein of 340 amino acids (Morris 1992). The presegment functions as a signal peptide directing prorenin to the secretory pathway. Recently, a splice-variant of the renin gene was discovered which lacks the signal peptide and part of the prosegment. This truncated prorenin displays enzymatic activity because the truncated prosegment only partially covers the enzymatic cleft. It is thought to remain intracellular (Clausmeyer et al 2000), although truncated prorenin has also been demonstrated extracellularly (Shinagawa et al 1992).

Mice lacking the ren-1^d gene are characterized by sexually dimorphic hypotension (leading to a significant reduction of blood pressure in female mice), absence of dense secretory/storage granule formation in juxta-glomerular cells, altered morphology of the kidney, and a significant increase of plasma prorenin levels (Clark et al 1997). Deletion of the ren-2 gene resulted in increased renin and decreased prorenin levels (Sharp et al 1996), but no changes in blood pressure, nor morphological changes occurred.

Transgenic mice overexpressing human renin did not develop hypertension whereas transgenic mice expressing both human renin and human angiotensinogen showed a significantly increased blood pressure (Fukamizu et al 1993). The plasma concentrations of Ang I and Ang II were 3-5-fold increased in double transgenic mice as compared to either control mice or transgenic mice overexpressing human renin. These results demonstrate that human renin does not crossreact with mouse angiotensinogen, thereby illustrating the unique species specifity of the RAS.

Prorenin can be activated through cleavage of the prosegment (proteolytic activation) or via a conformational change induced by low pH or low temperature (non-proteolytic activation) (Danser and Deinum 2005) (Fig. 1). Proteolytic activation is an irreversible process in which the prosegment is cleaved, e.g., by kallikrein, trypsin or plasmin. In vivo, proteolytic activation is probably mediated by a proconvertase in the renin-producing cells of the juxta-glomerular apparatus of the kidney. Non-proteolytic activation of prorenin is a reversible process in which prorenin is converted from the 'closed' (inactive) to the 'open' (active) conformation by unfolding of the prosegment from the enzymatic cleft (Suzuki et al 2003). Acid activation leads to complete activation of prorenin whereas exposure to cold ('cryoactivation') only leads to partial activation ($\sim$15%). Kinetic studies have shown that an equilibrium exists between the closed and open conformations of prorenin, and that under physiological conditions (pH 7.4, 37°C) <2% of prorenin is in the open conformation (Danser and Deinum 2005).

The kidneys are the main source of circulating (pro)renin. However, following a bilateral nephrectomy, prorenin, in contrast with renin, remains detectable. This suggests that prorenin is also produced outside the kidney. Potential extrarenal prorenin-producing tissues are the eye, adrenal, ovary and testis (Sealey et al 1988; Danser et al 1989; Itskovitz et al 1992; Clausmeyer et al 2000). Normally, the concentration of prorenin in human plasma is 10 times higher than that of renin. The reasons for this excess are unknown, as prorenin does not seem to be activated

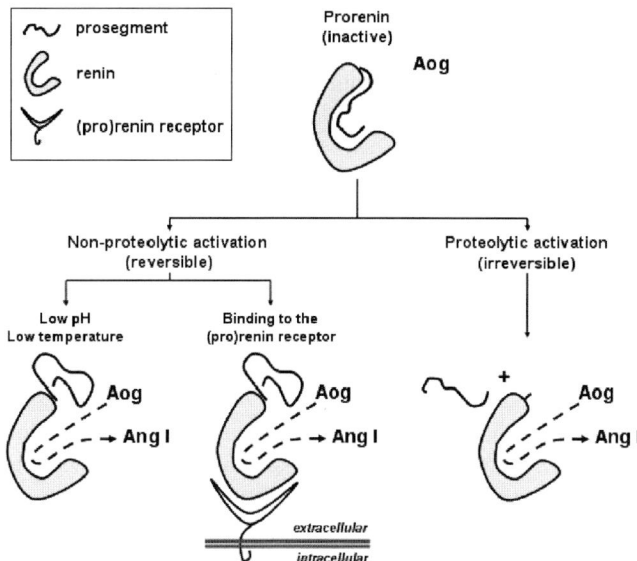

Figure 1. Proteolytic and non-proteolytic activation of prorenin. Aog, angiotensinogen; Ang, angiotensin. See text for explanation

outside the kidney (Lenz *et al* 1990). One possibility is that prorenin has functions unrelated to angiotensin generation. In this regard, it is of interest to note that it has recently been suggested that prorenin binds to a '(pro)renin receptor', thereby activating second messenger pathways in a manner that is independent of Ang II (Nguyen *et al* 2002; Saris *et al* 2006). (Pro)renin receptors may also mediate the uptake of renin and/or prorenin into tissues that do not synthesize renin and prorenin themselves, like the heart and the vessel wall.

To date, two (pro)renin-binding receptors have been identified: the mannose-6-phosphate (M6P) receptor (Saris *et al* 2001) and the above-mentioned (pro)renin receptor. The M6P receptor is identical to the insulin-like growth factor II (IGFII) receptor and binds IGFII, M6P-containing proteins such as prorenin and renin, and retinoic acid at distinct sites (Kornfeld 1992; Kang *et al* 1997). Prorenin and renin are both rapidly internalized after binding to this receptor, and internalized prorenin is proteolytically converted to renin. However, binding to this receptor did not result in angiotensin generation, either intra- or extracellularly. This, in combination with the fact that intracellularly generated renin was found to be degraded within a few hours, suggests that M6P/IGFII receptors function as clearance receptors for (pro)renin. Alternatively, since binding of M6P-containing proteins to M6P/IGFII receptors results in the activation of second messenger pathways involving G-proteins (Di Bacco and Gill 2003), (pro)renin may act as an M6P/IGFII receptor agonist.

The (pro)renin receptor was cloned by Nguyen and co-workers (Nguyen *et al* 2002). Prorenin and renin bind equally well to this receptor, without being internalized or degraded. Interestingly, the catalytic activity of bound renin was increased

5-fold, and receptor-bound prorenin became fully active in a non-proteolytic manner. Thus, apparently, this receptor allows prorenin to generate angiotensins at tissue sites. Importantly, binding of (pro)renin to the (pro)renin receptor in human mesangial cells also induced Ang II-independent effects, such as an increase in DNA synthesis, activation of the mitogen-activated protein kinases (MAPKs) extracellular signal-regulated kinase (ERK)1 (p44)/ERK2 (p42), and plasminogen-activator inhibitor-1 release. Furthermore, in cardiomyocytes, prorenin activated the p38 MAPK/heat shock protein 27 pathway, resulting in changes of actin filament dynamics (Saris et al 2006). These non-angiotensin-mediated effects may underlie the blood pressure-independent cardiac hypertrophy in rats with a hepatic prorenin overexpression (Véniant et al 1996).

Finally, Peters and co-workers demonstrated ren-2 prorenin internalization in cardiomyocytes of transgenic rats expressing the mouse ren-2 gene in the liver (Peters et al 2002). Since ren-2 prorenin is nonglycosylated, this phenomenon cannot be mediated by M6P/IGFII receptors. The internalization contrasts with the observations on the recently cloned (pro)renin receptor. Thus, there may be a third (pro)renin receptor, the identity of which is currently unclear.

2.2.   Angiotensinogen

Angiotensinogen, the precursor of all angiotensin metabolites, is the only known substrate for renin. The angiotensinogen gene encodes for a glycoprotein of 453 amino acids with a molecular weight of $\sim$60 kDa. The gene is located as a single copy on, respectively, chromosome 19 in rats, chromosome 8 in mice and chromosome 1 in humans. In 1983, Doolittle reported a significant sequence homology of angiotensinogen to α_1-antitrypsin (23%), ovalbumin (21%) and antithrombin III (18%) (Doolittle 1983). These proteins are members of the serine proteinase inhibitor family and are closely associated with acute inflammation reactions. Acute inflammation induces gene expression via acute-response which increases the angiotensinogen concentration in plasma (Kageyama et al 1985). The similarity between the structural organization of the angiotensinogen and α_1-antitrypsin genes suggests that both genes have evolved from a common ancestor (Kitamura et al 1987).

Although angiotensinogen mRNA has been detected in brain, adipocytes, heart and the reproductive system, its main source is the liver (Paul et al 2006). Hepatocytes constitutively secrete angiotensinogen into the extracellular fluid, without intracellular storage. Blood plasma/extracellular fluid functions as the major reservoir for angiotensinogen. Angiotensinogen plasma concentrations ($\sim$1 µM) approximate the Michaelis-Menten constant of the renin reaction, which makes RAS activity sensitive to small changes in angiotensinogen concentration. Deletion of the angiotensinogen gene in mice leads to hypotension, low body weight gain after birth, and an abnormal morphology of kidney and heart (Niimura et al 1995). In turn, overexpression of angiotensinogen led to the development of hypertension (Kimura et al 1992).

2.3.   ACE and ACE2

Two isoforms of ACE exist: somatic ACE and testis (germinal) ACE. Somatic ACE is abundantly expressed throughout the body, whereas testis ACE is exclusively expressed in the testis. Cloning of the ACE gene provided a better understanding of the relationship between somatic and testis ACE. Both forms are transcribed from the same gene by using different promoters (Hubert *et al* 1991). In humans the ACE gene is located on chromosome 17. Somatic ACE has 2 homologous domains which share 60% sequence homology. Both domains contain a catalytically active site (Wei *et al* 1991a) and are situated at the N- and C-terminal side of ACE. According to their position they are designated as N- and C-domain. The majority of somatic ACE is membrane-bound on endothelial cells. Circulating ACE is derived from ACE-expressing cells by proteolytic cleavage at the juxta-membrane stalk region (Wei *et al* 1991b). Testis ACE possesses only one catalytic domain which is identical to the C-domain of somatic ACE. Studies selectively blocking the C- and N-domain of somatic ACE revealed that conversion of Ang I to Ang II by membrane-bound ACE depends on the C-domain, whereas both domains contribute to this conversion in soluble ACE (van Esch *et al* 2005). Degradation of bradykinin at tissue sites also required both domains (Tom *et al* 2001). Deletion of both somatic and testis ACE (ACE$^{-/-}$) in mice led to hypotension, male infertility and changes in kidney morphology (Esther *et al* 1996). Vascular expression of germinal ACE in Ace null mice restored renal morphology but did not normalize blood pressure, thus demonstrating that germinal ACE cannot functionally substitute for somatic ACE (Kessler *et al* 2007).

Recently, a homologue of somatic ACE called ACE2 was discovered (Donoghue *et al* 2000). ACE2 shares 42% homology with the C- and N-terminal domains of somatic ACE. The gene encoding ACE2 is located on the X chromosome and ACE2 is mainly expressed in endothelial cells of heart, kidney and testis. Like somatic ACE, ACE2 can be released into the circulation after proteolytic cleavage (Turner and Hooper 2002). Unlike somatic ACE, ACE2 has only one catalytically active site which can convert Ang I and Ang II to Ang (1-9) and Ang (1-7), respectively (Donoghue *et al* 2000; Vickers *et al* 2002). These data suggest a potential role of ACE2 in the counterregulation of high blood pressure by inactivation of Ang II. Indeed, in a model of Ang II-dependent hypertension, blood pressures were substantially higher in ACE2-deficient mice than in wildtype controls (Gurley *et al* 2006). Mice lacking the ACE2 gene were originally described to develop an abnormal heart function with severely impaired contractility (Crackower *et al* 2002), but this was not confirmed in a follow-up study (Gurley *et al* 2006). Remarkably, ACE2 also functions as a receptor for the virus causing severe acute respiratory syndrome, thereby stressing the importance of ACE2 in a manner unrelated to the RAS (Li *et al* 2003).

2.4.   Angiotensin II Receptors

Initially, it was thought that the responses to Ang II were mediated by a single Ang II receptor. At the end of the 1980s, the discovery of specific Ang II receptor ligands such as losartan, PD12377, PD123319 and CGP42112 made it possible to identify several Ang II receptor subtypes. We now know that the biological actions of Ang II in man are mediated by at least two types of Ang II receptors: Ang II type 1 (AT_1) and AT_2 receptors (Fig. 3).

2.4.1. AT_1 receptor

AT_1 receptors mediate virtually all the known physiological actions of Ang II, such as vasoconstriction, inotropy, chronotropy, aldosterone release, noradrenaline release and growth stimulation. The AT_1 receptor gene encodes for a protein of 359 amino acids with a molecular weight of 41 kDa. The gene was first cloned in 1991 from rat vascular smooth muscle cells (Murphy *et al* 1991) and bovine adrenal gland (Sasaki *et al* 1991). Cloning and genetic analysis of the human AT_1 receptor gene revealed that the human AT_1 receptor gene is located on chromosome 3 and can produce two isoforms by alternative splicing. Both isoforms have similar binding - and functional properties.

In rodents two subtypes of the AT_1 receptor have been identified: AT_{1A} and AT_{1B} (Elton *et al* 1992). The origin of these subtypes lies in a gene duplication which occurred after the divergence of rodents from the human/artiodactyls group about 24 million years ago. AT_{1A} and AT_{1B} share 94% sequence homology and are located on chromosome 17 and 2 in rat and chromosome 13 and 3 in mice, respectively. Not surprisingly, both subtypes have similar ligand binding affinities and signal transduction properties but varying expression levels in different tissues. The AT_{1A} receptor predominates in heart, kidney, lung, liver and vascular smooth muscle, whereas the AT_{1B} receptor is mainly expressed in the adrenal and pituitary gland (Burson *et al* 1994). To date, there are no pharmacological antagonists which clearly discriminate AT_{1A} and AT_{1B} receptors.

Studies in mice using targeted gene manipulation provided more insight in the functional role of both subtypes *in vivo*. Deletion of the AT_{1A} receptor gene significantly decreased resting blood pressure in both heterozygous $AT_{1A}^{+/-}$ and homozygous $AT_{1A}^{-/-}$ receptor mice (Ito *et al* 1995). Ang II infusions resulted in a diminished pressor response in $AT_{1A}^{+/-}$ receptor mutants whereas this response was virtually abolished in $AT_{1A}^{-/-}$ mutants. Additionally, both the expression levels of renin mRNA and plasma renin activity were markedly increased in AT_{1A} receptor knockout mice (Sugaya *et al* 1995). Deletion of the AT_{1B} receptor gene did not affect resting blood pressure, nor altered the pressure response to Ang II (Chen *et al* 1997). Taken together, these findings indicate the important role of the AT_{1A} receptor in mediating the pressure response in mice. AT_{1A} or AT_{1B} receptor deficiency is not associated with an impaired development or survival, but double knockout mice lacking both receptors display a phenotype similar to that observed in angiotensinogen knockout mice (Tsuchida *et al* 1998). These observations, together with the fact that Ang II does cause a pressor response in AT_{1A} knockout mice after enalapril pretreatment (Oliverio *et al* 1997), suggest a compensatory role for the AT_{1B} receptor. Additionally, *in vitro* studies demonstrated that the AT_{1B} receptor is the most important regulator of Ang II contractile responses in the mouse aorta and femoral artery (Zhou *et al* 2003).

The AT_1 receptor belongs to the seven-transmembrane G-protein-coupled receptor superfamily, and couples to a wide variety of second messenger systems, including the phospholipase C/inositol-1,4,5-triphosphate/diacylglycerol/protein kinase C pathway, the phospholipase A_2/arachidonic acid pathway, the phospholipase D/phosphatidylcholine/phosphatidic acid pathway, and tyrosine kinases such as the MAP kinases ERK1/2, p38 and c-jun N-terminal kinase (Mehta and Griendling 2007).

AT_1 receptor stimulation results in a rapid internalization of the Ang II-AT_1 receptor complex, followed by either receptor degradation in lysosomes or receptor recycling to the cell surface (Mehta and Griendling 2007). Internalized Ang II has been proposed to activate cytoplasmic or nuclear receptors prior to its intracellular degradation (Thomas *et al* 1996). Furthermore, Zou and co-workers recently demonstrated that mechanical stretch resulted in AT_1 receptor activation in a ligand-independent manner. Interestingly, the consequences of such activation could be prevented by an AT_1 receptor blocker (Zou *et al* 2004).

Several reports have described crosstalk between AT_1 receptor and other receptors, e.g. the bradykinin type 2 (B_2) receptor, the AT_2 receptor, and the α_1–adrenoceptor. AT_1 and B_2 receptors form stable heterodimers with an enhanced G-protein activation and altered receptor sequestration (AbdAlla *et al* 2000). AT_1 receptor-α_1-adrenoceptor crosstalk enhances the response to α_1-adrenoceptor agonists (Purdy and Weber 1988). Interestingly, although the postjunctional AT_1 receptor interacting with the α_1–adrenoceptor is of the AT_{1A} subtype, the prejunctional AT_1 receptor which facilitates noradrenaline release from sympathetic nerve endings is of the AT_{1B} subtype (Guimaraes and Pinheiro 2005).

2.4.2.   *AT₂ receptor*

In contrast to the well-characterized AT_1 receptor, the function of the AT_2 receptor is much less understood. In general, it is assumed that AT_2 receptors counteract the responses mediated by the AT_1 receptor (Hein *et al* 1995; Ichiki *et al* 1995; AbdAlla *et al* 2001; Schuijt *et al* 2001; Batenburg *et al* 2004). AT_2 receptors are involved in physiological processes like development and tissue remodeling (by inhibiting cell growth and by stimulating apoptosis), regulation of blood pressure (vasodilatation), natriuresis and neuronal activity.

Evidence for AT_2 receptor mediated vasodilatation is largely based on two approaches: an indirect approach, showing an enhanced response to Ang II in the presence of AT_2 receptor blockade or gene disruption (Hein *et al* 1995; Ichiki *et al* 1995; Batenburg *et al* 2004; van Esch *et al* 2006), and a direct approach showing AT_2 receptor-induced responses by applying either the (partial) AT_2 receptor agonist CGP42112A or Ang II in the presence of an AT_1 receptor blocker (Widdop *et al* 2002; Li and Widdop 2004).

The AT_2 receptor gene was first cloned in 1993 (Mukoyama *et al* 1993). The AT_2 receptor gene shares 34% sequence homology with its AT_1 receptor counterpart and encodes for a protein of 363 amino acids with a molecular mass of 41 kDa. It is located on the X chromosome in both humans and rodents. In fetal tissues the AT_2 receptor is the predominant subtype. This situation changes rapidly after birth, resulting in the AT_1 receptor becoming the dominant subtype in most adult tissues (Widdop et al 2003). Yet, in adults, AT_2 receptors can still be detected in a variety of tissues, including uterus, ovary, adrenal medulla, heart, blood vessels and brain (Bottari et al 1993). Here it is important to consider that the distribution of the AT_2 receptor depends on age and species, but is also subject to changes in expression during pregnancy and pathological conditions such as hypertension, heart failure and vascular injury (see below) (Bottari et al 1993; de Gasparo et al 2000).

In 1995, two groups reported that deletion of the AT_2 receptor in mice led to an increased pressor response to Ang II (Hein et al 1995; Ichiki et al 1995). Additionally, Ichiki et al reported a significant increased blood pressure in hemizygous $AT_2^{-/Y}$ receptor mice whereas blood pressure was not significantly increased in a similar model described by Hein and co-workers. Mutants lacking the AT_2 receptor gene showed a lower body temperature and impaired exploratory behavior. Remarkably, despite its wide expression in the fetus, the AT_2 receptor does not seem to be required for embryonic development, as no morphological and developmental differences were found between homozygous $AT_2^{-/-}$ or hemizygous $AT_2^{-/Y}$ receptor mice and their wildtype controls. Possibly, AT_2 receptor knockout mice display a delayed expression of calponin and h-caldesmon after birth (Yamada et al 1999). During pregnancy, Ang II levels are elevated. Because the fetus is also exposed to these high Ang II levels, it has been postulated that the AT_2 receptor plays a role in the regulation of Ang II responsiveness in order to prevent fetal hypertension (Perlegas et al 2005).

Like AT_1 receptors, AT_2 receptors belong to the G protein-coupled receptor superfamily. However, in contrast to the AT_1 receptor, the AT_2 receptor is not internalized upon binding of Ang II (Widdop et al 2003). Two major pathways have been described for AT_2 receptor signaling (Nouet and Nahmias 2000): (a) activation of protein phosphatases causing protein dephosphorylation and (b) activation of the nitric oxide (NO)/guanosine cyclic 3', 5'-monophosphate (cGMP) pathway. Up to now, three specific phosphatases have been linked to AT_2 receptor activation: MAPK phosphatase 1, SH2-domain-containing phosphatase 1 and protein phosphatase 2A. Growth factors, including Ang II via the AT_1 receptor, mediate their growth promoting actions through tyrosine kinase receptors and several kinase-driven phosphorylation steps. Activation of the AT_2 receptor counteracts these growth-promoting actions by dephosphorylation through subsequent activation of phosphatases. In addition to the inhibitory effect on growth, dephosphorylation (e.g., of ERK1/2) also seems to play an important role in the stimulation of apoptosis (Horiuchi et al 1998).

Several studies have shown that AT_2 receptor-mediated vasodilation is an endothelium-dependent phenomenon involving B_2 receptors, NO and cGMP (Wiemer et al 1993; Siragy and Carey 1997) (Fig. 2). Initially, in vitro studies using endothelial cells showed that the stimulatory effect of Ang II on cGMP production,

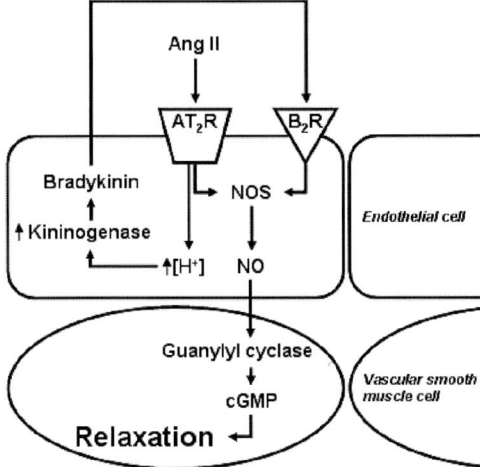

Figure 2. AT$_2$ receptor-mediated relaxation involves either intracellular activation of kininogenase and subsequent bradykinin type 2 (B_2) receptor activation, or a direct activation of NO synthase (NOS)

a downstream signaling product of NO production, was abolished by blocking both B$_2$ receptors and nitric oxide synthase (NOS) (Wiemer *et al* 1993). Subsequent *in vivo* studies confirmed that the AT$_2$ receptor-induced rise in cGMP involves bradykinin and NO (Siragy and Carey 1997). *In vitro* studies in endothelial cells reported that intracellular acidosis, as a result of AT$_2$ receptor activation, stimulates bradykinin formation by activating kininogenases (Tsutsumi *et al* 1999). Katada and Majima were able to show production of bradykinin after AT$_2$ activation in rat mesenteric arteries, suggesting that the B$_2$ receptor mediates vasodilatation by endogenous bradykinin released upon AT$_2$ receptor activation (Katada and Majima 2002). In agreement with this concept, deletion of the B$_2$ receptor enhanced the Ang II-induced hypertensive response *in vivo* (Cervenka *et al* 2001). Additional studies concluded that NO production following AT$_2$ receptor stimulation may also occur independently of B$_2$ receptors, through direct NOS activation (Abadir *et al* 2003), possibly involving the calcineurin/nuclear factor of activated T cells pathway (Ritter *et al* 2003).

As both AT$_2$ and B$_2$ receptors are co-expressed in various tissues, the hypothesis was raised that both receptors form heterodimers which can interact through receptor crosstalk. Recent studies in rat pheochromocytoma cells, applying fluorescence resonance energy transfer, confirmed this hypothesis (Abadir *et al* 2006). Heterodimer formation appeared to be dependent on the receptor number that was expressed, but also required AT$_2$ receptor stimulation. As a consequence of heterodimer formation, it is possible that AT$_2$ receptor activation results in B$_2$ receptor activation without intermediate bradykinin synthesis (Batenburg *et al* 2004).

In addition to its interaction with the B$_2$ receptor, AT$_2$ receptors are also known to interact with their AT$_1$ counterpart. Transfection studies in fetal fibroblasts showed that AT_1 and AT_2 receptors form heterodimers in which the AT_2 receptor functions as a specific AT_1 receptor antagonist (AbdAlla et al 2001). Possibly, AT_2 receptor-induced vasodilatation depends on simultaneous AT_1 receptor activation, as no AT_2 receptor-mediated responses were noted in the absence of AT_1 receptors (van Esch et al 2006).

Furthermore, it is important to consider that data obtained in absence of the AT_2 receptor are complex because AT_2 receptors downregulate AT_1 receptors in a ligand-independent manner (Jin et al 2002) and AT_2 receptor knockout mice display an increased AT_1 receptor expression (Tanaka et al 1999). In addition to its interaction with AT_1 receptors, the AT_2 receptor also downregulates renin biosynthesis, thereby inhibiting the formation of Ang II (Siragy et al 2005).

2.5.   Angiotensin-Derived Metabolites and Their Receptors

Ang I and II are metabolized by a whole range of peptidases ('angiotensinases'). Although initially it was thought that all metabolites other than Ang II were inactive, it is now clear that at least several of these metabolites have functions of their own, which are sometimes mediated via non-AT_1/AT_2 receptors. The most important of these peptides are Ang (1-7), Ang (2-8) (Ang III) and Ang (3-8) (Ang IV) (Fig. 3).

Ang (1-7) can be formed from Ang I by the action of neutral endopeptidase or prolyl endopeptidase but also from the Ang I degradation products Ang (1-9) and Ang II (Vickers et al 2002). Ang (1-7) is generally believed to counteract the response of Ang II although there are reports of similar or distinct actions from Ang II (Santos et al 2000). Ang (1-7) induces relaxation in several vascular beds. The fact that this relaxation could be blocked by the selective Ang (1-7) antagonist A-779 [D-Ala^7-Ang (1-7)] suggested the involvement of a specific Ang (1-7) receptor (Santos et al 2000). Indeed, in 2003 the Mas proto-oncogene, a G protein-coupled receptor, was proposed to be the receptor for Ang (1-7) (Santos et al 2003). Ang (1-7) potentiates bradykinin-induced responses (Tom et al 2001) and releases NO (Brosnihan et al 1996) via Mas receptor stimulation. Mas receptor mRNA expression has been detected in heart, testis, kidney and brain (Metzger et al 1995). Mice deficient for the Mas-receptor lack the antidiuretic action of Ang (1-7) after an acute water load, and their aortas no longer relax in response to Ang (1-7) (Santos et al 2003). Mas$^{-/-}$ mice are also characterized by an impaired heart function, indicating an important role of the Mas receptor in the maintenance of the structure and function of the heart (Santos et al 2006).

Although the Mas-receptor is now held responsible for most of the responses to Ang (1-7), there are several other pharmacological mechanisms and receptors that are affected by Ang (1-7). As a slow substrate for ACE, Ang (1-7) may also function as an ACE inhibitor, resulting in decreased Ang II formation and potentiation of bradykinin-induced vasodilatation (Tom et al 2001). Furthermore, Ang (1-7) acts as an AT_1 receptor antagonist at low concentrations (Stegbauer et al 2003), and exerts AT_1 receptor agonistic effects at high concentrations (van Rodijnen et al 2002). A link between Ang (1-7) and the AT_2 receptor has recently been

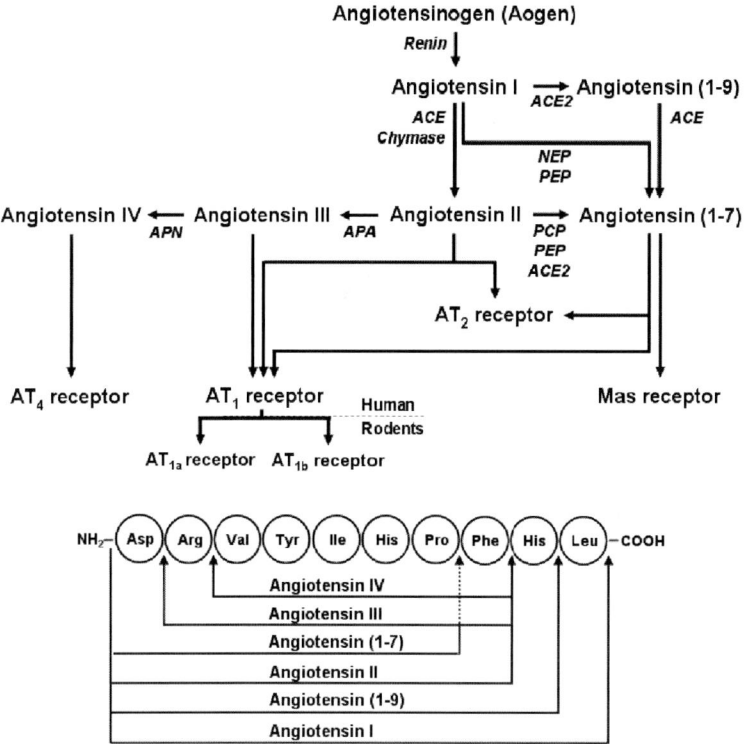

Figure 3. Schematical overview of the generation of angiotensin I and its metabolites. NEP, neutral endopeptidase; PEP, prolyl endopeptidase; PCP, prolyl carboxypeptidase; APA, aminopeptidase A; APN, aminopeptidase N

proposed, because infusion of Ang (1-7) during AT$_1$ receptor blockade unmasked a vasodepressor response in conscious SHR rats that could be attenuated by blockade of AT$_2$ receptors, B$_2$ receptors and NOS (Walters *et al* 2005). Possibly, Mas-AT$_1$ and/or Mas-AT$_2$ receptor heterodimers exist (Castro *et al* 2005; Lemos *et al* 2005).

Through the action of aminopeptidase A, Ang II is converted to Ang III, which in turn can be converted to Ang IV by aminopeptidase N (Ardaillou and Chansel 1997). Ang III mediates some of the classical responses of Ang II (such as stimulation of aldosterone secretion and vasoconstriction) and this most likely involves binding to AT$_1$ and AT$_2$ receptors. The affinity of Ang III for these receptors is somewhat lower than that of Ang II (Wright and Harding 1995). The responses to Ang III are less efficacious than those of Ang II, possibly due to its accelerated metabolism in the circulation. The latter relates to the wide distribution of aminopeptidase N that initiates the hydrolysis of Ang III but not Ang II. It is thought that Ang III might be the final mediator of some of the actions of Ang II. For example, the central action of Ang II on vasopressin secretion in rats is dependent on Ang III, as this effect was absent after specific blockade of aminopeptidase A (Zini *et al* 1996).

Additionally, Ang III, and not Ang II, mediates the excretion of Na^+ excretion through AT_2 receptors in the presence of AT_1 receptor blockade (Padia *et al* 2006).

Ang IV was initially believed to have no biological activity. This was based on two important findings: both AT_1 and AT_2 receptors display a poor affinity for Ang IV, and Ang IV does not elicit the characteristic Ang II responses like Ang III. The discovery of a specific Ang IV binding site, designated as the AT_4 receptor, changed this view (Swanson *et al* 1992). After purification, the receptor was identified as insulin-regulated aminopeptidase (Albiston *et al* 2001), a protein which is abundantly found in vesicles containing the insulin-sensitive glucose transporter (GLUT4) (Keller *et al* 1995). AT_4 receptor expression occurs in brain, spinal cord, heart, kidney, colon, prostate, adrenal gland, bladder and vascular smooth muscle cells (Wright and Harding 1995; de Gasparo *et al* 2000). Ang IV and the AT_4 receptor appear to be involved in the facilitation of memory and learning (Wright *et al* 1999). Ang IV infusions cause vasorelaxation in cerebral and renal vascular beds, possibly by increasing NOS activity (Patel *et al* 1998). On the other hand, there are also studies showing that Ang IV, because of its weak agonistic activity towards the AT_1 receptor, induces vasoconstriction (van Rodijnen *et al* 2002). The close association of the AT_4 receptor with GLUT4 suggests that Ang IV might modulate glucose uptake.

3.   TISSUE ANGIOTENSIN GENERATION

As soon as it was realized that angiotensin production at tissue sites is of greater importance than angiotensin generation in the circulation, many investigators started to unravel how and where such local angiotensin production might occur. Initially, it was thought that all components required for local Ang II production (i.e., renin, angiotensinogen and ACE) would be produced at tissue sites. Infusions of radiolabeled angiotensins, allowing the quantification of uptake of blood-derived angiotensin in tissues, confirmed that the majority of tissue Ang I and II is produced at tissue sites, and not derived from blood (Schuijt and Danser 2002).

ACE is well-known to be abundantly expressed in virtually every tissue of the body, its main site being the surface of endothelial cells. Thus, its local synthesis is beyond doubt. Although angiotensinogen mRNA has been detected outside the liver, direct proof for actual angiotensinogen synthesis at important sites of local angiotensin production (e.g., heart and vessel wall) is lacking. For instance, the isolated perfused heart does not release angiotensinogen (de Lannoy *et al* 1997). Therefore, the majority of tissue angiotensinogen is probably of hepatic origin. The fact that angiotensinogen is neither internalized, nor binds to membranes, combined with the observation that angiotensinogen-synthesizing cells release angiotensinogen to the extracellular space (Klett *et al* 1993), rather than storing it intracellularly, indicates that angiotensin generation must occurs extracellularly. Thus, tissue angiotensin generation is restricted to the interstitial space and/or the cell surface (Fig. 4).

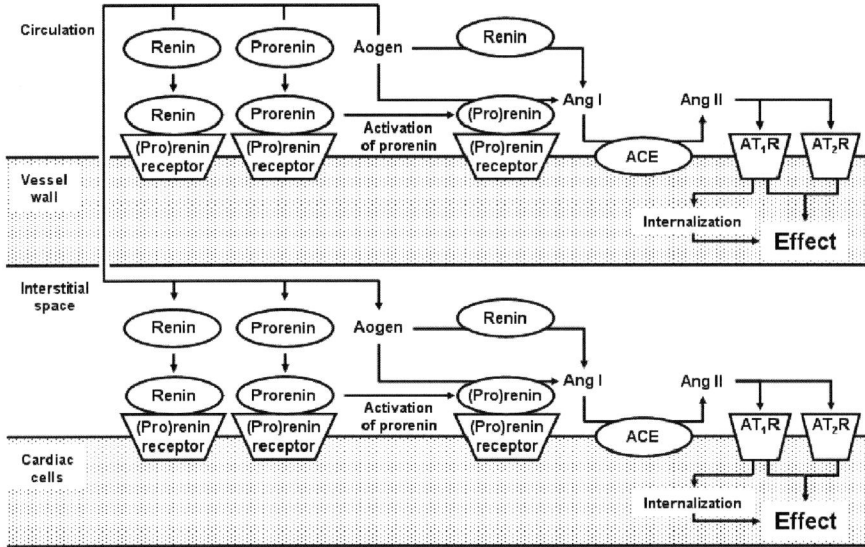

Figure 4. Model of angiotensin generation at cardiac tissue sites

Following a bilateral nephrectomy, tissue renin and angiotensin levels drop to levels at or below the detection limit (Campbell *et al* 1993; Danser *et al* 1994; Katz *et al* 1997). This suggests that the majority of tissue renin is not locally produced, but kidney-derived, and that without renin, there is no angiotensin production. The presence of renin in cardiac membrane fractions (Danser *et al* 1994) suggested that circulating renin, in addition to its diffusion into the interstitial space (Katz *et al* 1997; van den Eijnden *et al* 2002), may bind to renin-binding proteins or receptors at tissue sites. The recent discovery of several of such receptors, as discussed above, supports this concept. An interesting additional observation is that these receptors also bind prorenin, and that prorenin, upon binding, becomes catalytically active. In view of the much higher prorenin than renin levels, an attractive concept is that prorenin rather than renin contributes to tissue angiotensin generation. Studies with (pro)renin receptor blockers in diabetic rats confirmed this concept (Ichihara *et al* 2004). Unexpectedly however, these blockers did not affect tissue angiotensin levels in control rats, although the prorenin levels of the latter rats were only ≈2-fold lower than those of the diabetic rats. Moreover, despite the fact that prorenin is still present in circulating blood after a nephrectomy (Danser *et al* 1994), tissue angiotensin levels are close to zero. This suggests that, if prorenin contributes to tissue angiotensin production, this involves prorenin of renal rather than extrarenal origin. Currently, the only known difference between renal and extrarenal prorenin relates to their degree of glycosylation.

In vitro studies using the isolated perfused rat Langendorff heart fully confirmed the idea of renin and angiotensinogen uptake underlying tissue angiotensin production. During buffer perfusion, no release of RAS components could be demonstrated in the coronary effluent or interstitial fluid (de Lannoy *et al* 1997). After adding renin to the perfusion fluid, renin started to accumulate in the interstitial fluid, reaching steady-state levels in this compartment that were identical to its levels in the coronary circulation. Findings on angiotensinogen were similar. Stopping the exposure to renin revealed a biphasic washout curve, in agreement with the concept that renin is not only present in extracellular fluid but also binds to receptors. Angiotensinogen washout was mono-phasic. Angiotensin synthesis only occurred during simultaneous perfusion with renin and angiotensinogen. Interestingly, in hearts of transgenic rats overexpressing angiotensinogen, angiotensin release continued after stopping the renin perfusion, i.e., when renin was no longer present in the coronary circulation (Müller *et al* 1998). This was due to the fact that receptor-bound renin continued to generate Ang I.

At steady state, the cardiac tissue levels of Ang I were as high as expected assuming that Ang I is restricted to the extracellular fluid (de Lannoy *et al* 1998; Schuijt *et al* 1999). In contrast, the tissue Ang II levels were much higher. Pretreatment with an AT_1 receptor antagonist greatly reduced the cardiac tissue Ang II levels during renin + angiotensinogen perfusion. This suggests that locally generated Ang II accumulates at tissue sites through binding to AT_1 receptors. Subsequent subcellular fractionation studies confirmed that tissue Ang II, but not Ang I, is located intracellularly (Schuijt *et al* 1999; van Kats *et al* 2001). This is due to the fact that AT_1 receptor-bound Ang II is rapidly internalized, after which intracellular degradation occurs. Based on these observations, it is not surprising that the tissue Ang II content correlates directly with tissue AT_1 receptor density (van Kats *et al* 1997).

A wide range of in vitro studies has provided evidence for the existence of enzymes other than renin and ACE generating Ang I and II, including cathepsin D, kallikrein, tonin and chymase (Hackenthal *et al* 1978; Urata *et al* 1990). The *in vivo* importance of these alternative pathways is questionable. The fact that Ang I and II are virtually absent in plasma and tissue of nephrectomized animals (including humans) argue against a role of non-renin angiotensinogen-converting enzymes *in vivo*. A similar situation exists for chymase which is present in the cardiac interstitium, mast cells and endothelial cells. *In vitro* studies have provided evidence for an important role of chymase in the conversion of Ang I to Ang II (Urata *et al* 1990; Tom *et al* 2003), but *in vivo* evidence for chymase-dependent Ang II generation could not be obtained (Saris *et al* 2000). Moreover, angiotensinogen and ACE knockout mice have similar phenotypes (Tanimoto *et al* 1994; Krege *et al* 1995), and ACE deletion reduced the Ang II levels in both tissue and circulation by up to 99% (Campbell *et al* 2004). Thus, at least in mice, ACE is the main, if not only Ang II-generating enzyme *in vivo*.

4. AT_2 RECEPTORS AND PATHOPHYSIOLOGY

As discussed above, AT_2 receptor expression is low or undetectable in adult tissues, in contrast with its high expression in fetal tissues. However, AT_2 receptors reappear under pathophysiological conditions.

For instance, in the kidney, AT$_2$ receptor expression increases when inflammation, apoptosis, and proteinuria occur (Ruiz-Ortega *et al* 2003). Interestingly, transgenic AT$_2$ receptor-overexpressing mice displayed less glomerular injury, proteinuria and transforming growth factor β expression in a subtotal nephrectomy model (Hashimoto *et al* 2004). This suggests that the re-appearance of AT$_2$ receptors under pathological conditions is part of a protective mechanism, for instance related to enhanced NO production (Hiyoshi *et al* 2005). However, not all studies confirm the counterregulatory, protective actions of AT$_2$ receptors in the kidney. Duke and co-workers report that AT$_2$ receptors mediate vasoconstriction in the renal medulla of 2-kidney, 1-clip rats, as opposed to the vasodilator effects mediated by AT$_1$ receptors in this model (Duke *et al* 2005).

In the heart, a wide range of animal studies revealed increased AT$_2$ receptor expression under pathological conditions, e.g. during pressure overload, hypertension and ischemia, and post-myocardial infarction (Wiemer *et al* 1993; Wu *et al* 1994; Schuijt *et al* 2001; Yayama *et al* 2004). Studies in failing human hearts confirmed the animal data, and simultaneously showed a downregulation of AT$_1$ receptors (Asano *et al* 1997; Wharton *et al* 1998). From studies with AT$_1$ receptor antagonists it is widely accepted that AT$_1$ receptors play a major role in the post-myocardial remodeling process, mediating both fibrosis and hypertrophy (Schieffer *et al* 1994). Since the beneficial effects of AT$_1$ receptor blockade following myocardial infarction were diminished in AT$^{-/Y}$ receptor mice (Xu *et al* 2002), it is reasonable to assume that the increased Ang II levels that will occur during AT$_1$ receptor blockade (see below) exert beneficial effects via AT$_2$ receptor stimulation. Indeed, transgenic mice overexpressing AT$_2$ receptors in the heart displayed improved cardiac hemodynamics post-myocardial infarction in an NO-dependent manner (Yang *et al* 2002; Bove *et al* 2004). Furthermore, treatment with either an AT$_2$ receptor antagonist or a B$_2$ receptor antagonist reduced the beneficial effects of AT$_1$ receptor blockade in wildtype mice following myocardial infarction (Liu *et al* 2002). Therefore, the beneficial effects of AT$_2$ receptors in the heart involve the B$_2$ receptor/NO/cGMP pathway.

In contrast with these observations, a few studies have shown that AT$_2$ receptors, like AT$_1$ receptors, induce cardiac hypertrophy and fibrosis (Senbonmatsu *et al* 2000; Ichihara *et al* 2001). To explain these discrepant data, it has been hypothesized that AT$_2$ receptor upregulation is beneficial in the early pathological phase, by counteracting hypertrophy and fibrosis, but that chronic stimulation of the AT$_2$ receptor (for instance by the high Ang II levels that will occur during AT$_1$ receptor blockade) has deleterious effects on cardiac recovery (Schneider and Lorell 2001).

Knowledge on the effects of AT$_2$ receptors in the human heart comes from polymorphism studies, although the data are often contradictory. AT$_2$ receptor gene variants have been linked to both cardiac hypertrophy and coronary ischemia (Schmieder *et al* 2001; Herrmann *et al* 2002; Alfakih *et al* 2005), without knowing however whether this is based on inceased or decreased AT$_2$ receptor density. AT$_2$ receptor-mediated vasodilation in isolated human coronary microarteries increases with age (Batenburg *et al* 2004). Since endothelial function decreases with age, this could point to increased AT$_2$ receptor expression in the face of decreased endothelial function, again in agreement with the concept that AT_2 receptor density increases under pathological conditions. AT_2 receptor expression also increased in peripheral resistance arteries of hypertensive diabetic patients during treatment with an AT_1 receptor blocker, and this resulted in enhanced Ang II-induced vasodilation (Savoia *et al* 2007).

Recent studies have shown that AT_2 receptors are also expressed in various carcinomas (Deshayes and Nahmias 2005). Assuming that AT_1 receptors contribute to tumor growth and vascularization (Fujita *et al* 2002), one may predict that, here too, AT_2 receptors will counteract the effects of the AT_1 receptor stimulation, thus inhibiting growth and vascularization (Silvestre *et al* 2002). However, proangiogenic effects of AT_2 receptors have also been described, occurring in conjunction with AT_1 receptor activation (Walther *et al* 2003).

5.   RAS BLOCKADE AND AT_2 RECEPTOR STIMULATION

Blocking the RAS is possible at three levels: renin, ACE and the AT receptors. Beta-adrenoceptor blockers, by antagonizing the renin-releasing β_1-adrenoceptors in the juxta-glomerular cells, were the first drugs to suppress the RAS. These drugs will lower renin (Campbell *et al* 2001), Ang I and Ang II, thereby reducing the degree of AT_1 and AT_2 receptor stimulation (Table 1).

Subsequently, the ACE inhibitors were introduced. These drugs will lower Ang II. Given the wide variety of available angiotensinases, this will not lead to substantial Ang I accumulation, but rather result in metabolism of Ang I through different (compensatory) pathways, e.g. by neutral endopeptidase. As a consequence, Ang-(1-7) levels will rise during ACE inhibition, thereby allowing Ang-(1-7) to contribute to the beneficial effects of ACE inhibitors (Tom *et al* 2001). Simultaneously, due to the interference with Ang II generation, the negative feedback loop system regulating renin release is affected, and thus, the kidneys will release more renin. Therefore, depending on the degree of ACE inhibition, Ang II levels may rise again, sometimes to levels above baseline (Campbell *et al* 1993; van Kats *et al* 2000). For instance, at 90% ACE inhibition, a 10-fold rise in renin is sufficient to fully restore Ang II levels, whereas a 20-fold rise in renin would increase Ang II twofold above its baseline levels. In addition, prolonged ACE inhibition is known to upregulate ACE. Given these compensatory mechanisms, it

Table 1. Effects of various RAS blockers on renin, angiotensins and AT receptor stimulation

	Renin		Ang formation		Receptor stimulation	
	[Protein]	Activity	[Ang I]	[Ang II]	AT_1	AT_2
β blocker	↓	↓	↓	↓	↓	↓
Renin inhibitor	↑	↓	↓	↓	↓	↓
ACE inhibitor	↑	↑	↑	↓=	↓	↓
AT_1 receptor blocker	↑	↑	↑	↑	↓	↑

is not surprising that it has proven difficult to show that blood plasma and tissue Ang II levels remain suppressed during continuous ACE inhibition (van Kats *et al* 2000).

Indeed, in pigs treated with captopril for 3 weeks post-myocardial infarction, cardiac Ang II levels were increased as compared to untreated control pigs (Fig. 5). Although this Ang II may theoretically stimulate AT$_1$ and AT$_2$ receptors, it must be kept in mind that such receptor stimulation may occur less efficiently than normal. Without ACE inhibitor treatment, ACE generates Ang II in a highly efficient manner, in close proximity of AT receptors. During chronic ACE inhibition, the increase in Ang I generation will still allow Ang II generation, either by non-inhibited ACE or by non-ACE converting enzymes like chymase (van Kats *et al* 2005). However, this type of Ang II generation is less efficient, because it does not result in a high level of regional AT receptor stimulation. In particular, Ang II generated by chymase (which is localized in the adventitia) will be subject to rapid metabolism in the interstitial space on its way to AT receptors (Schuijt *et al* 1999; de Lannoy *et al* 2001) and thus is less likely to result in a high regional AT receptor occupancy. Therefore, a low overall AT receptor occupancy will occur, below the minimum per cell required to induce an effect.

AT$_1$ receptor blockers, available since the early 1990s, will also cause a rise in renin. Ang I and II in blood and tissues (as well as their metabolites) will increase in parallel with renin, and although this will not result in AT$_1$ receptor stimulation, non-AT$_1$ receptors (including AT$_2$ receptors and Mas) may now be stimulated excessively. As discussed above, it is feasible that, at least part of the beneficial effect of AT$_1$ receptor blockers is due to such AT$_2$ receptor stimulation (Widdop *et al* 2002).

Finally, renin inhibitors will soon be clinically available. These drugs lower both Ang I and II, and evidence for this, at least in blood plasma, is already available (Nussberger *et al* 2002; Azizi *et al* 2004). Whether renin inhibitors also decrease tissue Ang I and II levels is not yet known. This relates to the fact

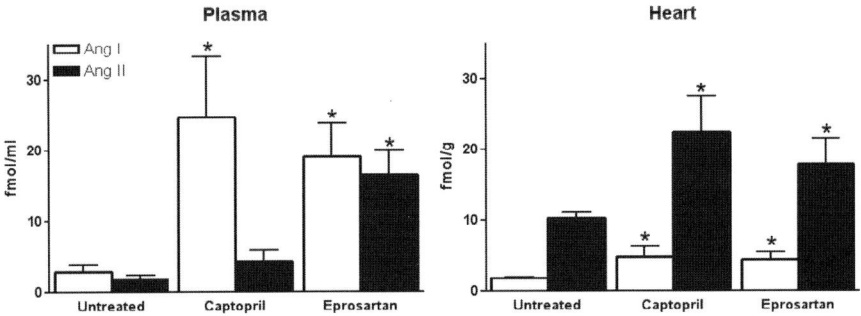

*Figure 5. Plasma and cardiac tissue angiotensin levels in pigs that were either untreated or treated with the ACE inhibitor captopril or the AT$_1$ receptor antagonist eprosartan for 3 weeks after a myocardial infarction. *P<0.05 vs. untreated. Data are derived from (van Kats et al 2000)*

that renin inhibitors primarily block human renin, and not (or to a much lesser degree) rat, mouse or porcine renin. Thus, renin inhibitors cannot be tested easily in well-established animal models. Theoretically, the decreased Ang I and II levels during renin inhibition will prevent AT_1 and AT_2 receptor stimulation, as well as the stimulation of any other receptor by angiotensin metabolites. Although renin will rise during renin inhibitor treatment (like it does during any RAS blocker treatment), this renin cannot be enzymatically active due to the presence of the renin inhibitor. Thus, renin inhibitors may offer a more complete suppression of the RAS, although this also implies that the putative beneficial effects mediated by AT_2 or Mas receptors will now no longer occur. So far, this does not appear to diminish the effects of renin inhibitors, at least on blood pressure (Gradman *et al* 2005).

6.   CONCLUSIONS

Ang II generated at tissue sites stimulates both AT_1 and AT_2 receptors. This local generation depends largely on angiotensinogen and renin and/or prorenin taken up from blood, the latter uptake possibly involving the recently discovered (pro)renin receptor. ACE is generated locally, and appears to be the main, if not the only, Ang II-generating enzyme. Ang II has a whole range of metabolites, the most important of which are Ang (1-7), Ang III and Ang IV. The enzymes generating these metabolites, including ACE2, have recently been characterized, as well as their putative (non-AT_1/AT_2) receptors, like the Mas and AT_4 receptor. Stimulation of AT_2 receptors most likely contributes to the beneficial effect of RAS blockers, in particular during AT_1 receptor antagonism. These receptors are upregulated under pathophysiological conditions, and are generally believed to counteract the effects of AT_1 receptor stimulation. However, not all studies agree on this aspect, and thus it remains to be seen how the effect of drugs that completely suppress the RAS, i.e., renin inhibitors, compare to those that allow/require AT_2 receptor stimulation, like ACE inhibitors and AT_1 receptor antagonists.

REFERENCES

Abadir, P. M., Carey, R. M. and Siragy, H. M., 2003, Angiotensin AT2 receptors directly stimulate renal nitric oxide in bradykinin B2-receptor-null mice. *Hypertension*. **42:** 600–604.

Abadir, P. M., Periasamy, A., Carey, R. M. and Siragy, H. M., 2006, Angiotensin II type 2 receptor-bradykinin B2 receptor functional heterodimerization. *Hypertension*. **48:** 316–322.

AbdAlla, S., Lother, H., Abdel-tawab, A. M. and Quitterer, U., 2001, The angiotensin II AT2 receptor is an AT1 receptor antagonist. *J Biol Chem*. **276:** 39721–39726.

AbdAlla, S., Lother, H. and Quitterer, U., 2000, AT1-receptor heterodimers show enhanced G-protein activation and altered receptor sequestration. *Nature*. **407:** 94–98.

Albiston, A. L., McDowall, S. G., Matsacos, D., Sim, P., Clune, E., Mustafa, T., Lee, J., Mendelsohn, F. A., Simpson, R. J., Connolly, L. M. and Chai, S. Y., 2001, Evidence that the angiotensin IV (AT(4)) receptor is the enzyme insulin-regulated aminopeptidase. *J Biol Chem*. **276:** 48623–48626.

Alfakih, K., Lawrance, R. A., Maqbool, A., Walters, K., Ball, S. G., Balmforth, A. J. and Hall, A. S., 2005, The clinical significance of a common, functional, X-linked angiotensin II type 2-receptor gene polymorphism (-1332 G/A) in a cohort of 509 families with premature coronary artery disease. *Eur Heart J*. **26**: 584–589.

Ardaillou, R. and Chansel, D., 1997, Synthesis and effects of active fragments of angiotensin II. *Kidney Int*. **52**: 1458–1468.

Asano, K., Dutcher, D. L., Port, J. D., Minobe, W. A., Tremmel, K. D., Roden, R. L., Bohlmeyer, T. J., Bush, E. W., Jenkin, M. J., Abraham, W. T., Raynolds, M. V., Zisman, L. S., Perryman, M. B. and Bristow, M. R., 1997, Selective downregulation of the angiotensin II AT1-receptor subtype in failing human ventricular myocardium. *Circulation*. **95**: 1193–1200.

Azizi, M., Menard, J., Bissery, A., Guyenne, T. T., Bura-Riviere, A., Vaidyanathan, S. and Camisasca, R. P., 2004, Pharmacologic demonstration of the synergistic effects of a combination of the renin inhibitor aliskiren and the AT1 receptor antagonist valsartan on the angiotensin II-renin feedback interruption. *J Am Soc Nephrol*. **15**: 3126–3133.

Batenburg, W. W., Garrelds, I. M., Bernasconi, C. C., Juillerat-Jeanneret, L., van Kats, J. P., Saxena, P. R. and Danser, A. H. J., 2004, Angiotensin II type 2 receptor-mediated vasodilation in human coronary microarteries. *Circulation*. **109**: 2296–2301.

Bottari, S. P., de Gasparo, M., Steckelings, U. M. and Levens, N. R., 1993, Angiotensin II receptor subtypes: characterization, signalling mechanisms, and possible physiological implications. *Front Neuroendocrinol*. **14**: 123–171.

Bove, C. M., Yang, Z., Gilson, W. D., Epstein, F. H., French, B. A., Berr, S. S., Bishop, S. P., Matsubara, H., Carey, R. M. and Kramer, C. M., 2004, Nitric oxide mediates benefits of angiotensin II type 2 receptor overexpression during post-infarct remodeling. *Hypertension*. **43**: 680–685.

Brosnihan, K. B., Li, P. and Ferrario, C. M., 1996, Angiotensin-(1-7) dilates canine coronary arteries through kinins and nitric oxide. *Hypertension*. **27**: 523–528.

Burson, J. M., Aguilera, G., Gross, K. W. and Sigmund, C. D., 1994, Differential expression of angiotensin receptor 1A and 1B in mouse. *Am J Physiol*. **267**: E260–267.

Campbell, D. J., Aggarwal, A., Esler, M. and Kaye, D., 2001, beta-blockers, angiotensin II, and ACE inhibitors in patients with heart failure. *Lancet*. **358**: 1609–1610.

Campbell, D. J., Alexiou, T., Xiao, H. D., Fuchs, S., McKinley, M. J., Corvol, P. and Bernstein, K. E., 2004, Effect of reduced angiotensin-converting enzyme gene expression and angiotensin-converting enzyme inhibition on angiotensin and bradykinin peptide levels in mice. *Hypertension*. **43**: 854–859.

Campbell, D. J., Kladis, A. and Duncan, A. M., 1993, Nephrectomy, converting enzyme inhibition, and angiotensin peptides. *Hypertension*. **22**: 513–522.

Castro, C. H., Santos, R. A., Ferreira, A. J., Bader, M., Alenina, N. and Almeida, A. P., 2005, Evidence for a functional interaction of the angiotensin-(1-7) receptor Mas with AT1 and AT2 receptors in the mouse heart. *Hypertension*. **46**: 937–942.

Cervenka, L., Maly, J., Karasova, L., Simova, M., Vitko, S., Hellerova, S., Heller, J. and El-Dahr, S. S., 2001, Angiotensin II-induced hypertension in bradykinin B2 receptor knockout mice. *Hypertension*. **37**: 967–973.

Chen, X., Li, W., Yoshida, H., Tsuchida, S., Nishimura, H., Takemoto, F., Okubo, S., Fogo, A., Matsusaka, T. and Ichikawa, I., 1997, Targeting deletion of angiotensin type 1B receptor gene in the mouse. *Am J Physiol*. **272**: F299–304.

Clark, A. F., Sharp, M. G., Morley, S. D., Fleming, S., Peters, J. and Mullins, J. J., 1997, Renin-1 is essential for normal renal juxtaglomerular cell granulation and macula densa morphology. *J Biol Chem*. **272**: 18185–18190.

Clausmeyer, S., Reinecke, A., Farrenkopf, R., Unger, T. and Peters, J., 2000, Tissue-specific expression of a rat renin transcript lacking the coding sequence for the prefragment and its stimulation by myocardial infarction. *Endocrinology*. **141**: 2963–2970.

Crackower, M. A., Sarao, R., Oudit, G. Y., Yagil, C., Kozieradzki, I., Scanga, S. E., Oliveira-dos-Santos, A. J., da Costa, J., Zhang, L., Pei, Y., Scholey, J., Ferrario, C. M., Manoukian, A. S., Chappell, M. C., Backx, P. H., Yagil, Y. and Penninger, J. M., 2002, Angiotensin-converting enzyme 2 is an essential regulator of heart function. *Nature*. **417**: 822–828.

Danser, A. H. J. and Deinum, J., 2005, Renin, prorenin and the putative (pro)renin receptor. *Hypertension.* **46:** 1069–1076.

Danser, A. H. J., van den Dorpel, M. A., Deinum, J., Derkx, F. H., Franken, A. A., Peperkamp, E., de Jong, P. T. and Schalekamp, M. A. D. H., 1989, Renin, prorenin, and immunoreactive renin in vitreous fluid from eyes with and without diabetic retinopathy. *J Clin Endocrinol Metab.* **68:** 160–167.

Danser, A. H. J., van Kats, J. P., Admiraal, P. J., Derkx, F. H., Lamers, J. M., Verdouw, P. D., Saxena, P. R. and Schalekamp, M. A. D. H., 1994, Cardiac renin and angiotensins. Uptake from plasma versus in situ synthesis. *Hypertension.* **24:** 37–48.

de Gasparo, M., Catt, K. J., Inagami, T., Wright, J. W. and Unger, T., 2000, International union of pharmacology. XXIII. The angiotensin II receptors. *Pharmacol Rev.* **52:** 415–472.

de Lannoy, L. M., Danser, A. H. J., Bouhuizen, A. M., Saxena, P. R. and Schalekamp, M. A. D. H., 1998, Localization and production of angiotensin II in the isolated perfused rat heart. *Hypertension.* **31:** 1111–1117.

de Lannoy, L. M., Danser, A. H. J., van Kats, J. P., Schoemaker, R. G., Saxena, P. R. and Schalekamp, M. A. D. H., 1997, Renin-angiotensin system components in the interstitial fluid of the isolated perfused rat heart. Local production of angiotensin I. *Hypertension.* **29:** 1240–1251.

de Lannoy, L. M., Schuijt, M. P., Saxena, P. R., Schalekamp, M. A. D. H. and Danser, A. H. J., 2001, Angiotensin converting enzyme is the main contributor to angiotensin I-II conversion in the interstitium of the isolated perfused rat heart. *J Hypertens.* **19:** 959–965.

Deshayes, F. and Nahmias, C., 2005, Angiotensin receptors: a new role in cancer?, *Trends Endocrinol Metab.* **16:** 293–299.

Di Bacco, A. and Gill, G., 2003, The secreted glycoprotein CREG inhibits cell growth dependent on the mannose-6-phosphate/insulin-like growth factor II receptor. *Oncogene.* **22:** 5436–5445.

Donoghue, M., Hsieh, F., Baronas, E., Godbout, K., Gosselin, M., Stagliano, N., Donovan, M., Woolf, B., Robison, K., Jeyaseelan, R., Breitbart, R. E. and Acton, S., 2000, A novel angiotensin-converting enzyme-related carboxypeptidase (ACE2) converts angiotensin I to angiotensin 1–9. *Circ Res.* **87:** E1–9.

Doolittle, R. F., 1983, Angiotensinogen is related to the antitrypsin-antithrombin-ovalbumin family. *Science.* **222:** 417–419.

Duke, L. M., Widdop, R. E., Kett, M. M. and Evans, R. G., 2005, AT(2) receptors mediate tonic renal medullary vasoconstriction in renovascular hypertension. *Br J Pharmacol.* **144:** 486–492.

Elton, T. S., Stephan, C. C., Taylor, G. R., Kimball, M. G., Martin, M. M., Durand, J. N. and Oparil, S., 1992, Isolation of two distinct type I angiotensin II receptor genes. *Biochem Biophys Res Commun.* **184:** 1067–1073.

Esther, C. R., Jr., Howard, T. E., Marino, E. M., Goddard, J. M., Capecchi, M. R. and Bernstein, K. E., 1996, Mice lacking angiotensin-converting enzyme have low blood pressure, renal pathology, and reduced male fertility. *Lab Invest.* **74:** 953–965.

Fujita, M., Hayashi, I., Yamashina, S., Itoman, M. and Majima, M., 2002, Blockade of angiotensin AT1a receptor signaling reduces tumor growth, angiogenesis, and metastasis. *Biochem Biophys Res Commun.* **294:** 441–447.

Fukamizu, A., Sugimura, K., Takimoto, E., Sugiyama, F., Seo, M. S., Takahashi, S., Hatae, T., Kajiwara, N., Yagami, K. and Murakami, K., 1993, Chimeric renin-angiotensin system demonstrates sustained increase in blood pressure of transgenic mice carrying both human renin and human angiotensinogen genes. *J Biol Chem.* **268:** 11617–11621.

Gradman, A. H., Schmieder, R. E., Lins, R. L., Nussberger, J., Chiang, Y. and Bedigian, M. P., 2005, Aliskiren, a novel orally effective renin inhibitor, provides dose-dependent antihypertensive efficacy and placebo-like tolerability in hypertensive patients. *Circulation.* **111:** 1012–1018.

Guimaraes, S. and Pinheiro, H., 2005, Functional evidence that in the cardiovascular system AT1 angiotensin II receptors are AT1B prejunctionally and AT1A postjunctionally. *Cardiovasc Res.* **67:** 208–215.

Gurley, S. B., Allred, A., Le, T. H., Griffiths, R., Mao, L., Philip, N., Haystead, T. A., Donoghue, M., Breitbart, R. E., Acton, S. L., Rockman, H. A. and Coffman, T. M., 2006, Altered blood pressure responses and normal cardiac phenotype in ACE2-null mice. *J Clin Invest*. 116: 2218–2225.

Hackenthal, E., Hackenthal, R. and Hilgenfeldt, U., 1978, Isorenin, pseudorenin, cathepsin D and renin. A comparative enzymatic study of angiotensin-forming enzymes. *Biochim Biophys Acta*. 522: 574–588.

Hashimoto, N., Maeshima, Y., Satoh, M., Odawara, M., Sugiyama, H., Kashihara, N., Matsubara, H., Yamasaki, Y. and Makino, H., 2004, Overexpression of angiotensin type 2 receptor ameliorates glomerular injury in a mouse remnant kidney model. *Am J Physiol Renal Physiol*. 286: F516–525.

Hein, L., Barsh, G. S., Pratt, R. E., Dzau, V. J. and Kobilka, B. K., 1995, Behavioural and cardiovascular effects of disrupting the angiotensin II type-2 receptor in mice. *Nature*. 377: 744–747.

Herrmann, S. M., Nicaud, V., Schmidt-Petersen, K., Pfeifer, J., Erdmann, J., McDonagh, T., Dargie, H. J., Paul, M. and Regitz-Zagrosek, V., 2002, Angiotensin II type 2 receptor gene polymorphism and cardiovascular phenotypes: the GLAECO and GLAOLD studies. *Eur J Heart Fail*. 4: 707–712.

Hiyoshi, H., Yayama, K., Takano, M. and Okamoto, H., 2005, Angiotensin type 2 receptor-mediated phosphorylation of eNOS in the aortas of mice with 2-kidney, 1-clip hypertension. *Hypertension*. 45: 967–973.

Horiuchi, M., Akishita, M. and Dzau, V. J., 1998, Molecular and cellular mechanism of angiotensin II-mediated apoptosis. *Endocr Res*. 24: 307–314.

Hubert, C., Houot, A. M., Corvol, P. and Soubrier, F., 1991, Structure of the angiotensin I-converting enzyme gene. Two alternate promoters correspond to evolutionary steps of a duplicated gene. *J Biol Chem*. 266: 15377–15383.

Ichihara, A., Hayashi, M., Kaneshiro, Y., Suzuki, F., Nakagawa, T., Tada, Y., Koura, Y., Nishiyama, A., Okada, H., Uddin, M. N., Nabi, A. H., Ishida, Y., Inagami, T. and Saruta, T., 2004, Inhibition of diabetic nephropathy by a decoy peptide corresponding to the "handle" region for nonproteolytic activation of prorenin. *J Clin Invest*. 114: 1128–1135.

Ichihara, S., Senbonmatsu, T., Price, E., Jr., Ichiki, T., Gaffney, F. A. and Inagami, T., 2001, Angiotensin II type 2 receptor is essential for left ventricular hypertrophy and cardiac fibrosis in chronic angiotensin II-induced hypertension. *Circulation*. 104: 346–351.

Ichiki, T., Labosky, P. A., Shiota, C., Okuyama, S., Imagawa, Y., Fogo, A., Niimura, F., Ichikawa, I., Hogan, B. L. and Inagami, T., 1995, Effects on blood pressure and exploratory behaviour of mice lacking angiotensin II type-2 receptor. *Nature*. 377: 748–750.

Ito, M., Oliverio, M. I., Mannon, P. J., Best, C. F., Maeda, N., Smithies, O. and Coffman, T. M., 1995, Regulation of blood pressure by the type 1A angiotensin II receptor gene. *Proc Natl Acad Sci U S A*. 92: 3521–3525.

Itskovitz, J., Rubattu, S., Levron, J. and Sealey, J. E., 1992, Highest concentrations of prorenin and human chorionic gonadotropin in gestational sacs during early human pregnancy. *J Clin Endocrinol Metab*. 75: 906–910.

Jin, X. Q., Fukuda, N., Su, J. Z., Lai, Y. M., Suzuki, R., Tahira, Y., Takagi, H., Ikeda, Y., Kanmatsuse, K. and Miyazaki, H., 2002, Angiotensin II type 2 receptor gene transfer downregulates angiotensin II type 1a receptor in vascular smooth muscle cells. *Hypertension*. 39: 1021–1027.

Kageyama, R., Ohkubo, H. and Nakanishi, S., 1985, Induction of rat liver angiotensinogen mRNA following acute inflammation. *Biochem Biophys Res Commun*. 129: 826–832.

Kang, J. X., Li, Y. and Leaf, A., 1997, Mannose-6-phosphate/insulin-like growth factor-II receptor is a receptor for retinoic acid. *Proc Natl Acad Sci U S A*. 94: 13671–13676.

Katada, J. and Majima, M., 2002, AT(2) receptor-dependent vasodilation is mediated by activation of vascular kinin generation under flow conditions. *Br J Pharmacol*. 136: 484–491.

Katz, S. A., Opsahl, J. A., Lunzer, M. M., Forbis, L. M. and Hirsch, A. T., 1997, Effect of bilateral nephrectomy on active renin, angiotensinogen, and renin glycoforms in plasma and myocardium. *Hypertension*. 30: 259–266.

Keller, S. R., Scott, H. M., Mastick, C. C., Aebersold, R. and Lienhard, G. E., 1995, Cloning and characterization of a novel insulin-regulated membrane aminopeptidase from Glut4 vesicles. *J Biol Chem*. 270: 23612–23618.

Kessler, S. P., Senanayake, P. D., Gaughan, C. and Sen, G. C., 2007, Vascular expression of germinal ACE fails to maintain normal blood pressure in ACE-/- mice. *FASEB J.* **21**: 156–166.

Kimura, S., Mullins, J. J., Bunnemann, B., Metzger, R., Hilgenfeldt, U., Zimmermann, F., Jacob, H., Fuxe, K., Ganten, D. and Kaling, M., 1992, High blood pressure in transgenic mice carrying the rat angiotensinogen gene. *EMBO J.* **11**: 821–827.

Kitamura, N., Ohkubo, H. and Nakanishi, S., 1987, Molecular biology of the angiotensinogen and kininogen genes. *J Cardiovasc Pharmacol.* **10** (suppl 7): S49–53.

Klett, C., Nobiling, R., Gierschik, P. and Hackenthal, E., 1993, Angiotensin II stimulates the synthesis of angiotensinogen in hepatocytes by inhibiting adenylylcyclase activity and stabilizing angiotensinogen mRNA. *J Biol Chem.* **268**: 25095–25107.

Kornfeld, S., 1992, Structure and function of the mannose 6-phosphate/insulinlike growth factor II receptors. *Annu Rev Biochem.* **61**: 307–330.

Krege, J. H., John, S. W., Langenbach, L. L., Hodgin, J. B., Hagaman, J. R., Bachman, E. S., Jennette, J. C., O'Brien, D. A. and Smithies, O., 1995, Male-female differences in fertility and blood pressure in ACE-deficient mice. *Nature.* **375**: 146–148.

Lemos, V. S., Silva, D. M., Walther, T., Alenina, N., Bader, M. and Santos, R. A., 2005, The endothelium-dependent vasodilator effect of the nonpeptide Ang(1-7) mimic AVE 0991 is abolished in the aorta of mas-knockout mice. *J Cardiovasc Pharmacol.* **46**: 274–279.

Lenz, T., Sealey, J. E., Lappe, R. W., Carilli, C., Oshiro, G. T., Baxter, J. D. and Laragh, J. H., 1990, Infusion of recombinant human prorenin into rhesus monkeys. Effects on hemodynamics, renin-angiotensin-aldosterone axis and plasma testosterone. *Am J Hypertens.* **3**: 257–261.

Li, W., Moore, M. J., Vasilieva, N., Sui, J., Wong, S. K., Berne, M. A., Somasundaran, M., Sullivan, J. L., Luzuriaga, K., Greenough, T. C., Choe, H. and Farzan, M., 2003, Angiotensin-converting enzyme 2 is a functional receptor for the SARS coronavirus. *Nature.* **426**: 450–454.

Li, X. C. and Widdop, R. E., 2004, AT2 receptor-mediated vasodilatation is unmasked by AT1 receptor blockade in conscious SHR. *Br J Pharmacol.* **142**: 821–830.

Liu, Y. H., Xu, J., Yang, X. P., Yang, F., Shesely, E. and Carretero, O. A., 2002, Effect of ACE inhibitors and angiotensin II type 1 receptor antagonists on endothelial NO synthase knockout mice with heart failure. *Hypertension.* **39**: 375–381.

Mehta, P. K. and Griendling, K. K., 2007, Angiotensin II cell signaling: physiological and pathological effects in the cardiovascular system. *Am J Physiol Cell Physiol.* **292**: C82–97.

Metzger, R., Bader, M., Ludwig, T., Berberich, C., Bunnemann, B. and Ganten, D., 1995, Expression of the mouse and rat mas proto-oncogene in the brain and peripheral tissues. *FEBS Lett.* **357**: 27–32.

Morris, B. J., 1992, Molecular biology of renin. I: Gene and protein structure, synthesis and processing. *J Hypertens.* **10**: 209–214.

Mukoyama, M., Nakajima, M., Horiuchi, M., Sasamura, H., Pratt, R. E. and Dzau, V. J., 1993, Expression cloning of type 2 angiotensin II receptor reveals a unique class of seven-transmembrane receptors. *J Biol Chem.* **268**: 24539–24542.

Müller, D. N., Fischli, W., Clozel, J. P., Hilgers, K. F., Bohlender, J., Menard, J., Busjahn, A., Ganten, D. and Luft, F. C., 1998, Local angiotensin II generation in the rat heart: role of renin uptake. *Circ Res.* **82**: 13–20.

Murphy, T. J., Alexander, R. W., Griendling, K. K., Runge, M. S. and Bernstein, K. E., 1991, Isolation of a cDNA encoding the vascular type-1 angiotensin II receptor. *Nature.* **351**: 233–236.

Nguyen, G., Delarue, F., Burckle, C., Bouzhir, L., Giller, T. and Sraer, J. D., 2002, Pivotal role of the renin/prorenin receptor in angiotensin II production and cellular responses to renin. *J Clin Invest.* **109**: 1417–1427.

Niimura, F., Labosky, P. A., Kakuchi, J., Okubo, S., Yoshida, H., Oikawa, T., Ichiki, T., Naftilan, A. J., Fogo, A., Inagami, T. and et al., 1995, Gene targeting in mice reveals a requirement for angiotensin in the development and maintenance of kidney morphology and growth factor regulation. *J Clin Invest.* **96**: 2947–2954.

Nouet, S. and Nahmias, C., 2000, Signal transduction from the angiotensin II AT2 receptor. *Trends Endocrinol Metab.* **11**: 1–6.

Nussberger, J., Wuerzner, G., Jensen, C. and Brunner, H. R., 2002, Angiotensin II suppression in humans by the orally active renin inhibitor Aliskiren (SPP100): comparison with enalapril. *Hypertension.* **39:** E1–8.

Oliverio, M. I., Best, C. F., Kim, H. S., Arendshorst, W. J., Smithies, O. and Coffman, T. M., 1997, Angiotensin II responses in AT1A receptor-deficient mice: a role for AT1B receptors in blood pressure regulation. *Am J Physiol.* **272:** F515–520.

Padia, S. H., Howell, N. L., Siragy, H. M. and Carey, R. M., 2006, Renal angiotensin type 2 receptors mediate natriuresis via angiotensin III in the angiotensin II type 1 receptor-blocked rat. *Hypertension.* **47:** 537–544.

Patel, J. M., Martens, J. R., Li, Y. D., Gelband, C. H., Raizada, M. K. and Block, E. R., 1998, Angiotensin IV receptor-mediated activation of lung endothelial NOS is associated with vasorelaxation. *Am J Physiol.* **275:** L1061–1068.

Paul, M., Poyan Mehr, A. and Kreutz, R., 2006, Physiology of local renin-angiotensin systems. *Physiol Rev.* **86:** 747–803.

Perlegas, D., Xie, H., Sinha, S., Somlyo, A. V. and Owens, G. K., 2005, ANG II type 2 receptor regulates smooth muscle growth and force generation in late fetal mouse development. *Am J Physiol Heart Circ Physiol.* **288:** H96–102.

Peters, J., Farrenkopf, R., Clausmeyer, S., Zimmer, J., Kantachuvesiri, S., Sharp, M. G. and Mullins, J. J., 2002, Functional significance of prorenin internalization in the rat heart. *Circ Res.* **90:** 1135–1141.

Purdy, R. E. and Weber, M. A., 1988, Angiotensin II amplification of alpha-adrenergic vasoconstriction: role of receptor reserve. *Circ Res.* **63:** 748–757.

Ritter, O., Schuh, K., Brede, M., Rothlein, N., Burkard, N., Hein, L. and Neyses, L., 2003, AT2 receptor activation regulates myocardial eNOS expression via the calcineurin-NF-AT pathway. *Faseb J.* **17:** 283–285.

Ruiz-Ortega, M., Esteban, V., Suzuki, Y., Ruperez, M., Mezzano, S., Ardiles, L., Justo, P., Ortiz, A. and Egido, J., 2003, Renal expression of angiotensin type 2 (AT2) receptors during kidney damage. *Kidn Int.* **86:** S21–26.

Santos, R. A. S., Campagnole-Santos, M. J. and Andrade, S. P., 2000, Angiotensin-(1–7): an update. *Regul Pept.* **91:** 45–62.

Santos, R. A. S., Castro, C. H., Gava, E., Pinheiro, S. V., Almeida, A. P., Paula, R. D., Cruz, J. S., Ramos, A. S., Rosa, K. T., Irigoyen, M. C., Bader, M., Alenina, N., Kitten, G. T. and Ferreira, A. J., 2006, Impairment of in vitro and in vivo heart function in angiotensin-(1–7) receptor MAS knockout mice. *Hypertension.* **47:** 996–1002.

Santos, R. A. S., Simoes e Silva, A. C., Maric, C., Silva, D. M., Machado, R. P., de Buhr, I., Heringer-Walther, S., Pinheiro, S. V., Lopes, M. T., Bader, M., Mendes, E. P., Lemos, V. S., Campagnole-Santos, M. J., Schultheiss, H. P., Speth, R. and Walther, T., 2003, Angiotensin-(1–7) is an endogenous ligand for the G protein-coupled receptor Mas. *Proc Natl Acad Sci U S A.* **100:** 8258–8263.

Saris, J. J., Derkx, F. H. M., de Bruin, R. J. A., Dekkers, D. H., Lamers, J. M., Saxena, P. R., Schalekamp, M. A. D. H. and Danser, A. H. J., 2001, High-affinity prorenin binding to cardiac man-6-P/IGF-II receptors precedes proteolytic activation to renin. *Am J Physiol Heart Circ Physiol.* **280:** H1706–1715.

Saris, J. J., t Hoen, P. A., Garrelds, I. M., Dekkers, D. H., den Dunnen, J. T., Lamers, J. M. and Danser, A. H. J., 2006, Prorenin induces intracellular signaling in cardiomyocytes independently of angiotensin II. *Hypertension.* **48:** 564–571.

Saris, J. J., van Dijk, M. A., Kroon, I., Schalekamp, M. A. D. H. and Danser, A. H. J., 2000, Functional importance of angiotensin-converting enzyme-dependent in situ angiotensin II generation in the human forearm. *Hypertension.* **35:** 764–768.

Sasaki, K., Yamano, Y., Bardhan, S., Iwai, N., Murray, J. J., Hasegawa, M., Matsuda, Y. and Inagami, T., 1991, Cloning and expression of a complementary DNA encoding a bovine adrenal angiotensin II type-1 receptor. *Nature.* **351:** 230–233.

Savoia, C., Touyz, R. M., Volpe, M. and Schiffrin, E. L., 2007, Angiotensin type 2 receptor in resistance arteries of type 2 diabetic hypertensive patients. *Hypertension.* **49:** 341–346.

Schieffer, B., Wirger, A., Meybrunn, M., Seitz, S., Holtz, J., Riede, U. N. and Drexler, H., 1994, Comparative effects of chronic angiotensin-converting enzyme inhibition and angiotensin II type 1 receptor blockade on cardiac remodeling after myocardial infarction in the rat. *Circulation.* **89:** 2273–2282.

Schmieder, R. E., Erdmann, J., Delles, C., Jacobi, J., Fleck, E., Hilgers, K. and Regitz-Zagrosek, V., 2001, Effect of the angiotensin II type 2-receptor gene (+1675 G/A) on left ventricular structure in humans. *J Am Coll Cardiol.* **37:** 175–182.

Schneider, M. D. and Lorell, B. H., 2001, AT(2), judgment day: which angiotensin receptor is the culprit in cardiac hypertrophy?, *Circulation.* **104:** 247–248.

Schuijt, M. P., Basdew, M., van Veghel, R., de Vries, R., Saxena, P. R., Schoemaker, R. G. and Danser, A. H. J., 2001, AT(2) receptor-mediated vasodilation in the heart: effect of myocardial infarction. *Am J Physiol Heart Circ Physiol.* **281:** H2590–2596.

Schuijt, M. P. and Danser, A. H. J., 2002, Cardiac angiotensin II: an intracrine hormone?, *Am J Hypertens.* **15:** 1109–1116.

Schuijt, M. P., van Kats, J. P., de Zeeuw, S., Duncker, D. J., Verdouw, P. D., Schalekamp, M. A. D. H. and Danser, A. H. J., 1999, Cardiac interstitial fluid levels of angiotensin I and II in the pig. *J Hypertens.* **17:** 1885–1891.

Sealey, J. E., Goldstein, M., Pitarresi, T., Kudlak, T. T., Glorioso, N., Fiamengo, S. A. and Laragh, J. H., 1988, Prorenin secretion from human testis: no evidence for secretion of active renin or angiotensinogen. *J Clin Endocrinol Metab.* **66:** 974–978.

Senbonmatsu, T., Ichihara, S., Price, E., Jr., Gaffney, F. A. and Inagami, T., 2000, Evidence for angiotensin II type 2 receptor-mediated cardiac myocyte enlargement during in vivo pressure overload. *J Clin Invest.* **106:** R25–29.

Sharp, M. G., Fettes, D., Brooker, G., Clark, A. F., Peters, J., Fleming, S. and Mullins, J. J., 1996, Targeted inactivation of the Ren-2 gene in mice. *Hypertension.* **28:** 1126–1131.

Shinagawa, T., Do, Y. S., Baxter, J. and Hsueh, W. A., 1992, Purification and characterization of human truncated prorenin. *Biochemistry.* **31:** 2758–2764.

Silvestre, J. S., Tamarat, R., Senbonmatsu, T., Icchiki, T., Ebrahimian, T., Iglarz, M., Besnard, S., Duriez, M., Inagami, T. and Levy, B. I., 2002, Antiangiogenic effect of angiotensin II type 2 receptor in ischemia-induced angiogenesis in mice hindlimb. *Circ Res.* **90:** 1072–1079.

Siragy, H. M. and Carey, R. M., 1997, The subtype 2 (AT2) angiotensin receptor mediates renal production of nitric oxide in conscious rats. *J Clin Invest.* **100:** 264–269.

Siragy, H. M., Xue, C., Abadir, P. and Carey, R. M., 2005, Angiotensin subtype-2 receptors inhibit renin biosynthesis and angiotensin II formation. *Hypertension.* **45:** 133–137.

Stegbauer, J., Vonend, O., Oberhauser, V. and Rump, L. C., 2003, Effects of angiotensin-(1–7) and other bioactive components of the renin-angiotensin system on vascular resistance and noradrenaline release in rat kidney. *J Hypertens.* **21:** 1391–1399.

Sugaya, T., Nishimatsu, S., Tanimoto, K., Takimoto, E., Yamagishi, T., Imamura, K., Goto, S., Imaizumi, K., Hisada, Y., Otsuka, A. and et al., 1995, Angiotensin II type 1a receptor-deficient mice with hypotension and hyperreninemia. *J Biol Chem.* **270:** 18719–18722.

Suzuki, F., Hayakawa, M., Nakagawa, T., Nasir, U. M., Ebihara, A., Iwasawa, A., Ishida, Y., Nakamura, Y. and Murakami, K., 2003, Human prorenin has "gate and handle" regions for its non-proteolytic activation. *J Biol Chem.* **278:** 22217–22222.

Swanson, G. N., Hanesworth, J. M., Sardinia, M. F., Coleman, J. K., Wright, J. W., Hall, K. L., Miller-Wing, A. V., Stobb, J. W., Cook, V. I., Harding, E. C. and et al., 1992, Discovery of a distinct binding site for angiotensin II (3–8), a putative angiotensin IV receptor. *Regul Pept.* **40:** 409–419.

Tanaka, M., Tsuchida, S., Imai, T., Fujii, N., Miyazaki, H., Ichiki, T., Naruse, M. and Inagami, T., 1999, Vascular response to angiotensin II is exaggerated through an upregulation of AT1 receptor in AT2 knockout mice. *Biochem Biophys Res Commun.* **258:** 194–198.

Tanimoto, K., Sugiyama, F., Goto, Y., Ishida, J., Takimoto, E., Yagami, K., Fukamizu, A. and Murakami, K., 1994, Angiotensinogen-deficient mice with hypotension. *J Biol Chem.* **269:** 31334–31337.

Thomas, W. G., Thekkumkara, T. J. and Baker, K. M., 1996, Molecular mechanisms of angiotensin II (AT1A) receptor endocytosis. *Clin Exp Pharmacol Physiol.* **3:** S74–80.

Tom, B., de Vries, R., Saxena, P. R. and Danser, A. H. J., 2001, Bradykinin potentiation by angiotensin-(1–7) and ACE inhibitors correlates with ACE C- and N-domain blockade. *Hypertension.* **38:** 95–99.

Tom, B., Garrelds, I. M., Scalbert, E., Stegmann, A. P., Boomsma, F., Saxena, P. R. and Danser, A. H. J., 2003, ACE-versus chymase-dependent angiotensin II generation in human coronary arteries: a matter of efficiency?, *Arterioscler Thromb Vasc Biol.* **23:** 251–256.

Tsuchida, S., Matsusaka, T., Chen, X., Okubo, S., Niimura, F., Nishimura, H., Fogo, A., Utsunomiya, H., Inagami, T. and Ichikawa, I., 1998, Murine double nullizygotes of the angiotensin type 1A and 1B receptor genes duplicate severe abnormal phenotypes of angiotensinogen nullizygotes. *J Clin Invest.* **101:** 755–760.

Tsutsumi, Y., Matsubara, H., Masaki, H., Kurihara, H., Murasawa, S., Takai, S., Miyazaki, M., Nozawa, Y., Ozono, R., Nakagawa, K., Miwa, T., Kawada, N., Mori, Y., Shibasaki, Y., Tanaka, Y., Fujiyama, S., Koyama, Y., Fujiyama, A., Takahashi, H. and Iwasaka, T., 1999, Angiotensin II type 2 receptor overexpression activates the vascular kinin system and causes vasodilation. *J Clin Invest.* **104:** 925–935.

Turner, A. J. and Hooper, N. M., 2002, The angiotensin-converting enzyme gene family: genomics and pharmacology. *Trends Pharmacol Sci.* **23:** 177–183.

Urata, H., Kinoshita, A., Misono, K. S., Bumpus, F. M. and Husain, A., 1990, Identification of a highly specific chymase as the major angiotensin II-forming enzyme in the human heart. *J Biol Chem.* **265:** 22348–22357.

van den Eijnden, M. M. E. D., de Bruin, R. J. A., de Wit, E., Sluiter, W., Deinum, J., Reudelhuber, T. L. and Danser, A. H. J., 2002, Transendothelial transport of renin-angiotensin system components. *J Hypertens.* **20:** 2029–2037.

van Esch, J. H. M., Schuijt, M. P., Sayed, J., Choudhry, Y., Walther, T. and Danser, A. H. J., 2006, AT(2) receptor-mediated vasodilation in the mouse heart depends on AT(1A) receptor activation. *Br J Pharmacol.* **148:** 452–458.

van Esch, J. H. M., Tom, B., Dive, V., Batenburg, W. W., Georgiadis, D., Yiotakis, A., van Gool, J. M., de Bruijn, R. J. A., de Vries, R. and Danser, A. H. J., 2005, Selective angiotensin-converting enzyme C-domain inhibition is sufficient to prevent angiotensin I-induced vasoconstriction. *Hypertension.* **45:** 120–125.

van Kats, J. P., Chai, W., Duncker, D. J., Schalekamp, M. A. D. H. and Danser, A. H. J., 2005, Adrenal angiotensin: origin and site of generation. *Am J Hypertens.* **18:** 1104–1110.

van Kats, J. P., de Lannoy, L. M., Danser, A. H. J., van Meegen, J. R., Verdouw, P. D. and Schalekamp, M. A. D. H., 1997, Angiotensin II type 1 (AT1) receptor-mediated accumulation of angiotensin II in tissues and its intracellular half-life in vivo. *Hypertension.* **30:** 42–49.

van Kats, J. P., Duncker, D. J., Haitsma, D. B., Schuijt, M. P., Niebuur, R., Stubenitsky, R., Boomsma, F., Schalekamp, M. A. D. H., Verdouw, P. D. and Danser, A. H. J., 2000, Angiotensin-converting enzyme inhibition and angiotensin II type 1 receptor blockade prevent cardiac remodeling in pigs after myocardial infarction: role of tissue angiotensin II. *Circulation.* **102:** 1556–1563.

van Kats, J. P., van Meegen, J. R., Verdouw, P. D., Duncker, D. J., Schalekamp, M. A. D. H. and Danser, A. H. J., 2001, Subcellular localization of angiotensin II in kidney and adrenal. *J Hypertens.* **19:** 583–589.

van Rodijnen, W. F., van Lambalgen, T. A., van Wijhe, M. H., Tangelder, G. J. and Ter Wee, P. M., 2002, Renal microvascular actions of angiotensin II fragments. *Am J Physiol Renal Physiol.* **283:** F86–92.

Véniant, M., Ménard, J., Bruneval, P., Morley, S., Gonzales, M. F. and Mullins, J. J., 1996, Vascular damage without hypertension in transgenic rats expressing prorenin exclusively in the liver. *J Clin Invest.* **98:** 1966–1970.

Vickers, C., Hales, P., Kaushik, V., Dick, L., Gavin, J., Tang, J., Godbout, K., Parsons, T., Baronas, E., Hsieh, F., Acton, S., Patane, M., Nichols, A. and Tummino, P., 2002, Hydrolysis of biological peptides by human angiotensin-converting enzyme-related carboxypeptidase. *J Biol Chem.* **277:** 14838–14843.

Walters, P. E., Gaspari, T. A. and Widdop, R. E., 2005, Angiotensin-(1–7) acts as a vasodepressor agent via angiotensin II type 2 receptors in conscious rats. *Hypertension.* **45**: 960–966.

Walther, T., Menrad, A., Orzechowski, H. D., Siemeister, G., Paul, M. and Schirner, M., 2003, Differential regulation of in vivo angiogenesis by angiotensin II receptors. *FASEB J.* **17**: 2061–2067.

Wei, L., Alhenc-Gelas, F., Corvol, P. and Clauser, E., 1991a, The two homologous domains of human angiotensin I-converting enzyme are both catalytically active. *J Biol Chem.* **266**: 9002–9008.

Wei, L., Alhenc-Gelas, F., Soubrier, F., Michaud, A., Corvol, P. and Clauser, E., 1991b, Expression and characterization of recombinant human angiotensin I-converting enzyme. Evidence for a C-terminal transmembrane anchor and for a proteolytic processing of the secreted recombinant and plasma enzymes. *J Biol Chem.* **266**: 5540–5546.

Wharton, J., Morgan, K., Rutherford, R. A., Catravas, J. D., Chester, A., Whitehead, B. F., De Leval, M. R., Yacoub, M. H. and Polak, J. M., 1998, Differential distribution of angiotensin AT2 receptors in the normal and failing human heart. *J Pharmacol Exp Ther.* **284**: 323–336.

Widdop, R. E., Jones, E. S., Hannan, R. E. and Gaspari, T. A., 2003, Angiotensin AT2 receptors: cardiovascular hope or hype?, *Br J Pharmacol.* **140**: 809–824.

Widdop, R. E., Matrougui, K., Levy, B. I. and Henrion, D., 2002, AT2 receptor-mediated relaxation is preserved after long-term AT1 receptor blockade. *Hypertension.* **40**: 516–520.

Wiemer, G., Schölkens, B. A., Wagner, A., Heitsch, H. and Linz, W., 1993, The possible role of angiotensin II subtype AT2 receptors in endothelial cells and isolated ischemic rat hearts. *J Hypertens.* **11**: S234–235.

Wright, J. W. and Harding, J. W., 1995, Brain angiotensin receptor subtypes AT1, AT2, and AT4 and their functions. *Regul Pept.* **59**: 269–295.

Wright, J. W., Stubley, L., Pederson, E. S., Kramar, E. A., Hanesworth, J. M. and Harding, J. W., 1999, Contributions of the brain angiotensin IV-AT4 receptor subtype system to spatial learning. *J Neurosci.* **19**: 3952–3961.

Wu, J. N., Edwards, D. and Berecek, K. H., 1994, Changes in renal angiotensin II receptors in spontaneously hypertensive rats by early treatment with the angiotensin-converting enzyme inhibitor captopril. *Hypertension.* **23**: 819–822.

Xu, J., Carretero, O.A., Liu, Y.H., Shesely, E.G., Yang, F., Kapke, A. and Yang, X.P., 2002, Role of AT2 receptors in the cardioprotective effect of AT1 antagonists in mice. *Hypertension.* **40**: 244–250.

Yamada, H., Akishita, M., Ito, M., Tamura, K., Daviet, L., Lehtonen, J. Y., Dzau, V. J. and Horiuchi, M., 1999, AT2 receptor and vascular smooth muscle cell differentiation in vascular development. *Hypertension.* **33**: 1414–1419.

Yang, Z., Bove, C. M., French, B. A., Epstein, F. H., Berr, S. S., DiMaria, J. M., Gibson, J. J., Carey, R. M. and Kramer, C. M., 2002, Angiotensin II type 2 receptor overexpression preserves left ventricular function after myocardial infarction. *Circulation.* **106**: 106–111.

Yayama, K., Horii, M., Hiyoshi, H., Takano, M., Okamoto, H., Kagota, S. and Kunitomo, M., 2004, Up-regulation of angiotensin II type 2 receptor in rat thoracic aorta by pressure-overload. *J Pharmacol Exp Ther.* **308**: 736–743.

Zhou, Y., Chen, Y., Dirksen, W. P., Morris, M. and Periasamy, M., 2003, AT1b receptor predominantly mediates contractions in major mouse blood vessels. *Circ Res.* **93**: 1089–1094.

Zini, S., Fournie-Zaluski, M. C., Chauvel, E., Roques, B. P., Corvol, P. and Llorens-Cortes, C., 1996, Identification of metabolic pathways of brain angiotensin II and III using specific aminopeptidase inhibitors: predominant role of angiotensin III in the control of vasopressin release. *Proc Natl Acad Sci U S A.* **93**: 11968–11973.

Zou, Y., Akazawa, H., Qin, Y., Sano, M., Takano, H., Minamino, T., Makita, N., Iwanaga, K., Zhu, W., Kudoh, S., Toko, H., Tamura, K., Kihara, M., Nagai, T., Fukamizu, A., Umemura, S., Iiri, T., Fujita, T. and Komuro, I., 2004, Mechanical stress activates angiotensin II type 1 receptor without the involvement of angiotensin II. *Nat Cell Biol.* **6**: 499–506.

CHAPTER 13

ADAMS AS MEDIATORS OF ANGIOTENSIN II ACTIONS

A.M. BOURNE[1,2] AND W.G. THOMAS[1]

[1]*Molecular Endocrinology, Baker Heart Research Institute, PO Box 6492 St Kilda Road Central, Melbourne 8008, Victoria, Australia*

[2]*Department of Biochemistry and Molecular Biology, Monash University, Melbourne 3800, Australia*

1. INTRODUCTION

Other chapters in this book focus on the role that proteolytic processing plays in the generation and degradation of angiotensin peptides. Such events are crucial to the initiation, modulation and/or termination of angiotensin actions at the type 1 angiotensin receptor (AT_1) and other atypical angiotensin receptors. In addition, there is increasing awareness that following AT_1 receptor activation specific, cell surface proteases are stimulated and that the cleavage products of these proteases make a fundamental contribution to downstream receptor actions. Thus, AT_1 receptors can promote a set of classical signals attributed to their cognate heterotrimeric guanine nucleotide-binding (G) proteins whilst simultaneously activating alternative signals based on the proteolytic shedding of extracellular ligands for other receptors. The most compelling – although still relatively poorly understood – example of such activity is the capacity of G protein-coupled receptors (GPCRs), such as the AT_1 receptor, to promote the shedding of epidermal growth factor (EGF) ligands which subsequently activate EGF receptors (EGFR) in a process termed EGFR transactivation. In this chapter, we focus on a major class of cell surface proteases called ADAMs (a disintegrin and metalloprotease) that have been strongly implicated in the shedding of growth factor ligands, and review the evidence that these important enzymes form a critical component of AT_1 receptor activity and contribute to disease.

Po Sing Leung (ed.), Frontiers in Research of the Renin-Angiotensin System on Human Disease, 273–301.
© 2007 *Springer.*

2.   AT$_1$ RECEPTOR SIGNALLING

2.1.   Classic GPCR Signalling

Activation of G proteins is the primary mechanism by which GPCRs, such the AT$_1$ receptor, induce intracellular signalling pathways. In the case of the AT$_1$ receptor, binding of AngII induces conformational changes in the receptor that enable it to interact with, and activate, the G protein G$_{q/11}$ (De Gasparo *et al* 2000). G$_{q/11}$ activation stimulates phospholipase C-β1 (PLCβ-1), which generates the second messengers inositol trisphosphate (IP$_3$) and diacylglycerol (DAG). These second messengers in turn promote intracellular release of calcium and protein kinase C (PKC) activation, which leads to a variety of cellular responses. Although most of the important cardiovascular, endocrine and metabolic actions of AngII can be explained by AT$_1$/G$_{q/11}$-mediated signals, AT$_1$ receptors have also been reported to couple to other G proteins, such as G$_i$, G$_o$, G$_{12/13}$, and G$_s$ and their downstream effectors, in various tissues and cell models.

2.2.   Alternative Receptor Signalling

In addition to the signalling mediated by classical G protein-dependent pathways, GPCRs also activate pathways that require the activity of receptor and non-receptor tyrosine kinases (Waters *et al* 2004). For the AT$_1$ receptor, these tyrosine kinase-related pathways appear to be important players in AngII-mediated growth (hypertrophy and/or proliferation) of cardiac, vascular and renal cells (Shah and Catt 2004; Shah *et al* 2004; Ohtsu *et al* 2006a; Shah and Catt 2006) and are especially important to the pathological actions of AngII in cardiovascular dysfunction. The exact molecular mechanisms that permit GPCRs to activate tyrosine kinases remain ill defined, but there is much experimental support for the idea that significant cross-talk exists between different families of cell surface receptors. There is little doubt that GPCRs can activate tyrosine kinase receptors and, conversely, that tyrosine kinase receptors modulate the activity of GPCRs. As an example, there is considerable evidence from multiple laboratories that stimulation of the AT$_1$ receptor leads to co-incident tyrosine phosphorylation and activation of the EGFR (see section 3.1). Conversely, activation of the EGFR also leads to phosphorylation of the AT$_1$ receptor (Olivares-Reyes *et al* 2005) and its decreased expression (Ullian *et al* 2004) (processes normally associated with AT$_1$ receptor desensitisation).

3.   EGFR ACTIVATION

The EGFR family consists of four main members (EGFR or HER1, HER2, HER3 and HER4; also known as ErbB1-4). These multi-domain receptors consist of an extracellular ligand-binding site, a single transmembrane spanning region and a cytoplasmic tyrosine kinase domain, and are implicated in controlling a number of cellular processes including cellular proliferation, cell cycle progression, cell metabolism, migration, apoptosis and differentiation (Burgess *et al* 2003). EGF receptors are activated by ligands including EGF, heparin-binding EGF (HB-EGF), transforming growth factor α (TGFα), the neuregulins, betacellulin, amphiregulin, epiregulin, and epigen (Harris *et al* 2003). Alternatively, EGFRs can also be activated by mutations, which occur in many types of cancers. Upon ligand-binding (or mutation), a conformational change in the receptor is induced that exposes a peptide loop (*the dimersation arm*) that enables the ligand-bound EGFR to bind to another EGFR in the same conformation to form back-to back dimers (Ferguson 2004). In the dimerised state, the cytoplasmic tyrosine kinase domains are brought into close proximity, allowing auto- and trans-phosphorylation of the respective carboxyl-termini. These phosphorylated residues then become docking/activation sites for downstream signalling molecules that promote growth and proliferation signalling cascades, such as the Ras/Raf/MAPK pathway (Schlessinger 2000). With the exception of HER2, which doesn't bind ligands with high affinity but instead acts as a preferred binding and signalling partner for other activated EGFR subtypes, and HER3, which lacks kinase activity and can not form an active homo-dimer, EGF receptors, in general, bind multiple ligands and form both homo- and hetero-dimers, which *flavour* the response to various stimuli (Garrett *et al* 2002; Cho *et al* 2003; Citri *et al* 2003).

3.1.   EGFR Transactivation

The first evidence that seven transmembrane-spanning, GPCRs can *transactivate* EGFRs was reported in 1996, when Ullrich and colleagues reported that thrombin, endothelin-1 and lysophosphatidic acid (LPA) (ligands that bind and activate GPCRs) could stimulate rapid tyrosine phosphorylation of both EGFR and HER2 in Rat-1 fibroblasts (Daub *et al* 1996). These GPCR ligands stimulated cellular growth (activated MAPK signalling pathways and DNA synthesis), which was blocked by a small molecule inhibitor of EGFR, AG1478, as well as a dominant/negative version of the EGFR, indicating that these processes were dependent upon activation of the EGFR. The transactivation of the EGFR was so rapid (tyrosine phospho-rylation of the EGFR occurred within minutes of GPCR ligand activation) that the authors doubted at the time whether EGF ligands could be involved. Ensuing studies indicated that the AT_1 receptor also displayed a facility to tyrosine phospho-rylate and transactivate the EGFR via cytoplasmic signals and/or second messengers emanating from the activated AT_1 receptor (such as increased cytoplasmic Ca^{2+}, protein kinase C (PKC) and the soluble tyrosine kinases, Src and Pyk) rather than the shedding of EGF ligands from the cell surface (Li *et al* 1998; Murasawa *et al* 1998b; Eguchi *et al* 1999; Moriguchi *et al* 1999). In particular, studies in vascular smooth muscle cells (VSMCs) and cardiac fibroblasts have shown a requirement for such molecules (Eguchi *et al* 1998; Murasawa *et al* 1998a).

However, in a landmark paper in 1999, Ullrich and colleagues reported a new paradigm for GPCR-mediated transactivation, which involved a metalloprotease-dependent cleavage of an EGF ligand (pro-HB-EGF) and its subsequent binding and activation of the EGFR (Prenzel *et al* 1999). Three main observations were used to support this model: 1) stimulation by GPCR ligands lead to the tyrosine phosphorylation of a chimeric receptor, consisting of the extracellular ligand binding domain of the EGFR fused to the cytoplasmic domain of the platelet-derived growth factor receptor (PDGFR) – importantly, the wild type PDGFR was not activated by the GPCR ligands. This indicated that the extracellular ligand-binding domain of the EGFR was crucial for transactivation (presumably by binding shed ligands); 2) EGFR transactivation was observed in co-cultures of cells expressing separately the activating GPCR or the EGFR, suggesting the release of a paracrine factor in response to GPCR activation; 3) GPCR ligands led to the proteolytic cleavage of the HB-EGF ligand precursor (pro-HB-EGF), which was prevented using a metalloproteinase inhibitor. In addition to the above evidence, they also showed that GPCR-induced EGFR transactivation was blocked by a metalloproteinase inhibitor or by specifically inhibiting the activity of released HB-EGF. Rather than dispelling the notion that EGFR transactivation can result exclusively from the intracellular actions of the GPCR, these data indicate that transactivation likely occurs via both metalloprotease-dependent (i.e. shedding) or independent mechanisms (Waters *et al* 2004).

This entire process of GPCR activation resulting in metalloprotease-mediated cleavage of an EGFR ligand and subsequent activation of the EGFR growth pathway is now known as the 'triple membrane passing signalling' (TMPS) paradigm (Prenzel *et al* 1999) (Fig. 1). Since its discovery, TMPS has been identified in a number of different cellular contexts and a number of GPCRs are now known to activate it. To date, GPCR-mediated EGFR transactivation has been identified in a number of cell types including rat-1 fibroblasts (Daub *et al* 1996), COS-7

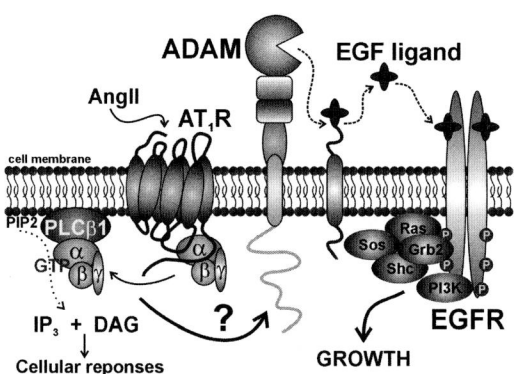

Figure 1. AT1R-mediated EGFR transactivation (TMPS). Interaction of AngII with the AT_1R activates its cognate G protein (Gq/11); the activated (GTP-bound) alpha subunits stimulate phospholipase C (PLCβ-1) to generate the second messengers, inositol trisphosphate (IP3) and diacylglyerol (DAG), which increase intracellular calcium and activate protein kinase C (PKC,) respectively. In the current model of TMPS, the activated AT_1R, via unresolved intracellular mechanisms, induces ADAM-mediated EGFR ligand shedding on the extracellular side of the cell membrane. The released ligand activates the EGFR, leading to dimerisation, phosphorylation, and recruitment of signalling complexes that stimulate growth-associated pathways

cells (Yan *et al* 2002), VSMCs (Eguchi *et al* 1999), liver epithelial cells (Li *et al* 1998), primary mouse astrocytes (Daub *et al* 1997), HaCaT keratinocytes (Daub *et al* 1997), rat pheochromocytoma cell line PC-12 cells (Zwick *et al* 1997), cardiac fibroblasts (Murasawa *et al* 1998a), cardiac endothelial cells (Fujiyama *et al* 2001) and cardiomyocytes (Asakura *et al* 2002; Kodama *et al* 2002; Thomas *et al* 2002). The prevalence of EGFR transactivation by the AT_1 receptor in different cell types (Bokemeyer *et al* 2000; Eguchi *et al* 2001; Fujiyama *et al* 2001; Uchiyama-Tanaka *et al* 2001; Ushio-Fukai *et al* 2001a; Asakura *et al* 2002; Kodama *et al* 2002; Saito *et al* 2002; Thomas *et al* 2002; Greco *et al* 2003; Lin and Freeman 2003; Suarez *et al* 2003; Shah *et al* 2004; Chiu *et al* 2005; Laurette *et al* 2005; Mifune *et al* 2005; Yang *et al* 2005; Flannery and Spurney 2006; Yahata *et al* 2006) likely indicates a conserved, key mechanism for usurping tyrosine kinase pathways, although the prevailing molecular mechanism seems to vary in different cellular contexts.

Recent evidence supports the emerging role for ADAMs as the key metal-loproteinases involved in EGF ligand shedding and EGFR transactivation given their ability to shed EGF-like ligands from the cell surface and their involvement in cardiac development/growth (Blobel 2005). The following sections review the structure and function of ADAMs as well as potential mechanisms of activation by the AT_1 receptor.

4. ADAMS

ADAMs are a family of zinc-dependent metalloproteases with high sequence homology to snake venom disintegrins (Blobel *et al* 1992; Weskamp and Blobel 1994; Wolfsberg *et al* 1995; Stone *et al* 1999). To date, about 40 ADAM family members have been identified (an up-to-date list of ADAMs in different species is maintained by Dr. Judith White.[1] Expression studies in mammals have shown that many of the ADAMs are expressed predominantly, or solely, in the testis and other reproductive structures and are thus thought to function mostly in fertilisation and spermatogenesis (Zhu *et al* 1999), whereas other family members have a more widespread somatic distribution (Seals and Courtneidge 2003).

As well as being involved in shedding membrane-bound proteins (such as EGFR ligands, receptors, cytokines, adhesion molecules), ADAMs are also involved in cleavage of extracellular matrix (ECM) proteins, amlyoid precursor protein and *Notch*, and thereby affect ECM communication, cell migration, cell proliferation and development (Blobel 2005). In addition to having important roles in various cellular processes, the activity of ADAMs is also associated with a number of human diseases including cancer, Alzheimer's disease, and asthma (Seals and Courtneidge 2003), as well as renal diseases (such as chronic kidney disease) (Laurette *et al* 2005; Shah and Catt 2006) and polycystic kidney disease (Dell *et al* 2001) and cardiovascular diseases (such as left ventricular hypertrophy and vascular remod-elling) (Shah and Catt 2004).

---

[1] http://www.people.virginia.edu/%7Ejw7g/Table_of_the_ADAMs.html

5.   ADAM STRUCTURE-FUNCTION

ADAMs are multi-domain proteins that contain an N-terminal signal sequence, prodomain, disintegrin domain, metalloprotease domain, cysteine-rich domain and an EGF-like domain (Fig. 2). ADAMs that are expressed at the cell surface also possess a transmembrane domain (that localises them to the plasma membrane) and a cytoplasmic domain (Blobel and White 1992; Wolfsberg *et al* 1995; Schlondorff and Blobel 1999). Each of these conserved domains plays an important role in the localisation, synthesis and function of the ADAMs (Wolfsberg and White 1996; Blobel 1997; Black and White 1998).

5.1.   The Metalloprotease Domain

ADAMs contain a metalloprotease domain that is believed to be the site of prote-olytic activity. Within this domain, half of the known ADAMs have the histidine-rich metalloprotease consensus sequence (HEXXH) in which the histidine residue binds zinc and the glutamic acid is the catalytic residue (Stocker *et al* 1995; Wolfsberg *et al* 1995; Jia *et al* 1996). In addition, the upstream Met-turn methionine

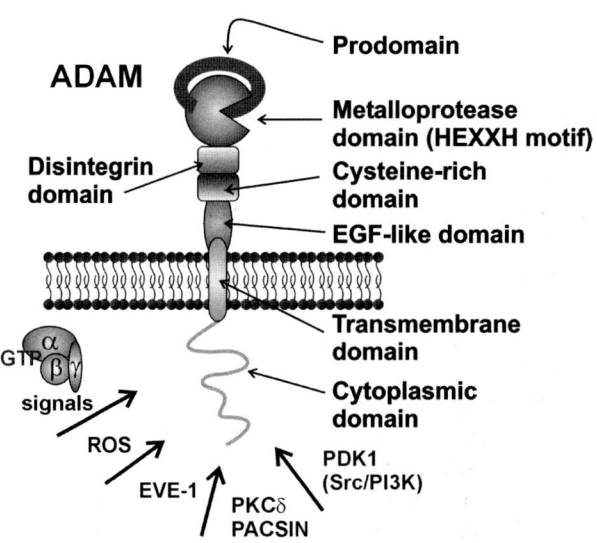

Figure 2. ADAM structure and potential regulation. ADAMs contain multiple functional domains, including: a prodomain, metalloprotease domain, disintegrin domain, cysteine-rich domain, EGF-like domain and can contain transmembrane and cytoplasmic domains when localised in the cell membrane as illustrated. Via these domains, ADAMs potentially mediate proteolysis, signalling, fusion and adhesion. GPCR-mediated transactivation (TMPS) presumably involve intracellular mechanisms that result in the activation of extracellular proteolysis by membrane-bound ADAMs. This is likely to involve interaction between the downstream signalling molecules of GPCRs and the cytoplasmic tail of ADAMs, which is thought to have important roles in signalling given the presence of putative proline-rich, SH3 binding sites and phosphorylation sites. Some putative modulators are shown

residue is thought to be involved in stabilising zinc binding (Bode *et al* 1993; Maskos *et al* 1998). ADAMs that contain this motif (including ADAMs 1, 8-10, 12, 13, 15, 16, 17, 19-21, 24-26, 28, 30, 33-40[1]) are therefore presumed to have the ability to cleave substrates (White 2003); although this has not yet been shown experimentally for all of the above (Howard *et al* 1996; Black *et al* 1997; Moss *et al* 1997; Loechel *et al* 1998; Chesneau *et al* 2003).

Catalytically-active ADAMs cleave membrane-bound proteins from the cell surface by cutting the protein near the plasma membrane (Pandiella *et al* 1992). Although studies have failed to find a consensus sequence, or a specific distance from the plasma membrane at which target proteins are cleaved by ADAMs (White 2003), substrate recognition may instead be via secondary and tertiary structure (Moss and Lambert 2002).

5.2.   The Disintegrin Domain

ADAMs also contain a disintegrin domain (named so because of its high sequence homology with snake-venom disintegrin) that is thought to have roles in cell adhesion and migration. Many proteins contain disintegrin domains and the conserved RGD motif that binds to integrins, such as $\alpha v\beta 3$ and $\alpha 5\beta 1$ (Blobel and White 1992; Niewiarowski *et al* 1994; Maskos *et al* 1998). However, despite displaying the ability to bind to integrins, only human ADAM15 contains the RGD motif (Kratzschmar *et al* 1996; Nath *et al* 1999). Other ADAMs are thought to interact with integrins that recognise the sequence RX_6DLPEF (Eto *et al* 2002). For example, the disintegrin and cysteine rich domains of ADAM12 interact with integrin $\alpha 7\beta 1$ (Zhao *et al* 2004).

5.3.   Cysteine-Rich and EGF-Like Domains

These domains are presumably involved in membrane fusion given that they contain motifs similar to those found in virus fusion peptides (Blobel and White 1992; Black and White 1998). Some ADAMs (including ADAMs 1, 3 and 12) have been shown to be involved in cell fusion reactions, (Seals and Courtneidge 2003). For example the cysteine-rich domain of ADAM12 is known to mediate myoblast and fibroblast adhesion (Yagami-Hiromasa *et al* 1995). In addition, these two domains may also be involved in increasing substrate binding efficiency by complementing that activity of the disintegrin domain (Stone *et al* 1999).

5.4.   ADAM Regulation and Trafficking- Key Roles for the Prodomain and Cytoplamic Carboxyl-Terminus

Given the key role of ADAMs in a number of signalling pathways including transactivation, it would seem likely that ADAMs are tightly regulated to ensure they are not over-active. Indeed, there is evidence to suggest that ADAM activity occurs (at least for ADAM17) at a basal level in unstimulated cells that is increased upon stimulation with a variety of pharmacological and physiological stimuli (Doedens *et al* 2003). However, details of how ADAMs are trafficked to the cell membrane and the regulation of their trafficking and/or activity is poorly understood at present.

In this regard, the trafficking and activation of ADAM17 has been studied more widely than other ADAMs, yet many questions still remain. Much of the research has focused on the potential role of the prodomain in controlling ADAM function by maintaining the ADAM in an inactive state either at the cell surface or prior to trafficking to the cell surface. The prodomain is thought to aid correct folding and localisation by acting as a chaperone (Milla *et al* 1999) and targeting ADAMs through the secretory pathway. Furin cleavage of the prodomain (presumably in the trans-Golgi network (Schafer *et al* 1995; Wouters *et al* 1998) has also been reported for several ADAMs and evidence suggests that prodomain removal is likely to be needed for metalloprotease activity (Lum *et al* 1998; Roghani *et al* 1999; Hougaard *et al* 2000; Howard *et al* 2000; Srour *et al* 2003) although the nature of the molecular switches involved in stimulating prodomain cleavage are unclear. Indeed, ADAM10 prodomain removal processing by furin and PC7 results in increased ADAM10 activity (Anders *et al* 2001).

The prodomain is postulated to keep the ADAM proteins inactive via a cysteine-switch mechanism that is later reversed when the prodomain is cleaved (Vanwart and Birkedalhansen 1990; Grams *et al* 1993). In this mechanism, it is thought that an unpaired cysteine residue within the prodomain blocks the active site by inter-acting with the zinc binding residues via a thiol link (Milla *et al* 1999). In line with this, other evidence to support the potentially important role of the prodomain have pointed to the cysteine-switch mechanism as being key, with modification of the cysteine-switch being suggested as a trigger for the cessation of ADAM activity inhibition. For example, there is evidence that sulphydral modifications induce shedding of cell surface proteins (Bennett *et al* 2000). In addition, since ADAM17 activity is able to be induced by nitric oxide and reactive oxygen (ROS), the inactivity of ADAM17 may be maintained by the cysteine-switch that is modified by these molecules to allow it to become active (Zhang *et al* 2000; Zhang *et al* 2001). There is also evidence to suggest that ADAM17 may be activated by alkylation, which may interrupt the cysteine switch and thus stop prodomain inhibition (Milla *et al* 1999).

A second possible mechanism for ADAM regulation that has been proposed is that ADAM activation may be controlled by the location/position of the sheddase and the substrate within the cell, particularly within the lipid rafts where ADAM activity has been reported (Wakatsuki *et al* 2004). Evidence has shown that basal shedding (at least) may be regulated by ADAM localisation within the plasma membrane given that depletion of cholesterol promotes the shedding of β-Amyloid precursor protein and L1 adhesion molecule (Kojro *et al* 2001; Mechtersheimer *et al* 2001). This is particularly relevant for the AT_1 receptor mediated transactivation pathway as both AT_1 receptor and EGFR activity has been reported to occur with lipid rafts/calveolin (Ushio-Fukai *et al* 2001b). Indeed, an important role of these micro-domains in transactivation in VSMCs has become evident with research showing that AT_1 receptor targeting into Caveolin1-enriched lipid rafts is necessary for the proper organisation of AT_1 receptor and EGFR during ROS-dependent Ang II signalling and VSMC hypertrophy (Zuo et al 2005).

There is also evidence that the ability of ADAMs to cleave substrates may be limited by substrate conformation. It has been proposed that intracellular signals may stimulate ADAM-mediated shedding by impinging on the ectodomain of the substrate, thus promoting a conformation in the substrate more favourable for shedding. As an example, a number of ectodomain shedding events are induced by sulfhydryl-modifying reagents that may cause not only ADAM activation, but may also induce such conformational changes in ADAM substrates (Zhang and Aggarwal 1994).

In addition to possible activation/inhibition by the prodomain, or sheddase/substrate interactions, the cytoplasmic tails of ADAMs have been proposed to act as regulators of metalloprotease activity. In transactivation, GPCRs activate the metalloprotease activity of ADAMs via a mechanism that might logically involve an intracellular signal emanating from the GPCR that impinges upon the cytoplasmic carboxyl-terminus of the ADAM (see Figs. 1 and 2). Given the membrane orientation of GPCRs and ADAMs, this intracellular mechanism most likely involves direct or indirect interaction between the cytoplasmic tail of ADAMs and signalling molecules that are activated by GPCRs (or the GPCRs themselves). Such direct or indirect interactions of signalling molecules and the cytoplasmic domain of ADAMs may induce proteolytic cleavage, affect disintegrin domain activity, or influence subcellular location/processing. Indeed, a variety of ADAM-protein interactions have been documented which may modulate ADAM function.

Accordingly, despite low sequence homology between ADAM family members, the cytoplasmic tail of many ADAMs is replete in potential serine-threonine and/or tyrosine kinase phosphorylation sites and protein:protein interaction motifs (e.g. PDZ, SH2 and SH3 binding domains that may be involved in signal trans-duction via the activation of SH3 domain containing proteins, such as Abl or Src (Weskamp and Blobel 1994; Wolfsberg and White 1996). Although the exact mechanism is yet to be determined, it seems possible that phosphorylation and/or binding of proteins to these sites in the ADAM tail may be the means by which GPCRs are able to either directly or indirectly intracellularly activate ADAMs and induce ADAM metalloprotease activity. Indeed, many well known, and several novel proteins, have been shown to bind to ADAM9 (Howard et al 1999; Nelson et al 1999), ADAM15 (Howard et al 1999), ADAM17 (Nelson et al 1999) and ADAM19 (Huang et al 2002) cytoplasmic domains in vitro and in vivo. For example ADAM12 has been found to interact with a number of SH3 domain containing proteins including p85α (Kang et al 2001), Src (Kang et al 2000) and Grb2 (Suzuki et al 2000) (although binding of these molecules has not been shown to induce substrate cleavage). In addition, proteins such as Eve-1 have been found to bind to the cytoplasmic tail of ADAM9, 10, 12, and 17 and induce HB-EGF shedding in response to AngII and phorbol ester (TPA) stimulation, as well as the shedding of amphiregulin, TGFα, and epiregulin in response to TPA (Tanaka et al 2004). Cytoplasmic binding of PACSIN3 to ADAM12 has also been shown to modulate metalloprotease activity since knockdown of endogenous PACSIN3 with small interfering RNA (siRNA) reduces the amount of TPA and AngII induced HB-EGF shedding (Mori *et al* 2003). As well as such protein:protein interactions, kinases have been shown to phosphorylate ADAMs including ADAM9 (Izumi *et al* 1998), ADAM12 (Suzuki *et al* 2000), ADAM15 (Poghosyan *et al* 2002) and ADAM17 (Diaz-Rodriguez *et al* 2000). In some cases, such phosphorylation events have been shown to regulate shedding under different conditions, which also might be important in stimulating/modulating ADAM enzymatic function. For example, PKCδ interaction with ADAM9 has been shown to regulate HB-EGF cleavage (Izumi *et al* 1998). Finally, a recent paper by Zhang *et al.* (Zhang *et al* 2006) reported that EGFR transactivation by the gastrin-releasing peptide receptor involved Src- and PI3-kinase-mediated activation of phosphoinositide-dependent kinase 1 (PDK1), which directly phosphorylated ADAM17 within this cytoplasmic domain and activated the shedding of the EGF ligand, amphiregulin. Whether such a mechanism is more widespread in GPCR transactivation, and for other ADAMs, awaits examination.

Despite a large amount of evidence for the cytoplasmic domain having a role in ADAM activation, there is also evidence that points to the contrary. For example, ADAM17 lacking the cytoplasmic domain was able to reconstitute phorbol ester (PMA)-induced shedding in ADAM17 deficient fibroblasts (Reddy *et al* 2000). Similar research using a peptide cleavage assay has also shown that the cytoplasmic domain of ADAM17 is not absolutely required for PMA induced shedding of p75-TNFR (Doedens *et al* 2003). Such evidence indicates that the ADAM cytoplasmic domain may not be the exclusive site of ADAM activation and points to extracellular protein:protein interactions and cell:cell contacts as possible alternatives.

6.   AT$_1$ RECEPTOR-MEDIATED EGFR TRANSACTIVATION

At present, most evidence points to an ADAM17/HB-EGF-driven EGFR transactivation for the activated AT$_1$R, although this more likely reflects the availability of experimental tools rather than representing the spectrum of actual TMPS scenarios in the various AngII target organs. Just as important as identifying in which cell can a particular GPCR couple to which ADAM and shed which EGF ligand to activate which EGFR isoform (discussed in more depth in later sections) is the need to understand the various molecular paths from AT$_1$R activation to ADAM shedding.

As mentioned above, the interaction of mediators such Eve-1, PACSIN3 with ADAMs and/or PDK1 phosphorylation are exciting possibilities that require further study and confirmation. In addition, other signalling molecules have been hypothesised to control GPCR-mediated ADAM stimulation, including Ca^{2+}, Pyk2, ROS, and even G$_q$ itself (Smith *et al* 2004). While this may be the case for certain cell types, research in cardiomyocytes indicates AngII-mediated transactivation is independent of calcium and PKC since pharmacological inhibition (BAPTA-AM and BIM respectively) does not reduce AngII-induced MAPK stimulation and/or cardiomyocyte hypertrophy *in vitro* (Thomas *et al* 2002).

In considering possible mechanisms for AT_1R coupling to ADAM activation and EGFR transactivation, a significant publication appeared in 2003 from Sadoshima and co-workers (Seta and Sadoshima 2003). These authors reported that the AngII-stimulated AT_1R was tyrosine phosphorylated within its proximal carboxyl-terminus at tyrosine[319] and that this modification of the receptor allowed it to form a higher-order complex with the EGFR, which initiated EGFR signalling, ERK1/2 activation and cell growth. Mutation of Y^{319} in the AT_1R abolished AngII-induced EGFR transactivation. In a follow-up study, these authors demonstrated that the cardiac-specific overexpression of a $Y^{319}F$ AT_1R mutant in transgenic mice prevented EGFR transactivation and AngII-mediated cardiac hypertrophy (Zhai *et al* 2006). Despite the fact that others have also reported the physical interaction between AT_1R and EGFR (Olivares-Reyes *et al* 2005; Ushio-Fukai *et al* 2005), unfortunately, the contribution of Y^{319} to AT_1R-mediated EGFR transactivation has not been replicated (Shah *et al* 2004; Mifune *et al* 2005). Eguchi and colleagues (Mifune *et al* 2005) demonstrated in both COS-7 and CHO-K1 cells that neither truncation of the AT_1R carboxyl-terminus after lysine[318] (thereby removing Y^{319}) nor point mutation at Y^{319} affected HB-EGF shedding or EGFR phosphorylation and transactivation. Instead, their data strongly supported a G protein-mediated activation of ADAM17, the shedding of HB-EGF and subsequent EGFR activation. Similarly, Catt and colleagues reported no difference between $Y^{319}F$ AT_1R and the wild type receptor in their capacity to activate ERK1/2 via AngII-mediated metalloprotease-dependent EGFR transactivation. Hence, in different laboratories under distinct conditions, there is no substantiation of the Y^{319} model of EGFR transactivation (Shah *et al* 2004).

7. A ROLE FOR EGFR TRANSACTIVATION IN AT_1 RECEPTOR-MEDIATED DISEASE

There is overwhelming experimental and clinical evidence that selective antagonism of the renin-angiotensin system, either by inhibiting angiotensin converting enzyme or via AT_1 receptor blockers, can lower blood pressure and reduce the morbidity and mortality associated with dysfunction and disease related to the inappropriate actions of AngII. Importantly, AngII (via the AT_1 receptor) contributes strongly to the growth of renal, vascular and cardiac cells and the remodelling and fibrosis associated with heart failure, atherosclerosis and chronic renal disease. The capacity to promote such growth and remodelling is closely aligned to tyrosine kinase signalling pathways activated by the AT_1 receptor and some recent cell-based and *in vivo* studies suggest that EGFR transactivation is the central conduit for this tyrosine kinase signalling.

7.1. Renal Disease

A variety of studies have now reported that AngII can transactivate the EGFR and promote growth in kidney cells (Bokemeyer *et al* 2000; Uchiyama-Tanaka *et al* 2001; Laurette *et al* 2005; Chen *et al* 2006; Yahata *et al* 2006). As reported by Lautrette *et al*. (2005) damage to the kidney (i.e., lesions, glomerulosclerosis, tubular atrophy, fibrosis, mononuclear cell infiltration and proteinuria) in response to chronic AngII infusion is significantly blunted in mice over-expressing a dominant-negative version of the EGFR (Lautrette *et al* 2005). The dominant-negative EGFR (CD533) is a truncated receptor lacking most of the cytoplasmic tail, suggesting that the inhibition resulted from sequestration of shed EGF-like ligands. Indeed, AngII stimulation promoted EGFR phosphorylation and the shedding of the EGF-like ligand transforming growth factor α (TGFα) and AngII-mediated ERK1/2 activation was inhibited by AG1478 (the EGFR antagonist) and TAPI-1 (an inhibitor with some selectivity towards ADAM17). Chronic AngII infusion resulted in up-regulated ADAM17 and TGFα, whereas AngII-induced renal damage was prevented in mice lacking TGFα or in which endogenous ADAM17 was inhibited. Together, these data strongly indicate that AngII-mediated kidney deterioration is closely associated with the activation of an ADAM (ADAM17) and the shedding of TGFα, and suggest that renal-specific antagonism of EGFR transactivation might be a useful therapeutic approach.

7.2.   Vascular Growth and Remodelling

Substantial evidence support a crucial role for AngII-mediated EGFR transactivation in vascular growth and dysfunction, much of which has been recently comprehensively reviewed (Nakashima *et al* 2006; Ohtsu *et al* 2006a; Mehta and Griendling 2007). Although a number of studies have directly observed EGFR phosphorylation as well as EGFR- and metalloprotease-dependent signals following AngII stimulation in various vascular cell models, the identity of the shed EGF ligand has variously been reported as betacellulin (Mifune *et al* 2004), HB-EGF (Yang *et al* 2005; Ohtsu *et al* 2006b), Epiregulin (Taylor *et al* 1999) or TGFα (Lemarie *et al* 2006). Little evidence exists as to the specific ADAM(s) involved, although Eguchi and colleagues favour ADAM17 based on reduced EGFR phosphorylation and HB-EGF shedding in vascular cells transduced with dominant-negative versions of ADAM17 (Ohtsu *et al* 2006b). An ADAM17-mediating shedding event would also correlate with the recent report that TGFα is an important player in mechanical stretch- and AngII-induced EGFR transactivation, NFκB signalling, vascular cell proliferation and wall thickening (Lemarie *et al* 2006). In their study, Lemarie (2006) reported that increased intraluminal pressure (from 80 mmHg to 150 mmHg) in isolated vessels resulted in an NAPDH oxidase-mediated generation of ROS and the subsequent activation of EGFR and the NFκB transcription factor. NFκB was not activated in vessels from mice bearing non-functional EGFRs or in mice lacking TGFα. In mice lacking TGFα, AngII induced vascular remodelling and NFκB were significantly reduced, indicating a key role for this EGF ligand in both AngII and strain-induced effects. Interestingly, whilst strain also activated ERK1/2 in an EGFR-dependent manner, this was not affected by the absence of TGFα suggesting that different effectors downstream of the EGFR are driven by distinct EGF ligands. It might well be that such selective EGFR transactivating systems are only evoked in the disease state where and when required. Indeed, AngII-mediated vasoreactivity appears to only become EGFR-dependent in a streptozotocin-model of diabetes, but not in non-diabetic controls (Benter *et al* 2005).

7.3.   Cardiac Hypertrophy and Failure

Cardiac hypertrophy is an important physiological mechanism that enables the heart to grow during post-natal development and to adapt to increases in workload and stress caused by tissue injury and cardiovascular diseases including hypertension, myocardial infarction and valvular diseases (Olson and Molkentin 1999). While initially a beneficial response, prolonged hypertrophy is maladaptive, and can lead to heart failure (Levy *et al* 1990). As for the renal and vascular systems, accumulating evidence also indicates that the AngII/AT$_1$ receptor axis, EGFRs, their ligands and ADAMs are major players in cardiac development and maintenance as well as the compensatory processes (hypertrophy and remodelling) that accompany stress or injury to the heart (Shah and Catt 2004; Smith *et al* 2004).

Studies from several groups, including our own, have implicated EGFR transactivation in AngII-mediated cardiac hypertrophy (Asakura *et al* 2002; Kagiyama *et al* 2002; Thomas *et al* 2002). We reported that AngII could promote EGFR phosphorylation in cultured cardiomyocytes and demonstrated that hypertrophy (and hypertrophic signalling) of these cells in response to AngII was blocked by AG1478 and by metalloprotease inhibitors (Thomas *et al* 2002). Kagiyama and colleagues reported that an EGFR antisense approach effectively blocked the development of left ventricular hypertrophy in an AngII-infusion model (Kagiyama *et al* 2002). Asakura and colleagues provided evidence that GPCR-mediated cardiomyocyte hypertrophy *in vitro* and *in vivo* results from an ADAM12-mediated HB-EGF shedding event (Asakura *et al* 2002), an idea that correlates well with the important role that HB-EGF plays in cardiac development (Iwamoto *et al* 2003). However, the ADAMs and EGF ligands (and EGFRs) involved in cardiac growth and development have not been systemically evaluated and, as outlined below, ADAMs in addition to ADAM 12 (including ADAMs 9, 10, 15, 17 and 19), either singly or in combination, are potential candidates. Indeed, in a recent study, Fedak and colleagues reported the differential expression and regulation of ADAMs 10, 12, 15 and 17 and their endogenous tissue inhibitor (TIMP-3) in human myocardium during various cardiac pathologies (Fedak *et al* 2006). Their data indicate complex interplay between multiple ADAMs, TIMPs and integrins in the heart. Moreover, the identity of the exact EGFR responsible for transactivation and the EGF-like ligand involved remains to be determined and indicates yet another gap in our current understanding of this process.

8.   ADAM CANDIDATES FOR EGFR TRANSACTIVATION IN HEART

While the exact ADAM(s) that mediate cardiac hypertrophy remain unknown, there is evidence to suggest the potential involvement of multiple ADAM family members.

ADAM 9 – shedding studies have implicated ADAM9 in the transactivation of EGFR since over-expressing ADAM9 leads to an increase in HB-EGF shedding (Izumi *et al* 1998). However, given that ADAM9 -/- mice are fertile, have no abnormalities and have stimulated and unstimulated HB-EGF shedding levels equal to that of wild type mice, ADAM9 is clearly not the sole ADAM responsible for HB-EGF release, although it may mediate HB-EGF-independent transactivation (Weskamp *et al* 2002).

ADAM10 (Kuzbanian) – ADAM10 is a potential key mediator of cardiac hypertrophy given its importance as an EGFR ligand sheddase, and its clear requirement for heart development. The ADAM10 homologue, Kuzbanian, was first identified in Drosophila as a protease of the Notch cell surface receptor required for neuronal development (Rooke *et al* 1996; Sotillos *et al* 1997). In mammals, ADAM10, is involved in proHB-EGF shedding in epithelial cells since LPA induced EGFR phosphorylation is inhibited by blocking ADAMs/MMPs with GM6001, or by blocking HB-EGF with it's inhibitor CRM197 (Lemjabbar and Basbaum 2002). It has also been implicated as a mediator of bombesin-induced proHB-EGF shedding in COS-7 cells (Yan *et al* 2002). ADAM10 also appears to be the main sheddase of betacellulin and EGF in mouse embryonic fibroblasts (Sahin *et al* 2004) and in mouse stomach epithelial mouse dermal fibroblast (Sanderson *et al* 2005). In addition to being an important sheddase in many cell types, ADAM10 may be involved in GPCR-induced cardiac hypertrophy given that ADAM10 is crucial for proper heart development in *Drosophila Melanogaster* (Albrecht *et al* 2006) and mice, since mice with a disrupted ADAM10 gene die early in embryogenesis due to neural and cardiovascular defects (Hartmann *et al* 2002).

ADAM12 (meltrin α) – ADAM12 was first studied in relation to its disintegrin domain that has a role in promoting C2C12 myoblast fusion into myotubes (Yagami-Hiromasa *et al* 1995). ADAM12 has been implicated in mediating AT_1 receptor activated transactivation given that it is known to shed important EGF ligands such as HB-EGF in a regulated manner (Mori *et al* 2003; Tanaka *et al* 2004). In addition, it has been implicated in cardiac hypertrophy primarily through the study of Asakura and colleagues. (Asakura *et al* 2002) (see section 10 for details).

ADAM15 – ADAM15 is expressed in the human myocardium and shows increased expression following dilated cardiomyopathy (Fedak *et al* 2006). This may be important in the progression of cardiac dysfunction as it may play a role in reducing cell-matrix interactions via cleavage of integrins, such as integrin β1D.

ADAM17 – ADAM17 (also known as TACE) is another strong candidate for mediating cardiac hypertrophy given its crucial role in cleaving EGFR ligands and in heart development. ADAM17 was first identified as the protease that cleaves the inflammatory cytokine TNFα from the plasma membrane (Black *et al* 1997; Moss *et al* 1997). Since then, ADAM17 has been shown to release EGFR ligands: TGF-α, amphiregulin, epiregulin, and HB-EGF in a variety of cells including mouse embryonic fibroblasts, squamous cell carcinoma cells and primary keratinocytes (Sunnarborg *et al* 2002; Gschwind *et al* 2003; Sahin *et al*

2004). In addition knockout studies also indicate that ADAM17 may play a major role in controlling cardiac development and hypertrophy. For example, ADAM17 has been implicated in fetal murine cardiac development and remodelling (Shi *et al* 2003) and ADAM17-/- mice are largely embryonic lethal, while those that survived have major epithelial developmental defects including open eyelids and thickened and misshapen hearts (Peschon *et al* 1998; Jackson *et al* 2003). This extreme cardiac phenotype is also seen in mice that lack EGFR-/- and/or HB-EGF-/- (or have an un-cleavable form of HB-EGF), indicating that ADAM17 may be involved in HB-EGF shedding and EGFR transactivation that is required for normal heart development (Miettinen *et al* 1995; Sibilia and Wagner 1995; Threadgill *et al* 1995; Iwamoto *et al* 2003; Yamazaki *et al* 2003). In addition, triple knockout studies have shown that deletion of ADAM17 alone results in malformed hearts, whereas ADAM9/12/15 triple knockout mice develop normal hearts (Sahin *et al* 2004) further supporting the potential role for ADAM17 in cardiac hypertrophy. On top of this, in the human heart, ADAM17 expression is increased during dilated cardiomyopathy and hypertrophy, further implicating ADAM17 in cardiac growth (Fedak *et al* 2006).

ADAM19 – Knockout studies have also indicated that ADAM19 may be involved in cardiac hypertrophy given that ADAM19 is essential for cardiovascular morphogenesis and development. ADAM19-/- mice have similar heart defects to ADAM17-/- mice(Kurohara *et al* 2004; Zhou *et al* 2004). However, ADAM19 is not likely to be involved in HB-EGF-mediated transactivation, as HB-EGF shedding is unaffected in ADAM19-/- mouse embryonic fibroblasts (Zhou *et al* 2004). Instead, like ADAM9, it may be involved mediating HB-EGF-independent transactivation by releasing other EGFR-ligands from the cell surface.

9.   ROLE OF EGFR SUBTYPES AND LIGANDS IN CARDIAC HYPERTROPHY

Any of the four EGFR subtypes (HER1-4) could theoretically be involved in EGFR transactivation and cardiac hypertrophy. Expression studies have revealed that the presence of all four family members is required for normal heart development, although the exact role of each receptor in cardiac hypertrophy is still under investigation (Chan *et al* 2006). Of the four subtypes, there is mounting evidence that transactivation could involve homo- or hetero-dimers of HER1, HER2 and HER4.

HER2 is a major candidate for mediating AngII-induced cardiac hypertrophy given that HER2 is activated by GPCR induced transactivation (Daub *et al* 1996; Lin and Freeman 2003). HER2 has also been implicated in heart development (Lee *et al* 1995) and HER2 conditional knockout mice have severe heart defects (Ozcelik *et al* 2002). Other evidence for the role of this receptor have come from anti-cancer clinical trials, where it was found that inhibiting HER2 with the anti-cancer drug Herceptin (that specifically inhibits HER2 activity) is associated with cardiomyopathy and heart failure (Crone *et al* 2002), indicating a key role for this receptor in the maintenance of cardiac integrity.

Like HER2, HER4 is another candidate for the key mediator of GPCR induced EGFR transactivation given that HER4 stimulation can result in hypertrophy in both adult and neonatal rat cardiomyocytes (Zhao *et al* 1998). HER4 is also activated by ligands that have been linked to transactivation (notably HB-EGF and the neuregulins) (Reise and Stern 1998; Zhao *et al* 1998). Knockout studies have also implicated this receptor as playing a major role in heart growth and development since HER4 knockout mice fail to develop myocardial trabeculae (Gassmann *et al* 1995).

Likewise HER1 could also be involved in transactivation in the heart given that inhibition of this receptor in cardiac fibroblasts with the HER1 specific antagonist AG1478 or with dominant-negative mutant versions of the receptor inhibit AngII-mediated transactivation (Murasawa *et al* 1998a). HER1 knockout studies also suggest a prominent role for this receptor subtype in heart growth and development given that HER1 knockout mice exhibit sever epithelial and vascular abnormalities (Miettinen *et al* 1995; Sibilia and Wagner 1995; Threadgill *et al* 1995). HER3 however is not likely to mediate hypertrophy in adult cardiomyocytes as expression levels drop to a very low level in the heart after embryogenesis (Zhao *et al* 1998). At present, the identification of the EGFR family member(s) that mediated cardiac hypertrophy under normal and pathological conditions remains to be determined.

Moreover, the specific EGFR ligand(s) that mediate transactivation in cardiomyocytes also remains unknown. As mentioned earlier, all EGFRs except HER2 are activated by ligands from the epidermal growth factor (EGF)/Neuregulin family, including EGF, HB-EGF, TGF-α, betacellulin, amphiregulin, epiregulin and epigen (Reise and Stern 1998). All EGFR ligands are synthesised as type I trans-membrane integral membrane-bound precursors that are able to be shed from the cell surface. However while shedding occurs, it may not be required for biological activity (Harris *et al* 2003). For example *in vitro* studies have shown that membrane bound precursors are able to have activity at the cell surface in a juxtacrine manner (Wong *et al* 1989). In most other instances, including those in *Drosophila* and mammals, it has been shown that the ligands require proteolytic cleavage from the membrane to form mature soluble proteins consisting mainly of the EGF-like domain (Freeman 1994; Dong *et al* 1999).

Most transactivation research has focused on HB-EGF as the ligand involved in GPCR mediated EGFR transactivation, as it was the first ligand identified in association with this phenomenon (Prenzel *et al* 1999). Evidence to support an important role for HB-EGF in transactivation in the heart comes from knockout studies, where HB-EGF-/- mice have cardiac defects similar to mice that lack EGFR (Iwamoto *et al* 2003). In cardiomyocyte hypertrophy, HB-EGF has also been implicated since blocking HB-EGF release via neutralising antibodies or catalytically inactive ADAM12 mutants blocks EGFR activation and hypertrophy of cardiomyocytes (Asakura *et al* 2002).

However, while HB-EGF may be involved in mediating transactivation in the heart, it may not be the sole ligand involved. Research has also shown that neuregulins have roles in heart growth and development (Garratt 2006). For example, neuregulin-1, knockout mice die of heart failure during mid-embryogenesis (Zhao *et al* 1998). In addition, neuregulin-1 has been implicated in cardiac hypertrophy (Baliga *et al* 1999), possibly via release from endothelial cells to activate HER4 and HER2 on cardiomyocytes (Lemmens *et al* 2006) to promote survival especially in situations where cardiac function is compromised (Liu *et al* 2006; Timolati *et al* 2006). The investigation of the role of these and other ligands is still being carried out.

10.   APPROACHES TO STUDY ADAMS IN THE EGFR TRANSACTIVATION PATHWAY

Traditionally, the involvement of a particular ADAM in a specific cellular process has been examined using over-expressed wild type ADAMs, catalytically-inactive "dominant-negatives" and/or pharmacological inhibitors of sometimes limited (or unknown) selectivity. The common approach for generating a dominant-negative ADAM is to introduce a point mutation in the catalytic motif of the metalloprotease domain that changes the key glutamate residue (responsible for binding the zinc ion needed for catalytic activity) to an alanine residue so that the ADAM is no longer able to bind zinc and thus no longer able to cleave ligands. While such E/A mutants have found some utility, results published from such studies should be viewed with some caution.

For example, ADAM17 was recently identified as the key ADAM involved in mediating transactivation in VSMCs. Ohtsu and colleagues showed that dominant-negative E/A ADAM17 was able to inhibit AngII mediated transactivation and growth in VSMCs, whereas ADAM10 dominant-negative wasn't able to inhibit AngII induced ERK1/2 activation (Ohtsu *et al* 2006b). While this indicates a potential role for ADAM17 in mediating this process, it is worth noting that the use of catalytically inactive mutants alone is questionable as these mutants may not act as true dominant-negatives, and may have other, unaccounted for, effects. Indeed, heterozygous ΔZn^+ mutants have a wild type phenotype, indicating that the protease inactive mutants do not act as dominant negative proteins, but rather act as loss of function mutants (Sunnarborg *et al* 2002). In addition, there has been concern raised about how such mutants may effect ligand expression. Dempsey has suggested that over-expression of protease-inactive ADAMs may perturb the processing and trafficking of EGF ligands and inhibit their cleavage and release, meaning that any inhibition seen in the presence of these mutants may reflect ligand, rather than ADAM, inhibition (Dempsey 2002). A final concern is that such mutations in the catalytic domain may alter ADAM structure and in fact may be insufficient to knock out ADAM metalloprotease activity. Indeed, there is evidence to suggest that the cysteine-rich domain *in vivo* regulates metalloprotease activity (Smith *et al* 2002) and thus complete metalloprotease inhibition via such mutants may not be achieved.

Pharmacological inhibition studies should likewise be viewed with some reservation. For example, ADAM12 was identified as being the key ADAM in mediating

AngII-induced cardiac hypertrophy in cardiomyocyte cultures (Asakura *et al* 2002). Using a reportedly ADAM12 specific inhibitor (KB-R7785), Asakura and colleagues demonstrated that blocking ADAM12 inhibited HB-EGF release, EGFR activation and cardiomyocyte hypertrophy. This led to the claim that ADAM12 was the primary ADAM involved in mediating GPCR agonist induced cardiac hypertrophy. However, doubts about the specificity of KB-R7785 for ADAM12 compared to other ADAMs were soon raised (Liao 2002), and indeed, since then it has been found that at concentrations of 10μM, KB-R7785 is able to inhibit both ADAM12 and ADAM17 (Ichikawa *et al* 2004).

Another interesting approach to understanding ADAM activity has relied on over-expressing the cytoplasmic domain of ADAMs alone to act as decoys. For example, over-expressing the cytoplasmic tail of ADAM12 is sufficient to act as a decoy to block myoblast fusion presumably by sequestering proteins that normally associate with the tail of ADAMs (Galliano *et al* 2000). There is also evidence that over-expressing the cytoplasmic tail of ADAM9 reduces TPA-induced HB-EGF shedding (Izumi *et al* 1998). Such a prominent role for the cytoplasmic domain blockers has yet to be shown for GPCR-mediated EFGR transactivation, but it worth considering.

Other attempts to elucidate the role of ADAMs in particular cellular functions have used RNA interference technology to reduce ADAM mRNA and therefore protein levels (Fischer *et al* 2006). While this approach is more likely to specifically inhibit a given ADAM, such studies are yet to be carried out for cardiomyocytes and have not yet been performed *in vivo*. More recently, the use of knockout mice for specific ADAMs, crossing between lines and derived cell lines from single or multiple ADAM knockouts has provided more compelling evidence for the involvement of a given ADAM in a specific shedding event (Sahin *et al* 2004). An obvious use of such tools will be to ascertain the involvement of particular ADAMs in GPCR-mediated transactivation.

Clearly, elucidating the contribution of particular ADAM family members to AngII-induced transactivation and their role in diseases, such as cardiac hypertrophy and remodelling, will require a multifaceted approach as well as the use of more specific ADAM inhibition/activation methods in a cell- and tissue-specific manner. For example, as an extension of the siRNA approach, microRNAs (which are more potent than siRNA sequences and can be driven by cell-specific promoters) could be used to reduce the expression of specific ADAMs in culture and *in vivo* to determine the effect of their inhibition on GPCR-mediated transactivation and cardiovascular disease.

11.   FUTURE DIRECTIONS FOR THE ROLE OF ADAMS AS MEDIATORS OF ANG II ACTIONS

Studies over the last decade have provided an explosion of interest in the idea that EGFR transactivation plays a significant role in the selective actions of GPCRs, like the AT_1 receptor. In particular, there has been much research into the deleterious effects of angiotensin on the growth and remodelling of cardiovascular tissues. For technical reasons, as well as the shear size, complexity and potential redundancy of the ADAM family, we still have many gaps in our knowledge about the role of ADAMs in AngII-induced transactivation that warrant investigation. Similarly, the presence of multiple EGFRs (that can homo- and hetero-dimerise) and numerous EGF-like ligands means correlating a specific ADAM with the shedding of a defined EGF ligand to activate a distinct EGFR complex in a particular cell type *in vivo* and perhaps relating that to a disease state is a significant challenge.

In addition, much remains to be done in delineating the mechanism(s) by which stimulated GPCRs lead to ADAM activation. Most current paradigms focus on the role of the ADAM carboxyl-terminus in this process and the next few years should see more examples of protein:protein interactions and regulatory events that mediate GPCR-ADAM linkages. In this regard, the view that the TMPS process of GPCR/ADAM/ligand/EGFR occurs *in cis* (i.e., the ADAM cleaves ligands and activates receptors located on the same cell as shown in Fig. 1) is probably too narrow and needs revision. Specifically, Lackmann and colleagues have recently shown that ADAM10 is able to cleave the ephrin ligand *in trans* (i.e. the ADAM cleaves ligands located on different cells) (Janes *et al* 2005). Does EGFR transactivation proceed in the same manner with AT_1 receptors and ADAM on one cell and the putative EGF ligand on another? This might make some sense in a situation like cardiac hypertrophy where cardiomyocytes, fibroblasts and endothelial cells all contribute to the remodelling phenotype. For example, Lemmens and colleagues have recently reported that the source of neuregulin 1 that appears to mediate cardiomyocyte survival pathways is from endothelial cells and that they activate HER2/HER4 heterotrimers on the cardiomyocyte cell to affect their function (Lemmens *et al* 2006). Whether GPCRs that induce hypertrophy (like the AT_1 receptor) and specific ADAMs are able to promote neuregulin release/shedding from endothelial cells is unknown, but is worthy of some consideration, as is the possible separate, cellular localisation of the various components of TMPS in heart.

12. CONCLUSIONS

The renin-angiotensin system is an important biological system that contributes to human health and disease. While many of the effects of the AngII via the AT_1 receptor can be explained by current theories of $G_{q/11}$ activation and classical signalling in various target tissues, it is now clear that many of the growth and remodelling effects associated with AngII-mediated disease involve the transactivation of EGFRs. As protagonists of EGF ligand shedding, ADAMs are central players in EGFR transactivation. Although the EGF receptor subtype, ligand and ADAM(s) involved in this complex pathway are yet to be fully determined, further understanding the mechanism through which this transactivation pathway occurs will support efforts to develop new and alternative therapeutics to treat/manage cardiovascular diseases and will provide insight into the mechanisms that allow cross-talk between GPCRs and receptor tyrosine kinases.

ACKNOWLEDGEMENTS

A.M.B is supported by an Australian Postgraduate Award, Monash University and the Baker Heart Research Institute. W.G.T is a Senior Research Fellow of the National Health and Medical Research Council of Australia.

REFERENCES

Albrecht, S, Wang, S, Holz, A, Bergter, A, Paululat, A, 2006, The ADAM metalloprotease Kuzbanian is crucial for proper heart formation in Drosophila melanogaster. *Mechanisms of Development.* **123**: 372–387.

Anders, A, Gilbert, S, Garten, W, Postina, R, Fahrenholz, F, 2001, Regulation of the {alpha}-secretase ADAM10 by its prodomain and proprotein convertases. *FASEB J.* **15**: 1837–1839.

Asakura, M, Kitakaze, M, Takashima, S, Liao, Y, Ishikura, F, Yoshinaka, T, Ohmoto, H, Node, K, Yoshino, K, Ishiguro, H, Asanuma, H, Sanada, S, Matsumura, Y, Takeda, H, Beppu, S, Tada, M, Hori, H, Higashiyama, S, 2002, Cardiac hypertrophy is inhibited by antagonism of ADAM12 processing of HB-EGF: Metalloproteinase inhibitors as a new therapy. *Nature Medicine.* **8**: 35–40.

Baliga, RR, Pimental, DR, Zhao, YY, Simmons, WW, Marchionni, MA, Sawyer, DB, Kelly, RA, 1999, NRG-1-induced cardiomyocyte hypertrophy. Role of PI-3-kinase, p70(S6K), and MEK-MAPK-RSK. *American Journal of Physiology-Heart and Circulatory Physiology.* **277**: H2026–H2037.

Bennett, TA, Edwards, BS, Sklar, LA, Rogelj, S, 2000, Sulfhydryl Regulation of L-Selectin Shedding: Phenylarsine Oxide Promotes Activation-Independent L-Selectin Shedding from Leukocytes. *J Immunol.* **164**: 4120–4129.

Benter, IF, Yousif, MHM, Hollins, AJ, Griffiths, SM, Akhtar, S, 2005, Diabetes-induced renal vascular dysfunction is normalized by inhibition of epidermal growth factor receptor tyrosine kinase. *Journal of Vascular Research.* **42**: 284–291.

Black, RA, Jin, S-LC, Milla, ME, Burkhart, W, Carter, HL, Chen W.-, J, Clay, WC, Didsbury, JR, Hassler, D, Hoffman, CR, Kost, TA, Lambert, MH, Leesnitzer, MA, McCauley, P, McGeehan, G, Mitchell, J, Moyer, M, Pahel, G, Rocque, W, Overton, LK, Schoen, FJ, Seaton, T, Su, JL, Warner, J, Willard, D, Becherer, JD, 1997, A metalloproteinase disintegrin that releases tumour-necrosis factor alpha from cells. *Nature.* **385**: 729–733.

Black, RA, White, JM, 1998, ADAMs: Focus on the protease domain. *Current Opinion in Cell Biology.* **10**: 654–659.

Blobel, CP, 1997, Metalloprotease-disintegrins: Links to cell adhesion and cleavage of TNF alpha and notch. *Cell.* **90**: 589–592.

Blobel, CP, 2005, ADAMs: Key components in egfr signalling and development. *Nature Reviews Molecular Cell Biology.* **6**: 32–43.

Blobel, CP, White, JM, 1992, Structure, function and evolutionary relationship of proteins containing a disintegrin domain. *Current Opinion in Cell Biology.* **4**: 760–765.

Blobel, CP, Wolfsberg, TG, Turck, CW, Myles, DG, Primakoff, P, White, JM, 1992, A potential fusion peptide and an integrin ligand domain in a protein active in sperm-egg fusion. *Nature.* **356**: 248–252.

Bode, W, Gomisruth, FX, Stockler, W, 1993, Astacins, Serralysins, Snake-Venom and Matrix Metalloproteinases Exhibit Identical Zinc-Binding Environments (Hexxhxxgxxh and Met-Turn) and Topologies and Should Be Grouped into a Common Family, the Metzincins. *Febs Letters.* **331**: 134–140.

Bokemeyer, D, Schmitz, U, Kramer, HJ, 2000, Angiotensin II-induced growth of vascular smooth muscle cells requires an Src-dependent activation of the epidermal growth factor receptor. *Kidney International.* **58**: 549–558.

Burgess, AW, Cho, H-S, Eigenbrot, C, Ferguson, KM, Garrett, TPJ, Leahy, DJ, Lemmon, MA, Sliwkowski, MX, Ward, CW, Yokoyama, S, 2003, An open-and-shut case? Recent insights into the activation of EGF/ErbB receptors. *Molecular Cell.* **12**: 541–552.

Chan, HW, Jenkins, A, Pipolo, L, Hannan, RD, Thomas, WG, Smith, NJ, 2006, Effect of dominant-negative epidermal growth factor receptors on cardiomyocyte hypertrophy. *J Recept Signal Transduct Res.* **26**: 659–677.

Chen, J, Chen, J-K, Neilson, EG, Harris, RC, 2006, Role of EGF Receptor Activation in Angiotensin II-Induced Renal Epithelial Cell Hypertrophy. *J Am Soc Nephrol.* **17**: 1615–1623.

Chesneau, V, Becherer, JD, Zheng, YF, Erdjument-Bromage, H, Tempst, P, Blobel, CP, 2003, Catalytic properties of ADAM19. *Journal of Biological Chemistry.* **278**: 22331–22340.

Chiu, T, Santiskulvong, C, Rozengurt, E, 2005, EGF receptor transactivation mediates ANG II-stimulated mitogenesis in intestinal epithelial cells through the PI3-kinase/Akt/mTOR/p70S6K1 signaling pathway. *American Journal of Physiology-Gastrointestinal and Liver Physiology.* **288**: G182–G194.

Cho, HS, Mason, K, Ramyar, KX, Stanley, AM, Gabelli, SB, Denney, DW, Leahy, DJ, 2003, Structure of the extracellular region of HER2 alone and in complex with the Herceptin Fab. *Nature.* **421**: 756–760.

Citri, A, Skaria, KB, Yarden, Y, 2003, The deaf and the dumb: the biology of ErbB-2 and ErbB-3. *Experimental Cell Research.* **284**: 54–65.

Crone, SA, Zhao, YY, Fan, L, Gu, YS, Minamisawa, S, Liu, Y, Peterson, KL, Chen, J, Kahn, R, Condorelli, G, Ross, J, Chien, KR, Lee, KF, 2002, ErbB2 is essential in the prevention of dilated cardiomyopathy. *Nature Medicine.* **8**: 459–465.

Daub, H, Wallasch, C, Lankenau, A, Herrlich, A, Ullrich, A, 1997, Signal characteristics of G protein-transactivated EGF receptor. *EMBO J.* **16**: 7032–7044.

Daub, H, Weiss, FU, Wallasch, C, Ullrich, A, 1996, Role of transactivation of the EGF receptor in signalling by G-protein-coupled receptors. *Nature.* **379**: 557–560.

De Gasparo, M, Catt, KJ, Inagami, T, Wright, JW, Unger, T, 2000, International union of pharmacology. XXIII. The angiotensin II receptors. *Pharmacological Reviews.* **52**: 415–472.

Dell, KM, Nemo, R, Sweeney, WE, Levin, JI, Frost, P, Avner, ED, 2001, A novel inhibitor of tumor necrosis factor-alpha converting enzyme ameliorates polycystic kidney disease. *Kidney International.* **60**: 1240–1248.

Dempsey, PJ, 2002, Emerging roles of TACE as a key protease in ErbB ligand shedding. *Molecular Interventions.* **2**: 136–141.

Diaz-Rodriguez, F, Esparis-Ogando, A, Montero, JC, Yuste, L, Pandiella, A, 2000, Stimulation of cleavage of membrane proteins by calmodulin inhibitors. *Biochemical Journal.* **346**: 359–367.

Doedens, JR, Mahimkar, RM, Black, RA, 2003, TACE/ADAM-17 enzymatic activity is increased in response to cellular stimulation. *Biochemical and Biophysical Research Communications.* **308**: 331–338.

Dong, J, Opresko, LK, Dempsey, PJ, Lauffenburger, DA, Coffey, RJ, Wiley, HS, 1999, Metalloprotease-mediated ligand release regulates autocrine signaling through the epidermal growth factor receptor. *Proceedings of the National Academy of Sciences of the United States of America.* **96**: 6235–6240.

Eguchi, S, Dempsey, PJ, Frank, GD, Motley, ED, Inagami, T, 2001, Activation of MAPKs by angiotensin II in vascular smooth muscle cells - Metalloprotease-dependent EGF receptor activation is required for activation of ERK and p38 MAPK but not for JNK. *Journal of Biological Chemistry.* **276**: 7957–7962.

Eguchi, S, Iwasaki, H, Inagami, T, Numaguchi, K, Yamakawa, T, Motley, ED, Owada, KM, Marumo, F, Hirata, Y, 1999, Involvement of PYK2 in Angiotensin II Signaling of Vascular Smooth Muscle Cells. *Hypertension.* **33**: 201–206.

Eguchi, S, Numaguchi, K, Iwasaki, H, Matsumoto, T, Yamakawa, T, Utsunomiya, H, Motley, ED, Kawakatsu, H, Owada, KM, Hirata, Y, Marumo, F, Inagami, T, 1998, Calcium-dependent epidermal growth factor receptor transactivation mediates the angiotensin II-induced mitogen-activated protein kinase activation in vascular smooth muscle cells. *Journal of Biological Chemistry.* **273**: 8890–8896.

Eto, K, Huet, C, Tarui, T, Kupriyanov, S, Liu, HZ, Puzon-McLaughlin, W, Zhang, XP, Sheppard, D, Engvall, E, Takada, Y, 2002, Functional classification of ADAMs based on a conserved motif for binding to integrin alpha(9)beta(1) - Implications for sperm-egg binding and other cell interactions. *Journal of Biological Chemistry.* **277**: 17804–17810.

Fedak, PWM, Moravec, CS, McCarthy, PM, Altamentova, SM, Wong, AP, Skrtic, M, Verma, S, Weisel, RD, Li, RK, 2006, Altered expression of disintegrin metalloproteinases and their inhibitor in human dilated cardiomyopathy. *Circulation.* **113**: 238–245.

Ferguson, KM, 2004, Active and inactive conformations of the epidermal growth factor receptor. *Biochem Soc Trans.* **32**: 742–745.

Fischer, OM, Hart, S, Ullrich, A, 2006, Dissecting the epidermal growth factor receptor signal transactivation pathway. *Methods Mol Biol.* **327**: 85–97.

Flannery, PJ, Spurney, RF, 2006, Transactivation of the Epidermal Growth Factor Receptor by Angiotensin II in Glomerular Podocytes. *Nephron.* **103**: e109.

Freeman, M, 1994, The spitz gene is required for photoreceptor determination in the Drosophila eye where it interacts with the EGF receptor. *Mechanisms of Development.* **48**: 25–33.

Fujiyama, S, Matsubara, H, Nozawa, Y, Maruyama, K, Mori, Y, Tsutsumi, Y, Masaki, H, Uchiyama, Y, Koyama, Y, Nose, A, Iba, O, Tateishi, E, Ogata, N, Jyo, N, Higashiyama, S, Iwasaka, T, 2001, Angiotensin AT(1) and AT(2) receptors differentially regulate angiopoietin-2 and vascular endothelial growth factor expression and angiogenesis by modulating heparin binding-epidermal growth factor (EGF)-mediated EGF receptor transactivation. *Circulation Research.* **88**: 22–29.

Galliano, MF, Huet, C, Frygelius, J, Polgren, A, Wewer, UM, Engvall, E, 2000, Binding of ADAM12, a marker of skeletal muscle regeneration, to the muscle-specific actin-binding protein, alpha-actinin-2, is required for myoblast fusion. *Journal of Biological Chemistry.* **275**: 13933–13939.

Garratt, AN, 2006, "To erb-B or not to erb-B..." Neuregulin-1/ErbB signaling in heart development and function. *Journal of Molecular and Cellular Cardiology.* **41**: 215–218.

Garrett, TPJ, McKern, NM, Lou, MZ, Elleman, TC, Adams, TE, Lovrecz, GO, Zhu, HJ, Walker, F, Frenkel, MJ, Hoyne, PA, Jorissen, RN, Nice, EC, Burgess, AW, Ward, CW, 2002, Crystal structure of a truncated epidermal growth factor receptor extracellular domain bound to transforming growth factor alpha. *Cell.* **110**: 763–773.

Gassmann, M, Casagranda, F, Orioli, D, Simon, H, Lai, C, Klein, R, Lemke, G, 1995, Aberrant Neural and Cardiac Development in Mice Lacking the Erbb4 Neuregulin Receptor. *Nature.* **378**: 390–394.

Grams, F, Huber, R, Kress, LF, Moroder, L, Bode, W, 1993, Activation of Snake-Venom Metalloproteinases by a Cysteine Switch-Like Mechanism. *Febs Letters.* **335**: 76–80.

Greco, S, Muscella, A, Elia, MG, Salvatore, P, Storelli, C, Mazzotta, A, Manca, C, Marsigliante, S, 2003, Angiotensin II activates extracellular signal regulated kinases via protein kinase C and epidermal growth factor receptor in breast cancer cells. *Journal of Cellular Physiology.* **196**: 370–377.

Gschwind, A, Hart, S, Fischer, OM, Ullrich, A, 2003, TACE cleavage of proamphiregulin regulates GPCR-induced proliferation and motility of cancer cells. *EMBO Journal.* **22**: 2411–2421.

Harris, RC, Chung, E, Coffey, RJ, 2003, EGF receptor ligands. *Experimental Cell Research.* **284**: 2–13.

Hartmann, D, de Strooper, B, Serneels, L, Craessaerts, K, Herreman, A, Annaert, W, Umans, L, Lubke, T, Lena Illert, A, von Figura, K, Saftig, P, 2002, The disintegrin/metalloprotease ADAM 10 is essential for Notch signalling but not for {alpha}-secretase activity in fibroblasts. *Hum Mol Genet.* **11**: 2615–2624.

Hougaard, S, Loechel, F, Xu, XF, Tajima, R, Albrechtsen, R, Wewer, UM, 2000, Trafficking of human ADAM 12-L: Retention in the trans-Golgi network. *Biochemical and Biophysical Research Communications.* **275**: 261–267.

Howard, L, Lu, XH, Mitchell, S, Griffiths, S, Glynn, P, 1996, Molecular cloning of MADM: A catalytically active mammalian disintegrin-metalloprotease expressed in various cell types. *Biochemical Journal.* **317**: 45–50.

Howard, L, Maciewicz, RA, Blobel, CP, 2000, Cloning and characterization of ADAM28: evidence for autocatalytic pro-domain removal and for cell surface localization of mature ADAM28. *Biochemical Journal.* **348**: 21–27.

Howard, L, Nelson, KK, Maciewicz, RA, Blobel, CP, 1999, Interaction of the metalloprotease disintegrins MDC9 and MDC15 with two SH3 domain-containing proteins, endophilin I and SH3PX1. *Journal of Biological Chemistry.* **274**: 31693–31699.

Huang, L, Feng, L, Yang, L, Zhou, W, Zhao, S, Li, C, 2002, Screen and identification of proteins interacting with ADAM19 cytoplasmic tail. *Molecular biology reports.* **29**: 317–323.

Ichikawa, Y, Miura, T, Nakano, A, Miki, T, Nakamura, Y, Tsuchihashi, K, Shimamoto, K, 2004, The role of ADAM protease in the tyrosine kinase-mediated trigger mechanism of ischemic preconditioning. *Cardiovascular Research.* **62**: 167–175.

Iwamoto, R, Yamazaki, S, Asakura, M, Takashima, S, Hasuwa, H, Miyado, K, Adachi, S, Kitakaze, M, Hashimoto, K, Raab, G, Nanba, D, Higashiyama, S, Hori, M, Klagsbrun, M, Mekada, E, 2003, Heparin-binding EGF-like growth factor and ErbB signaling is essential for heart function. *Proceedings of the National Academy of Sciences of the United States of America.* **100**: 3221–3226.

Izumi, Y, Hirata, M, Hasuwa, H, Iwamoto, R, Umata, T, Miyado, K, Tamai, Y, Kurisaki, T, Sehara-Fujisawa, A, Ohno, S, Mekada, E, 1998, A metalloprotease-disintegrin, MDC9/meltrin-(gamma)/ADAM9 and PKC(delta) are involved in TPA-induced ectodomain shedding of membrane-anchored heparin-binding EGF-like growth factor. *EMBO Journal.* **17**: 7260–7272.

Jackson, LF, Qiu, TH, Sunnarborg, SW, Chang, A, Zhang, C, Patterson, C, Lee, DC, 2003, Defective valvulogenesis in HB-EGF and TACE-null mice is associated with aberrant BMP signaling. *EMBO Journal.* **22**: 2704–2716.

Janes, PW, Saha, N, Barton, WA, Kolev, MV, Wimmer-Kleikamp, SH, Nievergall, E, Blobel, CP, Himanen, J-P, Lackmann, M, Nikolov, DB, 2005, Adam Meets Eph: An ADAM Substrate Recognition Module Acts as a Molecular Switch for Ephrin Cleavage In trans. *Cell.* **123**: 291–304.

Jia, LG, Shimokawa, KI, Bjarnason, JB, Fox, JW, 1996, Snake venom metalloproteinases: Structure, function and relationship to the Adams family of proteins. *Toxicon.* **34**: 1269–1276.

Kagiyama, S, Eguchi, S, Frank, GD, Inagami, T, Zhang, YC, Phillips, MI, 2002, Angiotensin II-induced cardiac hypertrophy and hypertension are attenuated by epidermal growth factor receptor antisense. *Circulation.* **106**: 909–912.

Kang, Q, Cao, Y, Zolkiewska, A, 2000, Metalloprotease-disintegrin ADAM 12 binds to the SH3 domain of Src and activates Src tyrosine kinase in C2C12 cells. *Biochemical Journal.* **352**: 883–892.

Kang, Q, Cao, Y, Zolkiewska, A, 2001, Direct interaction between the cytoplasmic tail of ADAM 12 and the Src homology 3 domain of p85 alpha activates phosphatidylinositol 3-kinase in C2C12 cells. *Journal of Biological Chemistry.* **276**: 24466–24472.

Kodama, H, Fukuda, K, Takahashi, T, Sano, M, Kato, T, Tahara, S, Hakuno, D, Sato, T, Manabe, T, Konishi, F, Ogawa, S, 2002, Role of EGF Receptor and Pyk2 in Endothelin-1-induced ERK Activation in Rat Cardiomyocytes. *Journal of Molecular and Cellular Cardiology.* **34**: 139–150.

Kojro, E, Gimpl, G, Lammich, S, Marz, W, Fahrenholz, F, 2001, Low cholesterol stimulates the nonamyloidogenic pathway by its effect on the alpha-secretase ADAM 10. *Proceedings of the National Academy of Sciences of the United States of America.* **98**: 5815–5820.

Kratzschmar, J, Lum, L, Blobel, CP, 1996, Metargidin, a membrane-anchored metalloprotease disintegrin protein with an RGD integrin binding sequence. *Journal of Biological Chemistry.* **271**: 4593–4596.

Kurohara, K, Komatsu, K, Kurisaki, T, Masuda, A, Irie, N, Asano, M, Sudo, K, Nabeshima, Y-i, Iwakura, Y, Sehara-Fujisawa, A, 2004, Essential roles of Meltrin [beta] (ADAM19) in heart development. *Developmental Biology.* **267**: 14–28.

Laurette, A, Li, S, Alili, R, Sunnarborg, SW, Burtin, M, Lee, DC, Freidlander, G, Terzi, F, 2005, Angiotensin II and EGF Receptor cross-talk in chronic kidney diseases: a new therapeutic approach. *Nature Medicine.* **11**: 867–874.

Lautrette, A, Li, SQ, Alili, R, Sunnarborg, SW, Burtin, M, Lee, DC, Friedlander, G, Terzi, F, 2005, Angiotensin II and EGF receptor cross-talk in chronic kidney diseases: a new therapeutic approach. *Nature Medicine.* **11**: 867–874.

Lee, KF, Simon, H, Chen, H, Bates, B, Hung, MC, Hauser, C, 1995, Requirement for Neuregulin Receptor Erbb2 in Neural and Cardiac Development. *Nature.* **378**: 394–398.

Lemarie, CA, Tharaux, PL, Esposito, B, Tedgui, A, Lehoux, S, 2006, Transforming growth factor-alpha mediates nuclear factor kappaB activation in strained arteries. *Circ Res.* **99**: 434–441.

Lemjabbar, H, Basbaum, C, 2002, Platelet-activating factor receptor and ADAM10 mediate responses to Staphylococcus aureus in epithelial cells. *Nature Medicine.* **8**: 41–46.

Lemmens, K, Segers, VFM, Demolder, M, De Keulenaer, GW, 2006, Role of Neuregulin-1/ErbB2 Signaling in Endothelium-Cardiomyocyte Cross-talk. *J Biol Chem.* **281**: 19469–19477.

Levy, D, Garrison, RJ, Kannel, WB, Castelli, WP, 1990, Prognostic Implications of Echocardiograph-ically Determined Left-Ventricular Mass in the Framingham Heart-Study - Reply. *New England Journal of Medicine.* **323**: 1706–1707.

Li, X, Lee, JW, Graves, LM, Earp, HS, 1998, Angiotensin II stimulates ERK via two pathways in epithelial cells: protein kinase C suppresses a G-protein coupled receptor EGF receptor transactivation pathway. *Embo Journal.* **17**: 2574–2583.

Liao, JK, 2002, Shedding growth factors in cardiac hypertrophy. *Nature Medicine.* **8**: 20–21.

Lin, JQ, Freeman, MR, 2003, Transactivation of ErbBl and ErbB2 receptors by angiotensin II in normal human prostate stromal cells. *Prostate.* **54**: 1–7.

Liu, X, Gu, X, Li, Z, Li, X, Li, H, Chang, J, Chen, P, Jin, J, Xi, B, Chen, D, Lai, D, Graham, RM, Zhou, M, 2006, Neuregulin-1/erbB-Activation Improves Cardiac Function and Survival in Models of Ischemic, Dilated, and Viral Cardiomyopathy. *Journal of the American College of Cardiology.* **48**: 1438–1447.

Loechel, F, Gilpin, BJ, Engvall, E, Albrechtsen, R, Wewer, UM, 1998, Human ADAM 12 (meltrin alpha) is an active metalloprotease. *Journal of Biological Chemistry.* **273**: 16993–16997.

Lum, L, Reid, MS, Blobel, CP, 1998, Intracellular maturation of the mouse metalloprotease disintegrin MDC15. *Journal of Biological Chemistry.* **273**: 26236–26247.

Maskos, K, Fernandez-Catalan, C, Huber, R, Bourenkov, GP, Bartunik, H, Ellestad, GA, Reddy, P, Wolfson, MF, Rauch, CT, Castner, BJ, Davis, R, Clarke, HRG, Petersen, M, Fitzner, JN, Cerretti, DP, March, CJ, Paxton, RJ, Black, RA, Bode, W, 1998, Crystal structure of the catalytic domain of human tumor necrosis factor-alpha-converting enzyme. *Proceedings of the National Academy of Sciences of the United States of America.* **95**: 3408–3412.

Mechtersheimer, S, Gutwein, P, Agmon-Levin, N, Stoeck, A, Oleszewski, M, Riedle, S, Postina, R, Fahrenholz, F, Fogel, M, Lemmon, V, Altevogt, P, 2001, Ectodomain shedding of L1 adhesion molecule promotes cell migration by autocrine binding to integrins. *J Cell Biol.* **155**: 661–674.

Mehta, PK, Griendling, KK, 2007, Angiotensin II cell signaling: physiological and pathological effects in the cardiovascular system. *Am J Physiol Cell Physiol.* **292**: C82–97.

Miettinen, PJ, Berger, JE, Meneses, J, Phung, Y, Pedersen, RA, Werb, Z, Derynck, R, 1995, Epithelial Immaturity and Multiorgan Failure in Mice Lacking Epidermal Growth-Factor Receptor. *Nature.* **376**: 337–341.

Mifune, M, Ohtsu, H, Suzuki, H, Frank, GD, Inagami, T, Utsunomiya, H, Dempsey, PJ, Eguchi, S, 2004, Signal transduction of betacellulin in growth and migration of vascular smooth muscle cells. *American Journal of Physiology - Cell Physiology.* **287**: C807–C813.

Mifune, M, Ohtsu, H, Suzuki, H, Nakashima, H, Brailoiu, E, Dun, NJ, Frank, GD, Inagami, T, Higashiyamii, S, Thomas, WG, Eckhart, AD, Dempsey, PJ, Eguchi, S, 2005, G protein coupling and second messenger generation are indispensable for metalloprotease-dependent, heparin-binding epidermal growth factor shedding through angiotensin II type-1 receptor. *Journal of Biological Chemistry.* **280**: 26592–26599.

Milla, ME, Leesnitzer, MA, Moss, ML, Clay, WC, Carter, HL, Miller, AB, Su, JL, Lambert, MH, Willard, DH, Sheeley, DM, Kost, TA, Burkhart, W, Moyer, M, Blackburn, RK, Pahel, GL, Mitchell, JL, Hoffmann, R, Becherer, JD, 1999, Specific sequence elements are required for the expression of functional tumor necrosis factor-alpha-converting enzyme (TACE). *Journal of Biological Chemistry.* **274**: 30563–30570.

Mori, S, Tanaka, M, Nanba, D, E, N, Ishiguro, H, Higashiyama, S, Matsuura, N, 2003, PACSIN3 Binds ADAM12/Meltrin alpha and Up-regulates Ectodomain Shedding of Heparin-binding Epidermal Growth Factor-like Growth Factor. *Journal of Biological Chemistry.* **278**: 46029–46034.

Moriguchi, Y, Matsubara, H, Mori, Y, Murasawa, S, Masaki, H, Maruyama, K, Tsutsumi, Y, Shibasaki, Y, Tanaka, Y, Nakajima, T, Oda, K, Iwasaka, T, 1999, Angiotensin II-induced transac-tivation of epidermal growth factor receptor regulates fibronectin and transforming growth factor-beta synthesis via transcriptional and posttranscriptional mechanisms. *Circulation Research.* **84**: 1073–1084.

Moss, ML, Jin, S-LC, Milla, ME, Burkhart, W, Carter, HL, Chen W.-, J, Clay, WC, Didsbury, JR, Hassler, D, Hoffman, CR, Kost, TA, Lambert, MH, Leesnitzer, MA, McCauley, P, Mageehan, G, Mitchell, J, Moyer, M, Pahel, G, Rocque, W, Overton, LK, Schoenen, F, Seaton, T, Su, J-L, Warner, J,

Willard, D, Becherer, JD, 1997, Cloning of a disintegrin metalloproteinase that processes precursor tumour-necrosis factor-(alpha). *Nature.* **385**: 733–736.

Moss, ML, Lambert, MH. (2002). Shedding of membrane proteins by ADAM family proteases. In *Proteases in Biology and Medicine* (Vol. 38, pp. 141–153).

Murasawa, S, Mori, Y, Nozawa, Y, Gotoh, N, Shibuya, M, Masaki, H, Maruyama, K, Tsutsumi, Y, Moriguchi, Y, Shibazaki, Y, Tanaka, Y, Iwasaka, T, Inada, M, Matsubara, H, 1998a, Angiotensin II type 1 receptor-induced extracellular signal-regulated protein kinase activation is mediated by Ca2+/calmodulin-dependent transactivation of epidermal growth factor receptor. *Circulation Research.* **82**: 1338–1348.

Murasawa, S, Mori, Y, Nozawa, Y, Masaki, H, Maruyama, K, Tsutsumi, Y, Moriguchi, Y, Shibasaki, Y, Tanaka, Y, Iwasaka, T, Inada, M, Matsubara, H, 1998b, Role of Calcium-Sensitive Tyrosine Kinase Pyk2/CAKß/RAFTK in Angiotensin II–Induced Ras/ERK Signaling. *Hypertension.* **32**: 668–675.

Nakashima, H, Suzuki, H, Ohtsu, H, Chao, JY, Utsunomiya, H, Frank, GD, Eguchi, S, 2006, Angiotensin II regulates vascular and endothelial dysfunction: recent topics of Angiotensin II type-1 receptor signaling in the vasculature. *Curr Vasc Pharmacol.* **4**: 67–78.

Nath, D, Slocombe, PM, Stephens, PE, Warn, A, Hutchinson, GR, Yamada, KM, Docherty, AJP, Murphy, G, 1999, Interaction of metargidin (ADAM-15) with alpha(v)beta(3) and alpha(5)beta(1) integrins on different haemopoietic cells. *Journal of Cell Science.* **112**: 579–587.

Nelson, KK, Schlondorff, J, Blobel, CP, 1999, Evidence for an interaction of the metalloprotease-disintegrin tumour necrosis factor (alpha) convertase (TACE) with mitotic arrest deficient 2 (MAD2), and of the metalloprotease-disintegrin MDC9 with a novel MAD2-related protein, MAD2(beta). *Biochemical Journal.* **343**: 673–680.

Niewiarowski, S, McLane, MA, Kloczewiak, M, Stewart, GJ, 1994, Disintegrins and Other Naturally-Occurring Antagonists of Platelet Fibrinogen Receptors. *Seminars in Hematology.* **31**: 289–300.

Ohtsu, H, Dempsey, PJ, Eguchi, S, 2006a, ADAMs as mediators of EGF receptor transactivation by G protein-coupled receptors. *American Journal of Physiology-Cell Physiology.* **291**: C1–C10.

Ohtsu, H, Dempsey, PJ, Frank, GD, Brailoiu, E, Higuchi, S, Suzuki, H, Nakashima, H, Eguchi, K, Eguchi, S, 2006b, ADAM17 Mediates Epidermal Growth Factor Receptor Transactivation and Vascular Smooth Muscle Cell Hypertrophy Induced by Angiotensin II. *Arterioscler Thromb Vasc Biol.* **26**: e133–137.

Olivares-Reyes, JA, Shah, BH, Hernandez-Aranda, J, Garcia-Caballero, A, Farshori, MP, Garcia-Sainz, JA, Catt, KJ, 2005, Agonist-induced interactions between angiotensin AT1 and epidermal growth factor receptors. *Molecular Pharmacology.* **68**: 356–364.

Olson, EN, Molkentin, JD, 1999, Prevention of cardiac hypertrophy by calcineurin inhibition - Hope or hype? *Circulation Research.* **84**: 623–632.

Ozcelik, C, Erdmann, B, Pilz, B, Wettschureck, N, Britsch, S, Hubner, N, Chien, KR, Birchmeier, C, Garratt, AN, 2002, Conditional mutation of the ErbB2 (HER2) receptor in cardiomyocytes leads to dilated cardiomyopathy. *Proceedings of the National Academy of Sciences of the United States of America.* **99**: 8880–8885.

Pandiella, A, Bosenberg, M, Huang, E, Besmer, P, Massague, J, 1992, Cleavage of membrane-anchored growth factors involves distinct protease activities regulated through common mechanisms. *J Biol Chem.* **267**: 24028–24033.

Peschon, JJ, Slack, JL, Reddy, P, Stocking, KL, Sunnarborg, SW, Lee, DC, Russell, WE, Castner, BJ, Johnson, RS, Fitzner, JN, Boyce, RW, Nelson, N, Kozlosky, CJ, Wolfson, MF, Rauch, CT, Cerretti, DP, Paxton, RJ, March, CJ, Black, RA, 1998, An essential role for ectodomain shedding in mammalian development. *Science.* **282**: 1281–1284.

Poghosyan, Z, Robbins, SM, Houslay, MD, Webster, A, Murphy, G, Edwards, DR, 2002, Phosphorylation-dependent interactions between ADAM15 cytoplasmic domain and Src family protein-tyrosine kinases. *Journal of Biological Chemistry.* **277**: 4999–5007.

Prenzel, N, Zwick, E, Daub, H, Michael Leserer, RA, Christian Wallasch, Axel UllrichNorbert Prenzel, 1999, EGF receptor transactivation by G-protein-coupled receptors requires metalloproteinase cleavage of proHB-EGF.

Reddy, P, Slack, JL, Davis, R, Cerretti, DP, Kozlosky, CJ, Blanton, RA, Shows, D, Peschon, JJ, Black, RA, 2000, Functional Analysis of the Domain Structure of Tumor Necrosis Factor-alpha Converting Enzyme. *J Biol Chem.* **275**: 14608–14614.

Reise, DJ, Stern, DF, 1998, Specificity within the EGF family/ErB receptor family signalling network. *Bioessays.* **20**: 41–48.

Roghani, M, Becherer, JD, Moss, ML, Atherton, RE, Erdjument-Bromage, H, Arribas, J, Blackburn, RK, Weskamp, G, Tempst, P, Blobel, CP, 1999, Metalloprotease-disintegrin MDC9: Intracellular maturation and catalytic activity. *Journal of Biological Chemistry.* **274**: 3531–3540.

Rooke, J, Pan, D, Xu, T, Rubin, GM, 1996, KUZ, a conserved metalloprotease-disintegrin protein with two roles in Drosophila neurogenesis. *Science.* **273**: 1227–1231.

Sahin, U, Weskamp, G, Kelly, K, Zhou, H-M, Higashiyama, S, Peschon, J, Hartmann, D, Saftig, P, Blobel, CP, 2004, Distinct roles for ADAM10 and ADAM17 in ectodomain shedding of six EGFR ligands. *Journal of Cell Biology.* **164**: 769–779.

Saito, S, Frank, GD, Motley, ED, Dempsey, PJ, Utsunomiya, H, Inagami, T, Eguchi, S, 2002, Metalloprotease inhibitor blocks angiotensin II-induced migration through inhibition of epidermal growth factor receptor transactivation. *Biochemical and Biophysical Research Communications.* **294**: 1023–1029.

Sanderson, MP, Erickson, SN, Gough, PJ, Garton, KJ, Wille, PT, Raines, EW, Dunbar, AJ, Dempsey, PJ, 2005, ADAM10 Mediates Ectodomain Shedding of the Betacellulin Precursor Activated by p-Aminophenylmercuric Acetate and Extracellular Calcium Influx. *J Biol Chem.* **280**: 1826–1837.

Schafer, W, Stroh, A, Berghofer, S, Seiler, J, Vey, M, Kruse, ML, Kern, HF, Klenk, HD, Garten, W, 1995, 2 Independent Targeting Signals in the Cytoplasmic Domain Determine Trans-Golgi Network Localization and Endosomal Trafficking of the Proprotein Convertase Furin. *Embo Journal.* **14**: 2424–2435.

Schlessinger, J, 2000, Cell signaling by receptor tyrosine kinases. *Cell.* **103**: 211–225.

Schlondorff, J, Blobel, CP, 1999, Metalloprotease-disintegrins: modular proteins capable of promoting cell-cell interactions and triggering signals by protein-ectodomain shedding. *Journal of Cell Science.* **112**: 3603–3617.

Seals, DF, Courtneidge, SA, 2003, The ADAMs family of metalloproteases: Multidomain proteins with multiple functions. *Genes and Development.* **17**: 7–30.

Seta, K, Sadoshima, J, 2003, Phosphorylation of Tyrosine 319 of the Angiotensin II Type 1 Receptor Mediates Angiotensin II-induced Trans-activation of the Epidermal Growth Factor Receptor. *J Biol Chem.* **278**: 9019–9026.

Shah, BH, Catt, KJ, 2004, Matrix metalloproteinase-dependent EGF receptor activation in hypertension and left ventricular hypertrophy. *Trends in Endocrinology and Metabolism.* **15**: 241–243.

Shah, BH, Catt, KJ, 2006, TACE-dependent EGF receptor activation in angiotensin-II-induced kidney disease. *Trends in Pharmacological Sciences.* **27**: 235–237.

Shah, BH, Yesilkaya, A, Olivares-Reyes, JA, Chen, H-D, Hunyady, L, Catt, KJ, 2004, Differential Pathways of Angiotensin II-Induced Extracellularly Regulated Kinase 1/2 Phosphorylation in Specific Cell Types: Role of Heparin-Binding Epidermal Growth Factor. *Mol Endocrinol.* **18**: 2035–2048.

Shi, W, Chen, H, Sun, J, Buckley, S, Zhao, J, Anderson, KD, Williams, RG, Warburton, D, 2003, TACE is required for fetal murine cardiac development and modeling. *Developmental Biology.* **261**: 371–380.

Sibilia, M, Wagner, EF, 1995, Strain-Dependent Epithelial Defects in Mice Lacking the Egf Receptor. *Science.* **269**: 234–238.

Smith, KM, Gaultier, A, Cousin, H, Alfandari, D, White, JM, DeSimone, DW, 2002, The cysteine-rich domain regulates ADAM protease function in vivo. *J Cell Biol.* **159**: 893–902.

Smith, NJ, Chan, H-W, Osborne, JE, Thomas, WG, Hannan, RD, 2004, Hijacking epidermal growth factor receptors by angiotensin II: New possibilities for understanding and treating cardiac hypertrophy. *Cellular and Molecular Life Sciences.* **61**: 2695–2703.

Sotillos, S, Roch, F, Campuzano, S, 1997, The metalloprotease-disintegrin Kuzbanian participates in Notch activation during growth and patterning of Drosophila imaginal discs. *Development.* **124**: 4769–4779.

Srour, N, Lebel, A, McMahon, S, Fournier, I, Fugere, M, Day, R, Dubois, CM, 2003, TACE/ADAM-17 maturation and activation of sheddase activity require proprotein convertase activity. *Febs Letters.* **554**: 275–283.

Stocker, W, Grams, F, Baumann, U, Reinemer, P, Gomisruth, FX, McKay, DB, Bode, W, 1995, The Metzincins - Topological and Sequential Relations between the Astacins, Adamalysins, Serralysins, and Matrixins (Collagenases) Define a Superfamily of Zinc-Peptidases. *Protein Science.* **4**: 823–840.

Stone, AL, Kroeger, M, Xiang, Q, Sang, A, 1999, Structure-function analysis of the ADAM family of disintegrin-like and metalloproteinase-containing proteins (review). *Journal of Protein Chemistry.* **18**: 447–465.

Suarez, C, Diaz-Torga, G, Gonzalez-Iglesias, A, Vela, J, Mladovan, A, Baldi, A, Becu-Villalobos, D, 2003, Angiotensin II phosphorylation of extracellular signal-regulated kinases in rat anterior pituitary cells. *American Journal of Physiology-Endocrinology and Metabolism.* **285**: E645–E653.

Sunnarborg, SW, Hinkle, CL, Stevenson, M, Russell, WE, Raska, CS, Peschon, JJ, Castner, BJ, Gerhart, MJ, Paxton, RJ, Black, RA, Lee, DC, 2002, Tumor necrosis factor-alpha converting enzyme (TACE) regulates epidermal growth factor receptor ligand availability. *Journal of Biological Chemistry.* **277**: 12838–12845.

Suzuki, A, Kadota, N, Hara, T, Nakagami, Y, Izumi, T, Takenawa, T, Sabe, H, Endo, T, 2000, Meltrin alpha cytoplasmic domain interacts with SH3 domains of Src and Grb2 and is phosphorylated by v-Src. *Oncogene.* **19**: 5842–5850.

Tanaka, M, Nanba, D, Mori, S, Shiba, F, Ishiguro, H, Yoshino, K, Matsuura, N, Higashiyama, S, 2004, ADAM binding protein Eve-1 is required for ectodomain shedding of epidermal growth factor receptor ligands. *Journal of Biological Chemistry.* **279**: 41950–41959.

Taylor, DS, Cheng, X, Pawlowski, JE, Wallace, AR, Ferrer, P, Molloy, CJ, 1999, Epiregulin is a potent vascular smooth muscle cell-derived mitogen induced by angiotensin II, endothelin-1, and thrombin. *Proc Natl Acad Sci U S A.* **96**: 1633–1638.

Thomas, WG, Brandenburger, Y, Autelitano, DJ, Pham, T, Qian, H, Hannan, RD, 2002, Adenoviral-directed expression of the type 1A angiotensin receptor promotes cardiomyocyte hypertrophy via transactivation of the epidermal growth factor receptor. *Circulation Research.* **90**: 135–142.

Threadgill, DW, Dlugosz, AA, Hansen, LA, Tennenbaum, T, Lichti, U, Yee, D, Lamantia, C, Mourton, T, Herrup, K, Harris, RC, Barnard, JA, Yuspa, SH, Coffey, RJ, Magnuson, T, 1995, Targeted Disruption of Mouse Egf Receptor - Effect of Genetic Background on Mutant Phenotype. *Science.* **269**: 230–234.

Timolati, F, Ott, D, Pentassuglia, L, Giraud, MN, Perriard, JC, Suter, TM, Zuppinger, C, 2006, Neuregulin-1 beta attenuates doxorubicin-induced alterations of excitation-contraction coupling and reduces oxidative stress in adult rat cardiomyocytes. *J Mol Cell Cardiol.* **41**: 845–854.

Uchiyama-Tanaka, Y, Matsubara, H, Nozawa, Y, Murasawa, S, Mori, Y, Kosaki, A, Maruama, K, Masaki, H, Shibasaki, Y, Fujiyama, S, Nose, A, Iba, O, Hasagawa, T, Higashiyama, S, Iwasaka, T, 2001, Angiotensin II signaling and HB-EGF shedding via metalloproteinase in glomerular mesangial cells. *Kidney International.* **60**: 2153–2163.

Ullian, ME, Webb, JG, Chen, R, Paul, RV, Morinelli, TA, 2004, Mechanisms of vascular angiotensin II surface receptor regulation by epidermal growth factor. *J Cell Physiol.* **200**: 451–457.

Ushio-Fukai, M, Griendling, KK, Becker, PL, Hilenski, L, Halleran, S, Alexander, RW, 2001a, Epidermal Growth Factor Receptor Transactivation by Angiotensin II Requires Reactive Oxygen Species in Vascular Smooth Muscle Cells. *Arterioscler Thromb Vasc Biol.* **21**: 489–495.

Ushio-Fukai, M, Hilenski, L, Santanam, N, Becker, PL, Ma, Y, Griendling, KK, Alexander, RW, 2001b, Cholesterol depletion inhibits epidermal growth factor receptor transactivation by angiotensin II in vascular smooth muscle cells: role of cholesterol-rich microdomains and focal adhesions in angiotensin II signaling. *Journal of Biological Chemistry.* **276**: 48269–48275.

Ushio-Fukai, M, Zuo, L, Ikeda, S, Tojo, T, Patrushev, N, Alexander, R, 2005, cAbl Tyrosine Kinase Mediates Reactive Oxygen Species- and Caveolin-Dependent AT1 Receptor Signaling in Vascular Smooth Muscle. *Circulation Research.* **97**: 829–836.

Vanwart, HE, Birkedalhansen, H, 1990, The Cysteine Switch - a Principle of Regulation of Metallo-proteinase Activity with Potential Applicability to the Entire Matrix Metalloproteinase Gene Family. *Proceedings of the National Academy of Sciences of the United States of America.* **87**: 5578–5582.

Wakatsuki, S, Kurisaki, T, Sehara-Fujisawa, A, 2004, Lipid rafts identified as locations of ectodomain shedding mediated by ADAM19. *Journal of Neurochemistry.* **89**: 119–123.

Waters, C, Pyne, S, Pyne, NJ, 2004, The role of G-protein coupled receptors and associated proteins in receptor tyrosine kinase signal transduction. *Seminars in Cell & Developmental Biology.* **15**: 309–323.

Weskamp, G, Blobel, CP, 1994, A Family of Cellular Proteins Related to Snake-Venom Disintegrins. *Proceedings of the National Academy of Sciences of the United States of America.* **91**: 2748–2751.

Weskamp, G, Cai, H, Brodie, TA, Higashyama, S, Manova, K, Ludwig, T, Blobel, CP, 2002, Mice lacking the metalloprotease-disintegrin MDC9 (ADAM9) have no evident major abnormalities during development or adult life. *Molecular and Cellular Biology.* **22**: 1537–1544.

White, JM, 2003, ADAMs: Modulators of cell-cell and cell-matrix interactions. *Current Opinion in Cell Biology.* **15**: 598–606.

Wolfsberg, TG, Primakoff, P, Myles, DG, White, JM, 1995, Adam, a Novel Family of Membrane-Proteins Containing a Disintegrin and Metalloprotease Domain - Multipotential Functions in Cell-Cell and Cell-Matrix Interactions. *Journal of Cell Biology.* **131**: 275–278.

Wolfsberg, TG, White, JM, 1996, ADAMs in fertilization and development. *Developmental Biology.* **180**: 389–401.

Wong, ST, Winchell, LF, McCune, BK, Earp, HS, Teixido, J, Massague, J, Herman, B, Lee, DC, 1989, The TGF-[alpha] precursor expressed on the cell surface binds to the EGF receptor on adjacent cells, leading to signal transduction. *Cell.* **56**: 495–506.

Wouters, S, Leruth, M, Decroly, E, Vandenbranden, M, Creemers, JWM, Van de Loo, J, Ruysschaert, JM, Courtoy, PJ, 1998, Furin and proprotein convertase 7 (PC7) lymphoma PC endogenously expressed in rat liver can be resolved into distinct post-Golgi compartments. *Biochemical Journal.* **336**: 311–316.

Yagami-Hiromasa, T, Sato, T, Kurisaki, T, Kamijo, K, al, e, 1995, A metalloprotease-disintegrin participating in myoblast fusion. *Nature.* **377**: 652.

Yahata, Y, Shirakata, Y, Tokumaru, S, Yang, LJ, Dai, XJ, Tohyama, M, Tsuda, T, Sayama, K, Iwai, M, Horiuchi, M, Hashimoto, K, 2006, A novel function of angiotensin II in skin wound healing - Induction of fibroblast and keratinocyte migration by angiotensin II via heparin-binding epidermal growth factor (EGF)-like growth factor-mediated egf receptor transactivation. *Journal of Biological Chemistry.* **281**: 13209–13216.

Yamazaki, S, Iwamoto, R, Saeki, K, Asakura, M, Takashima, S, Yamazaki, A, Kimura, R, Mizushima, H, Moribe, H, Higashiyama, S, Endoh, M, Kaneda, Y, Takagi, S, Itami, S, Takeda, N, Yamada, G, Mekada, E, 2003, Mice with defects in HB-EGF ectodomain shedding show severe developmental abnormalities. *J Cell Biol.* **163**: 469–475.

Yan, Y, Shirakabe, K, Werb, Z, 2002, The metalloprotease Kuzbanian (ADAM10) mediates the transactivation of EGF receptor by G protein-coupled receptors. *Journal of Cell Biology.* **158**: 221–226.

Yang, X, Zhu, MJ, Sreejayan, N, Ren, J, Du, M, 2005, Angiotensin II promotes smooth muscle cells proliferation and migration through release of heparin-binding epidermal growth factor and activaiotn of EGF-receptor pathway. *Molecules and Cells.* **20**: 263–270.

Zhai, P, Galeotti, J, Liu, J, Holle, E, Yu, X, Wagner, T, Sadoshima, J, 2006, An Angiotensin II Type 1 Receptor Mutant Lacking Epidermal Growth Factor Receptor Transactivation Does Not Induce Angiotensin II-Mediated Cardiac Hypertrophy. *Circ Res.* **99**: 528–536.

Zhang, L, Aggarwal, B, 1994, Role of sulfhydryl groups in induction of cell surface down-modulation and shedding of extracellular domain of human TNF receptors in human histiocytic lymphoma U937 cells. *J Immunol.* **153**: 3745–3754.

Zhang, Q, Thomas, SM, Lui, VWY, Xi, S, Siegfried, JM, Fan, H, Smithgall, TE, Mills, GB, Grandis, JR, 2006, Phosphorylation of TNF-alpha converting enzyme by gastrin-releasing peptide induces amphiregulin release and EGF receptor activation. *Proceedings of the National Academy of Sciences of the United States of America.* **103**: 6901–6906.

Zhang, Z, Kolls, JK, Oliver, P, Good, D, Schwarzenberger, PO, Joshi, MS, Ponthier, JL, Lancaster, JR, Jr., 2000, Activation of Tumor Necrosis Factor-alpha -converting Enzyme-mediated Ectodomain Shedding by Nitric Oxide. *J Biol Chem.* **275**: 15839–15844.

Zhang, Z, Oliver, P, Lancaster, JJ, Schwarzenberger, PO, Joshi, MS, Cork, J, Kolls, JK, 2001, Reactive oxygen species mediate tumour necrosis factor alpha-converting, enzyme-dependent ectodomain shedding induced by phorbol myrustate acetate. *FASEB J.* **15**: 303–305.

Zhao, Y-y, Sawyer, DR, Baliga, RR, Opel, DJ, Han, X, Marchionni, MA, Kelly, RA, 1998, Neuregulins Promote Survival and Growth of Cardiac Myocytes. Persistence of ErbB2 and ErbB4 Expression in Neonatal and Adult Ventricular Myocytes. *J Biol Chem.* **273**: 10261–10269.

Zhao, Z, Gruszczynska-Biegala, J, Cheuvront, T, Yi, H, Von Der Mark, H, Von Der Mark, K, Kaufman, SJ, Zolkiewska, A, 2004, Interaction of the disintegrin and cysteine-rich domains of ADAM12 with integrin (alpha)7(beta)1. *Experimental Cell Research.* **298**: 28–37.

Zhou, H-M, Weskamp, G, Chesneau, V, Sahin, U, Vortkamp, A, Horiuchi, K, Chiusaroli, R, Hahn, R, Wilkes, D, Fisher, P, Baron, R, Manova, K, Basson, CT, Hempstead, B, Blobel, CP, 2004, Essential Role for ADAM19 in Cardiovascular Morphogenesis. *Molecular and Cellular Biology.* **24**: 96–104.

Zhu, GZ, Lin, Y, Myles, DG, Primakoff, P, 1999, Identification of four novel ADAMs with potential roles in spermatogenesis and fertilization. *Gene.* **234**: 227–237.

Zuo, L, Ushio-Fukai, M, Ikeda, S, Hilenski, L, Patrushev, N, Alexander, RW, 2005, Caveolin-1 Is Essential for Activation of Rac1 and NAD(P)H Oxidase After Angiotensin II Type 1 Receptor Stimulation in Vascular Smooth Muscle Cells: Role in Redox Signaling and Vascular Hypertrophy. *Arterioscler Thromb Vasc Biol.* **25**: 1824–1830.

Zwick, E, Daub, H, Aoki, N, Yamaguchi-Aoki, Y, Tinhofer, I, Maly, K, Ullrich, A, 1997, Critical Role of Calcium- dependent Epidermal Growth Factor Receptor Transactivation in PC12 Cell Membrane Depolarization and Bradykinin Signaling. *J Biol Chem.* **272**: 24767–24770.

Index

ACE, *see* Angiotensin-converting enzyme
ACE-2, *see* Angiotensin-converting enzyme-2
ACE-related carboxypeptidase, *see*
    angiotensin-converting enzyme-2
AcSDKP, 30
ADAM, *see* A Disintegrin and Metalloprotease
A Disintegrin and Metalloprotease
    characteristics, 277
    structure, 278–282
Alcoholic
    liver disease, 114, 122
Aminopeptidase, 158, 199, 209–211
Angiotensin
    cancer, 139–141
    processing, 7, 65
    receptor blocker, 99, 103, 122, 123, 158, 159
    receptors, 65, 117, 136, 137, 141, 159, 182,
        204, 273
Angiotensin-converting enzyme
    cancer, 203
    carotid body, 159
    heart, 21, 30
    inhibitors, 116, 207
    kidney, 2
    skeletal muscle, 222
Angiotensin-converting enzyme-2, 5–10
Apoptosis
    angiotensin II, 204, 253
    cancer, 203
    pancreatitis, 64, 65
    skeletal muscle, 229
Apnea, 158, 165, 170
Atherosclerosis
    ACE inhibition, 39
    RAS activation, 96–98

Blood pressure
    ACE inhibition, 34
    Ang-(1-7), 25
    AT_1 receptor, 164–165
    AT_2 receptor, 373

cardiometabolic syndrome, 133
hypoxia, 169
Bradykinin, 4, 5, 36–37, 222–223, 233, 255–256
Breast cycle, 145

Cardiometabolic syndrome
    diagnosis, 88
Carotid body, 155–157, 160–171
Cell proliferation, 30, 137, 144, 145, 201–203,
    206–208, 211, 277, 284
Chemoreceptor, 155–157, 159–168, 169–171
Chymase
    Ang II generation, 260
    mast cell, 24
Cirrhosis, 113, 114, 123, 127

Diabetes
    ACE inhibition, 40
    clinical trials on RAS blockade, 103, 106,
        159, 231
    pancreatic stellate cell activation, 67
    type 2 diabetes mellitus, 73, 87
Dysfunctional adipose tissue, 90

EGFR, *see* Epidermal growth factor receptor
Epidermal growth factor receptor, 95

Fibrosis
    cardiac, 12, 25, 38
    hepatic, 113–127
    islet, 74, 76

Heart failure
    ACE inhibition, 30–31
    carotid RAS, 170–171
    role of EGFR, 287–289
    skeletal muscle RAS, 228–230
Human cancer
    role of RAS, 200–201

Hyperglycemia, 99, 101, 102
Hypoxia
    chronic, 156, 157, 161, 162, 163–165, 166, 167, 168
    intermittent, 165–169

Insulin resistance
    adipose tissue, 90–92
    role of skeletal muscle RAS, 230–234
Ischaemic heart disease, 21–41

Kallidin
    formation, 26–27
Kidney
    renin-angiotensin-aldosterone system, 1, 164

Liver
    characteristics, 143
    studies on human liver diseases, 123
Losartan, 37, 63, 67, 74, 101, 121, 122, 123, 126, 139, 158, 159, 160, 164, 166, 168, 169, 179, 184, 191, 206, 252

Metastasis, 139, 140, 141, 145, 203, 205, 207
Mineralization
    osteoblast mineralization, 185–186

N-acetyl-seryl-aspartyl-lysyl -proline, 21
Neprilysin, 10–12

Osteolysis, 179, 189
Oxidative stress
    in carotid body, 166
    RAS activation, 96

Pancreatitis
    activated pancreatic stellate cells, 76
    acute, 56–67
    pathophysiology, 57–58

Performance
    role of skeletal muscle RAS, 225–228

Portal hypertension, 114, 120, 126

Prorenin
    activation, 248
    receptor, 208–209, 247
    source, 248
Proximal tubule
    distribution of NADPH subunits, 98
    localization of ACE, 7
    localization of ACE2, 7
RANKL, 188
RAS, see Renin-angiotensin system
Receptor antagonist
    AT$_1$, 9, 13, 65, 68, 139, 158, 159, 159, 170, 186, 191, 256, 260, 261
    kinin B$_2$, 4
    type 2 bradykinin, 25
Renin
    cardiac renin, 21
    characteristics, 202
    ren-1/ren-2 gene, 247, 248, 250
Renin-angiotensin system
    breast RAS, 135–145
    cardiac RAS, 34
    circulating RAS, 116, 117, 156, 161, 162, 201, 221, 247
    in hypoxia, 157–159
    local RAS, 222
    regulation, 158–159
    skeletal muscle RAS, 221–236
Skeletal muscle
    ACE, 222
    angiotensin II, 223, 224
    angiotensin II receptor, 223
Stellate cell
    hepatic, 115, 116, 120, 121
    pancreatic, 76

Therapeutics
    RAS blockade, 103–106
Transactivation
    of EGFR, 286, 291
Triple membrane passing signaling, 276

UMR-106 cell, 182, 184, 185, 188
    apoptosis, 185
    AT$_1$ receptor regulation, 184
    mineralization activity, 185
    proliferation, 184–185